Genetic Predisposition to Cancer

Guest Editors

KENNETH OFFIT, MD, MPH
MARK ROBSON, MD

HEMATOLOGY/ONCOLOGY CLINICS OF NORTH AMERICA

www.hemonc.theclinics.com

Consulting Editors
GEORGE P. CANELLOS, MD
NANCY BERLINER, MD

October 2010 • Volume 24 • Number 5

SAUNDERS an imprint of ELSEVIER, Inc.

W.B. SAUNDERS COMPANY
A Division of Elsevier Inc.

1600 John F. Kennedy Blvd. ● Suite 1800 ● Philadelphia, PA 19103-2899

http://www.theclinics.com

HEMATOLOGY/ONCOLOGY CLINICS OF NORTH AMERICA Volume 24, Number 5
October 2010 ISSN 0889-8588, ISBN 13: 978-1-4377-2204-8

Editor: Kerry Holland
Developmental Editor: Donald Mumford

Hematology/Oncology Clinics (ISSN 0889-8588) is published bimonthly by Elsevier Inc., 360 Park Avenue South, New York, NY 10010-1710. Months of issue are February, April, June, August, October, and December. Business and Editorial Offices: 1600 John F. Kennedy Blvd., Ste. 1800, Philadelphia, PA 19103–2899. Customer Service Office: 3251 Riverport Lane, Maryland Heights, MO 63043. Periodicals postage paid at New York, NY and at additional mailing offices. Subscription prices are $306.00 per year (domestic individuals), $483.00 per year (domestic institutions), $152.00 per year (domestic students/residents), $347.00 per year (Canadian individuals), $591.00 per year (Canadian institutions) $413.00 per year (international individuals), $591.00 per year (international institutions), and $206.00 per year (international and Canadian students/residents). International air speed delivery is included in all *Clinics* subscription prices. All prices are subject to change without notice. **POSTMASTER:** Send address changes to *Hematology/Oncology Clinics of North America*, Elsevier Health Sciences Division, Subscription Customer Service, 3251 Riverport Lane, Maryland Heights, MO 63043. Customer Service (orders, claims, online, change of address): Elsevier Health Sciences Division, Subscription Customer Service, 3251 Riverport Lane, Maryland Heights, MO 63043. Tel: 1-800-654-2452 (U.S. and Canada); 314-447-8871 (outside U.S. and Canada). Fax: 314-447-8029. E-mail: journalscustomerservice-usa@elsevier.com (for print support); journalsonlinesupport-usa@elsevier.com (for online support).

Reprints. For copies of 100 or more, of articles in this publication, please contact the Commercial Reprints Department, Elsevier Inc., 360 Park Avenue South, New York, New York 10010-1710; Tel.: 212-633-3813, Fax: 212-462-1935, E-mail: reprints@elsevier.com.

Hematology/Oncology Clinics of North America is covered in *MEDLINE/PubMed (Index Medicus), EMBASE/ Excerpta Medica, and BIOSIS.*

Printed and bound in the United Kingdom
Transferred to Digital Print 2011

Contributors

CONSULTING EDITORS

GEORGE P. CANELLOS, MD
William Rosenberg Professor of Medicine, Department of Medical Oncology, Dana-Farber Cancer Institute, Boston, Massachusetts

NANCY BERLINER, MD
Chief, Division of Hematology, Brigham and Women's Hospital; Professor of Medicine, Harvard Medical School, Boston, Massachusetts

GUEST EDITORS

KENNETH OFFIT, MD, MPH
Attending Physician, and Chief, Clinical Genetics Service, Department of Medicine, Memorial Sloan-Kettering Cancer Center; Cancer Biology and Genetics Program, Sloan-Kettering Institute; and Professor of Medicine and Public Health, Department of Medicine, Weill Cornell Medical College, New York, New York

MARK ROBSON, MD
Associate Attending Physician, and Clinic Director, Clinical Genetics Service, Department of Medicine, Memorial Sloan-Kettering Cancer Center; Cancer Biology and Genetics Program, Sloan-Kettering Institute; and Associate Professor of Medicine, Department of Medicine, Weill College of Medicine, Cornell University, New York, New York

AUTHORS

JANE E. CHURPEK, MD
Section of Hematology/Oncology, Department of Medicine, The University of Chicago, Chicago, Illinois

JONATHAN A. COLEMAN, MD
Attending, Urology Service, Department of Surgery, Memorial Sloan-Kettering Cancer Center, New York, New York

SUSAN M. DOMCHEK, MD
Associate Professor, Department of Medicine, Abramson Cancer Center, University of Pennsylvania, Philadelphia, Pennsylvania

ANDREW FEIFER, MD
Fellow, Urology Service, Department of Surgery, Memorial Sloan-Kettering Cancer Center, New York, New York

DAVID J. GALLAGHER, MB BCh, BAO
Fellow, Clinical Genetics Service; Genitourinary Oncology Service, Division of Solid Tumor Oncology, Department of Medicine, Memorial Sloan-Kettering Cancer Center, New York, New York

MEG R. GERSTENBLITH, MD
CRTA Fellow, Genetic Epidemiology Branch, Division of Cancer Epidemiology and
Genetics, National Cancer Institute, National Institutes of Health, Rockville, Maryland

EMILY GLOGLOWSKI, MS, MSc
Clinical Genetics Service, Department of Medicine, Memorial Sloan-Kettering Cancer
Center, New York, New York

ALISA M. GOLDSTEIN, PhD
Senior Investigator, Genetic Epidemiology Branch, Division of Cancer Epidemiology and
Genetics, National Cancer Institute, National Institutes of Health, Rockville, Maryland

NICHOLE A.L. HANSEN, BS
Clinical Genetics Service, Department of Medicine, Memorial Sloan-Kettering Cancer
Center, New York, New York

DEBORAH HEMEL, MD
Department of Medicine, Hospital of the University of Pennsylvania, Abramson Cancer
Center, University of Pennsylvania, Philadelphia, Pennsylvania

NOAH D. KAUFF, MD
Clinical Genetics Service, Department of Medicine, Memorial Sloan-Kettering Cancer
Center, New York, New York

TOMAS KIRCHHOFF, PhD
Clinical Genetics Service, Department of Medicine, Memorial Sloan-Kettering Cancer
Center, New York, New York

ROBERT C. KURTZ, MD
Gastroenterology and Nutrition Service, Department of Medicine, Memorial
Sloan-Kettering Cancer Center; Department of Medicine, Weill Medical College
of Cornell University, New York, New York

STEVEN M. LIPKIN, MD, PhD
Gastroenterology, Department of Medicine, Weill Cornell College of Medicine, New York,
New York

KENNETH OFFIT, MD, MPH
Attending Physician, and Chief, Clinical Genetics Service, Department of Medicine,
Memorial Sloan-Kettering Cancer Center; Cancer Biology and Genetics Program,
Sloan-Kettering Institute; and Professor of Medicine and Public Health, Department
of Medicine, Weill Cornell Medical College, New York, New York

KENAN ONEL, MD, PhD
Assistant Professor of Pediatrics, Section of Hematology/Oncology, Department of
Pediatrics; Director, Familial Cancer Clinic, The University of Chicago, Chicago, Illinois

DEREK G. POWER, MD
Clinical Genetics Service, Department of Medicine, Memorial Sloan-Kettering Cancer
Center, New York, New York

MARK ROBSON, MD
Associate Attending Physician, and Clinic Director, Clinical Genetics Service, Department of Medicine, Memorial Sloan-Kettering Cancer Center; Cancer Biology and Genetics Program, Sloan-Kettering Institute; and Associate Professor of Medicine, Department of Medicine, Weill College of Medicine, Cornell University, New York, New York

WENDY S. RUBINSTEIN, MD, PhD
Clinical Associate Professor, Department of Medicine, University of Chicago Pritzker School of Medicine, Chicago; Chief, Division of Medical Genetics, NorthShore University HealthSystem, Evanston, Illinois

MANISH A. SHAH, MD
Gastrointestinal Oncology Service, Department of Medicine, Memorial Sloan-Kettering Cancer Center; Department of Medicine, Weill Medical College of Cornell University, New York, New York

ZSOFIA K. STADLER, MD
Clinical Genetics Service, Department of Medicine, Memorial Sloan-Kettering Cancer Center, New York, New York

PETER THOM, MS
Clinical Genetics Service, Department of Medicine, Memorial Sloan-Kettering Cancer Center, New York, New York

MARGARET A. TUCKER, MD
Senior Investigator, Genetic Epidemiology Branch, Division of Cancer Epidemiology and Genetics, National Cancer Institute, National Institutes of Health, Rockville, Maryland

JOSEPH VIJAI, PhD
Clinical Genetics Service, Department of Medicine, Memorial Sloan-Kettering Cancer Center, New York, New York

Contents

The past three decades have witnessed an explosion in information regarding the genetic mutations underlying predisposition to common malignancies. Discoveries are now being made regarding genomic variants associated with disease risk for, and outcome following, treatment for cancer. Responsible translation of these discoveries to medical practice requires attention to principles of clinical utility as well as social and ethical aspects.

A small, but important, percentage of breast cancer cases is caused by the inheritance of a single copy of a mutated gene. BRCA1 and BRCA2 are the genes most commonly associated with inherited breast cancer; however, mutations in TP53 and PTEN cause Li-Fraumeni syndrome and Cowden syndrome, respectively, both of which are associated with high lifetime risks of breast cancer. Advances in the field of breast cancer genetics have led to an improved understanding of detection and prevention strategies. More recently, strategies to target the underlying genetic defects in BRCA1- and BRCA2-associated breast and ovarian cancers are emerging and may have implications for certain types of sporadic breast cancer.

Malignancies of the upper gastrointestinal tract form a heterogeneous group of cancers characterized by unique epidemiology and biology. Despite these differences, survival for advanced disease remains poor across the panel of diseases, from cancers of the esophagus, stomach, pancreas, and, until recently, even gastrointestinal stromal tumors. Genetic predisposition syndromes associated with these diseases comprise an emerging subset of these diseases that may provide valuable information on cause and etiology. They may provide insight into molecular drivers for the disease, or disease subtypes, and also insights into novel gene/environment interactions. This review summarizes the current understanding of genetic predisposition syndromes of cancers of the upper gastrointestinal tract.

Colorectal cancer (CRC) is a common disease, and approximately 25% of patients have a familial component. High-penetrance singlegene germline mutations conferring a true hereditary susceptibility account for around 5% to 6% of all cases. Lynch syndrome is the most common hereditary form of colorectal cancer. Much of the hereditary component in the remaining familial cases of CRC is likely polygenic, and many of the genetic changes involved are as yet unidentified. This article addresses the most clinically important CRC genetic syndromes.

that indicate its evolution, and the syndrome sheds light on the role of mitochondria and energy metabolism in cancer. This article delineates the clinical presentation and practical management issues and summarizes the history, gene discovery, and molecular insights for each syndrome.

Many hematologic malignancies have an underlying heritable component. Although not as well characterized as the acquired genetic abnormalities that define important prognostic and therapeutic subgroups of myeloid and lymphoid neoplasms, investigations are beginning to unravel the role of germline genetic variation in the predisposition to hematologic malignancies. Information gained from the study of striking family pedigrees, epidemiologic data, and candidate genes are now being combined with unbiased genome-wide investigations to outline the network of genetic abnormalities that contribute to hematologic malignancy risk. This article reviews the current understanding of the heritability of hematologic malignancies in the genomics era.

Genome-wide association studies (GWAS) have now been performed in nearly all common malignancies and have identified more than 100 common genetic risk variants that confer a modest increased risk of cancer. For most discovered germline risk variants, the per allele effect size is small (<1.5) and the biologic mechanism of the detected association remains unexplained. Exceptions are the risk variants identified in JAK2 in myeloproliferative neoplasm and in the KITLG gene in testicular cancer, which are each associated with nearly a 3-fold increased risk of disease. GWAS have provided an efficient approach to identifying common, low-penetrance risk variants, and have implicated several novel cancer susceptibility loci. However, the identified low-penetrance risk variants explain only a small fraction of the heritability of cancer and the clinical usefulness of using these variants for cancer-risk prediction is to date limited. Studies involving more heterogeneous populations, determination of the causal variants, and functional studies are now necessary to further elucidate the potential biologic and clinical significance of the observed associations.

THE CLINICS ARE NOW AVAILABLE ONLINE!

Access your subscription at:
www.theclinics.com

Preface

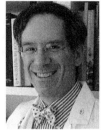 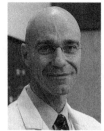

Kenneth Offit, MD, MPH   Mark Robson, MD
Guest Editors

There is now broad acceptance of the concept that hereditable factors are important determinants of cancer risk. Over a hundred genes have been associated with human cancer susceptibility. In this era of genome-wide association studies and next-generation sequencing, many groups are investigating the role of inherited suscepti-bility in the causation of apparently "sporadic" cancer. These exciting studies are the "new frontier" of cancer genetics, with potential to influence our understanding of the biology of cancer and to assist in the development of new therapeutics.

Have these new insights in cancer genetics made a meaningful impact in the care of patients and their families? In the early stages of the cancer genetics revolution, Fran-cis Collins quoted Sophocles, cautioning many of us that "It is but sorrow to be wise when wisdom profits not." Nearly two decades later, oncologists are beginning to utilize new therapies targeted to both the acquired as well as the inherited genetic defects in tumors. Increasingly, family history information augmented by genetic tests for cancer predisposition is being used to target screening, prevention, and treatment. Unaffected family members who share cancer predispositions have been shown to benefit from these interventions, providing the "profit" from genetic wisdom that was so elusive just two decades ago.

At the same time, the field of clinical cancer genetics has continued to grow in complexity. Numerous common and rare tumors are components of one or more human cancer predisposition syndromes. Although some of these syndromes are uncommon, recognizing them is of critical importance. Individuals with hereditary cancers are often at increased risk for second malignancies, often from a different primary site. Individuals with the same genetic mutation may develop a spectrum of associated tumors. Specific surveillance and preventive interventions may dramati-cally impact cancer morbidity in these families. Failing to recognize these syndromes and initiate appropriate measures may have a significant human (and potentially medi-colegal) cost.

The purpose of the current monograph is to provide the practicing clinical oncolo-gist with a state-of-the-art review of the cancer predisposition syndromes most likely to be encountered in practice, as well as a review of genomic research on the horizon. (Two articles will appear in the next issue of *Hematology/Oncology Clinics of North*

Hematol Oncol Clin N Am 24 (2010) xi–xii
doi:10.1016/j.hoc.2010.06.010   **hemonc.theclinics.com**

America (24:6) that were originally planned to publish in this issue; one article will review mouse models of human cancer susceptibility and the other will focus in-depth on colorectal cancer predisposition syndromes.) Each of the authors in this volume is a leader in clinical cancer genetics research, with a wealth of practical experience managing the syndromes about which they are writing. We hope that their willingness to share their expertise by contributing to this volume will improve the care of families affected by these syndromes and will further the important goal of translating advances in genetic research to clinical practice.

Kenneth Offit, MD, MPH
Clinical Genetics Service, Department of Medicine
Memorial Sloan-Kettering Cancer Center
Cancer Biology and Genetics Program
Sloan-Kettering Institute
1275 York Avenue
New York, NY 10065, USA

Mark Robson, MD
Clinical Genetics Service, Department of Medicine
Memorial Sloan-Kettering Cancer Center
1275 York Avenue
New York, NY 10065, USA

E-mail addresses:
offitk@mskcc.org (K. Offit)
robsonm@mskcc.org (M. Robson)

Inherited Predisposition to Cancer: Introduction and Overview

Mark Robson, MD[a,b], Kenneth Offit, MD, MPH[a,b,*]

KEYWORDS

• Genetic predisposition • History • High penetrance • Cancer

From the vantage point of 2010, it is hard to imagine a time when cancer was not widely accepted as a genetic disease, in the most basic sense of being caused by alterations in the structure and function of genes. It is also sometimes difficult to remember that the hereditable nature of some common cancers only became broadly understood in the second half of the 20th century. Broca[1] described a family with a strong predisposition to cancer as long ago as 1866, and Warthin[2] noted another such family in 1913. But it was not until the middle of the last century that clinical investigators began to ascertain significant numbers of families with what we would recognize today as familial adenomatous polyposis,[3] Lynch syndrome,[4] Li-Fraumeni syndrome,[5] and, of course, hereditary breast and ovarian cancer.[6]

Clinically, these kindreds seemed to be transmitting single, highly penetrant alleles in an autosomal dominant fashion. The technology of the day could not identify the causative genes, but Knudson[7] was able to provide empiric statistical support that at least one disorder, hereditary retinoblastoma, could be explained by a model in which disease resulted from an inherited mutation and a metachronous somatic mutation of the wild-type allele. In the 1980's, complex segregation analyses of colorectal and breast cancer kindreds provided further support for the idea that highly penetrant alleles cause a small but significant fraction of these common cancers.[8,9]

These genealogic and epidemiologic observations set the stage for a burst of scientific activity in the 1990s, when developments in positional cloning facilitated the discovery of the genes responsible for the most common cancer predisposition syndromes, and for several less common ones. These discoveries can rightly be

The authors have nothing to disclose.
ª Clinical Genetics Service, Department of Medicine, Memorial Sloan-Kettering Cancer Center, 1275 York Avenue, New York, NY 10065, USA
ᵇ Department of Medicine, Weill College of Medicine, Cornell University, New York, NY, USA
* Corresponding author. Clinical Genetics Service, Department of Medicine, Memorial Sloan-Kettering Cancer Center, 1275 York Avenue, New York, NY 10065.
E-mail address: offitk@mskcc.org

Hematol Oncol Clin N Am 24 (2010) 793–797
doi:10.1016/j.hoc.2010.06.005
0889-8588/10/$ – see front matter

considered triumphs of cancer genetics, providing important insights into the biology of not only inherited cancer but also sporadic disease.

However, at the time these discoveries were made, only a limited clinical evidence base was available to guide the management of individuals with an inherited predisposition. Guidelines were developed by various expert panels, but much of the clinical research to support and refine those guidelines had not been completed. The evidence base arose largely because of a firm commitment by those providing clinical genetic testing to do so mainly in the context of institutional review board–approved research studies, a commitment mirrored by the position statements of the American Society of Clinical Oncology and other groups.[10] Reviews of the results of these clinical investigations form a significant part of this issue. These results illustrate why genetic testing has become an accepted (even critical) element in the management of subsets of patients with certain cancers, some of which are very common (eg, breast, colorectal), whereas others are not (eg, retinoblastoma, paraganglioma, medullary thyroid cancer).[11]

Although genetic testing for cancer predisposition is broadly accepted for certain diseases, its clinical usefulness in others is less clear. For example, in this issue Gerstenblith and colleagues eloquently describe the limitations of testing for mutations in *CDKN2/p16* as part of an evaluation of melanoma predisposition. One group defines the clinical utility of a genetic test as "...its usefulness and added value to patient decision-making compared with current management without genetic testing."[12] In other words, a test has clinical utility if the result is likely to influence diagnosis or management. This clinical utility can manifest in several ways.

First, a genetic test may have clinical utility if it helps diagnose a condition, and this has certainly been a major role of testing in nononcologic clinical genetics. However, diagnostic testing is less directly relevant in cancer clinical genetics because neoplastic diagnoses are tissue-based and usually do not require germline information for interpretation. However, cancers that arise as the result of a strong germline predisposition may be managed differently from those that arise from sporadic disease. Patients may undergo more extensive local therapy if they are at increased risk for metachronous malignancy. Obvious examples include the consideration of bilateral mastectomy instead of breast conservation in patients with breast cancer carrying a *BRCA1* or *BRCA2* mutation, and subtotal colectomy instead of limited resection in patients with colorectal cancer who have Lynch syndrome. Although genetic testing is not absolutely necessary for consideration of more extensive surgery, it certainly informs patient decision-making about whether to undergo these preventive procedures.

Germline tests could also have clinical utility if the results were either prognostic or predictive of response to treatment. Although some predispositions may be associated with differential outcomes (eg, microsatellite instability and improved prognosis in colorectal cancer), germline testing has not yet found a place in prognostication for either early or advanced disease. Similarly, germline changes associated with susceptibility have not, until recently, been predictive of differential response to treatment approaches. Recent success of inhibitors of poly(ADP-ribose) polymerase inhibitors in *BRCA*-mutated breast and ovarian cancers indicates a possible role for this testing in the future,[13] as does the suggestion of sensitivity to cis-platinum in the neoadjuvant treatment of *BRCA1*-mutated breast cancer.[14] At the time of this writing, however, routine adjustment of systemic treatment is not based on germline status.

Although the role of germline testing in the treatment of established cancer is important to consider, the greatest clinical utility obviously flows from the ability of genetic testing to assess individual risk for developing cancer in the future. The usefulness of this genetically determined risk estimate depends on several factors. The estimate must be reasonably robust (clinically valid), in the sense that a mutation should be associated with a sufficiently consistent level of risk among individuals based on published absolute risk estimates which can be used to guide care for the patient being tested. If significant heterogeneity of risk exists among mutation carriers, then average estimates are difficult for patients to apply to their own situation, because their own risk may be either greater or less than the average. Even if the risk estimate is clinically valid, it must exceed an action threshold.

Although risk is a continuous variable, decisions about whether to pursue incremental screening or preventive surgeries are dichotomous. Modest elevations in risk may be perfectly reproducible and homogeneous, but not of sufficient magnitude to justify differential action. Similarly, effective interventions must be available to offer individuals at increased risk, which would not be offered without a documented genetic predisposition. The widespread acceptance of BRCA1 and BRCA2 testing is largely based on its ability to separate individuals into those who are or are not at increased risk for ovarian cancer, and the availability of effective and acceptable preventive surgery to address that risk. In other situations, such as Li-Fraumeni syndrome, the clinical utility of testing is limited because of the limited screening available for many of the component tumors of that syndrome.

Although highly penetrant genes are the ones most likely to be clinically relevant, they only explain a small portion of the hereditability of cancer. Several intermediate penetrance genes are associated with risks that do not clearly exceed an action threshold. And now, genome-wide association studies (GWAS) are identifying large numbers of genetic variants that are, individually, associated with very limited increases in risk. Notwithstanding the premature dissemination of "genomic profiles" of these variations by commercial entrepreneurs, the clinical utility of identifying these variants is completely unclear, and also poses real risks of false alarm and false reassurance.[15]

This limitation is not to deny the role genomic profiles will ultimately have in preventive and therapeutic oncology. In fact, we anticipate that a future Hematology/ Oncology Clinics volume on personalized cancer genomics will contain many articles on pathway analysis of the interplay of thousands of sequence and structural variants that will define the bulk of inherited cancer susceptibility and pharmacogenomic response. However, significant clinical and regulatory challenges remain as barriers to the effective integration of these new genomic discoveries into clinical care.[16]

Accompanying the accelerated pace of genetic discovery and clinical translation has been an equally rapid evolution in thinking about the legal, social, and ethical aspects of the genetics revolution. Two decades ago, at the dawn of clinical cancer genetics, there was broad apprehension about a range of adverse social implications. These untoward consequences were averted by legal judgments and timely legislation, and progressive policies. Foremost among these concerns was the risk of genetic discrimination by health insurers and employers, precluded by federal legislation in 2008. Rather than discriminate against BRCA mutation carriers, for example, insurers now use these tests to justify payment for risk-reducing surgeries. When our group described the most common BRCA2 mutation in Ashkenazi Jews in 1996, concern was expressed about the risk of group stigmatization. Instead, as other groups were noted to have "founder" mutations in disease predisposition genes, these discoveries were used to empower these groups to take preventive actions. Equally unimaginable two decades ago, the uses of cancer genetic tests are now routinely discussed in the context of reproductive planning through techniques such as preimplantation genetics.[17]

The further progress of clinical cancer genetics may also be influenced by recent and upcoming legal decisions that may result in loss or limitation of intellectual property protections afforded to patents on gene sequences. The outcome of those decisions, some argue, may dampen the pace of venture capital investment in needed biomedical research in the decades ahead, whereas others see the possibility that genomic information will become less expensive and more widely available. In any event, an intimate interplay exists among science, law, and medicine that will determine the ultimate future application of genomic information.

Following this introduction to the historical and societal context of two decades of discovery in cancer genetics, the articles in this issue provide the reader with expert and comprehensive reviews of the state of knowledge regarding genetic predisposition to cancer affecting several different sites. These reviews include detailed discussion of the genetics and management of individuals at risk for hereditary cancer of the breast and ovaries, upper and lower gastrointestinal tracts, genitourinary tract, genodermatoses, endocrine system, and pediatric tumors, breast and ovaries, upper and lower gastrointestinal tracts, genitourinary tract, genodermatoses, endocrine system, and pediatric tumors. A concluding article will review the emerging genomics of low-penetrance cancer susceptibility. Two articles will appear in the next issue of *Hematology/Oncology Clinics of North America* (24:6) that were originally planned to publish in this issue; one article will review mouse models of human cancer susceptibility and the other will focus in-depth on colorectal cancer predisposition syndromes. A common theme of these articles is that the clinical utility of testing for mutations in the genes described ranges widely, although this is an evolving field and new findings may well alter the perspective on the clinical utility of testing for different genes.

A detailed review of the current status of whole genome approaches to cancer predisposition concludes that it is not yet clear how newer findings from genomic profiling technologies should be used. Appropriate clinical research studies must be performed to answer that question. In this regard, the situation is not that different from what it was in the 1990s after discovery of *BRCA1*, *BRCA2*, and the mismatch repair genes responsible for Lynch syndrome. Currently, the major limitation to the clinical application of the new genomic results is that the magnitude of associated risk is insufficient to clearly justify differential action, although this may change with the advent of new screening technologies or biologically targeted pharmacologic prevention approaches. Furthermore, whole genome sequencing studies may identify less-common variants associated with sufficient risks to warrant intervention with available technologies. Much remains to be done to build on the 20th century successes of clinical cancer genetics so as to gain the maximum benefit from the genomic advances of the 21st century.

REFERENCES

1. Broca P. Traité des tumeurs: Tome Premier, Des tumeurs en général. In: Asselin P, editor. Paris; 1866. Available at: http://www.archive.org/stream/traitdestumeurs02brocgoog#page/n12/mode/1up. Accessed June 4, 2010.
2. Warthin AS. Heredity with reference to carcinoma as shown by the study of cases examined in the pathological laboratory of the University of Michigan, 1895–1913. Arch Intern Med 1913;12:546–55.
3. Dukes C, Lockhart-Mummery H. Familial intestinal polyposis. Surg Clin North Am 1955;1277–81.
4. Lynch HT, Krush AJ. Cancer family "G" revisited: 1895–1970. Cancer 1971;27(6): 1505–11.

5. Li FP, Fraumeni JF Jr. Rhabdomyosarcoma in children: epidemiologic study and identification of a familial cancer syndrome. J Natl Cancer Inst 1969;43(6): 1365–73.
6. Lynch HT, Krush AJ. Carcinoma of the breast and ovary in three families. Surg Gynecol Obstet 1971;133(4):644–8.
7. Knudson AG Jr. Mutation and cancer: statistical study of retinoblastoma. Proc Natl Acad Sci U S A 1971;68(4):820–3.
8. Bailey-Wilson JE, Elston RC, Schuelke GS, et al. Segregation analysis of hereditary nonpolyposis colorectal cancer. Genet Epidemiol 1986;3(1):27–38.
9. Newman B, Austin MA, Lee M, et al. Inheritance of human breast cancer: evidence for autosomal dominant transmission in high-risk families. Proc Natl Acad Sci U S A 1988;85(9):3044–8.
10. Offit K, Biesecker B, Burt R, et al. Statement of the American Society of Clinical Oncology: genetic testing for cancer susceptibility, Adopted on February 20, 1996. J Clin Oncol 1996;14(5):1730–6 [discussion: 1737–40].
11. Offit K. Clinical cancer genetics; risk counseling and management. New York: Wiley-Liss; 1998.
12. Teutsch SM, Bradley LA, Palomaki GE, et al. The Evaluation of Genomic Applications in Practice and Prevention (EGAPP) initiative: methods of the EGAPP Working Group. Genet Med 2009;11(1):3–14.
13. Fong PC, Boss DS, Yap TA, et al. Inhibition of poly(ADP-ribose) polymerase in tumors from BRCA mutation carriers. N Engl J Med 2009;361(2):123–34.
14. Byrski T, Gronwald J, Huzarski T, et al. Pathologic complete response rates in young women with BRCA1-positive breast cancers after neoadjuvant chemotherapy. J Clin Oncol 2010;28(3):375–9.
15. Offit K. Genomic profiles for disease risk: predictive or premature? JAMA 2008; 299(11):1353–5.
16. Robson ME, Storm CD, Weitzel J, et al. American Society of Clinical Oncology policy statement update: genetic and genomic testing for cancer susceptibility. J Clin Oncol 2010;28(5):893–901.
17. Offit K, Sagi M, Hurley K. Preimplantation genetic diagnosis for cancer syndromes: a new challenge for preventive medicine. JAMA 2006;296(22): 2727–30.

Breast Cancer Predisposition Syndromes

Deborah Hemel, MD[a], Susan M. Domchek, MD[b],*

KEYWORDS

- Li Fraumeni Syndrome • Cowden Syndrome
- Hereditary Breast and Ovarian Cancer Syndrome • *TP53*
- *PTEN* • *BRCA1* • *BRCA2*

Increasing numbers of genes have been implicated in the development of breast cancer. Some of these genes are highly penetrant, meaning that a significant proportion of individuals who carry mutations in these genes will develop cancer. Although only 5% to 10% of breast cancers are believed to be caused by mutations in single genes, such mutations predispose carriers to a very high lifetime risk of developing breast cancer. Additionally, women who carry such mutations are at disproportionate risk of developing breast cancer at a young age, before mammographic screening is recommended for the general population.[1]

This review article will focus on the autosomal-dominant, highly penetrant genes *TP53*, *PTEN*, *BRCA1*, and *BRCA2*. Mutations in these genes are responsible for the hereditary breast cancer syndromes known as Li Fraumeni syndrome (LFS), Cowden syndrome (CS), and hereditary breast and ovarian cancer syndrome (HBOC), respectively.

LFS

LFS is a rare cancer predisposition syndrome characterized by various early onset tumors including breast cancers, sarcomas, brain tumors, adrenal cortical tumors, and acute leukemias (**Table 1**).[2] Germline mutations in the *TP53* gene located on chromosome 17[3] are identified frequently in this syndrome, with 50% to 70% of families meeting the criteria for classic LFS having detectable mutations.[4–6] Many more

---

This work has been supported by a grant from the Cancer Genetics Network HHSN21620074400C to SMD.

[a] Department of Medicine, Hospital of the University of Pennsylvania, Abramson Cancer Center, University of Pennsylvania, 100 Centrex Building, 3400 Spruce Street, Philadelphia, PA 19104, USA

[b] Department of Medicine, Abramson Cancer Center, University of Pennsylvania, 3 West Perelman, 3400 Civic Center Boulevard, Philadelphia, PA 19104, USA

* Corresponding author.

E-mail address: susan.domchek@uphs.upenn.edu

Hematol Oncol Clin N Am 24 (2010) 799–814
doi:10.1016/j.hoc.2010.06.004

Table 1
Li Fraumeni, Cowden and hereditary breast and ovarian syndrome characteristics

	Li-Fraumeni Syndrome	Cowden Syndrome	Hereditary Breast and Ovarian Cancer Syndrome	
			BRCA1	BRCA2
Mutated Gene	TP53	PTEN	BRCA1	BRCA2
Gene Location	17p13.1	10q23.3	17q21	13q12–13
Gene Frequency	As high as 1 in 20,000[4]	Between 1/200,000 and 1/250,000[25]	Varies among ethnic groups: 1 in 40 among Ashkenazi Jews[32,33] Unselected breast cancer patients <5%[31]	
Associated, Nonbreast Cancer	Sarcomas Brain tumors Adrenal cortical tumors Acute leukemias Choroid plexus tumors[2]	Thyroid tumors (nonmedullary thyroid cancer) Endometrial cancer Genitourinary tumors, especially renal cell carcinoma[23]	Ovarian/fallopian tube/ primary peritoneal cancers Male breast cancer Prostate	Prostate Pancreatic Gall bladder Stomach Melanoma
Lifetime Risk of Developing Breast Cancer	90% by age 60	25%–50%	40%–80%	30%–60%
Associated Syndromes	N/A	Bannayan-Riley-Ruvalcaba syndrome Proteus syndrome[23]		Biallelic mutations in BRCA2: Fanconi anemia[85]

families do not meet the strict criteria for LFS, but meet looser criteria for Li-Fraumeni-like (LFL) syndrome (**Table 2**).[7,8] Depending on the criteria met, between 7% to 22% of LFL families have detectable *TP53* mutations.[5–7,9]

Inheritance and Penetrance

LFS is inherited in an autosomal-dominant pattern. Although most patients with documented *TP53* mutations have an extensive family history of cancer, including childhood cancer, de novo mutations are not infrequent. Approximately 7% to 20% of *TP53* mutations are thought to occur de novo.[10] Gonzalez and colleagues[4] estimated that the frequency of *TP53* mutations is 1 in 20,000 people, a frequency higher than previously estimated, although still very small. Founder mutations may exist in certain populations, most notably the R337H mutation in Brazil, which may be seen in up to 0.3% of the population.[11] Germline mutations in the *TP53* gene are thought to account for only a small fraction of hereditary breast cancers cases and for less than 1% of all breast cancer cases.[12,13]

LFS is associated with an extremely high lifetime risk of cancer. Women with documented *TP53* mutations are more likely to develop cancer than men, with a lifetime risk estimates of 93% and 68%, respectively. The most common cancer in women is early onset female breast cancer.[14] Unlike cases of sporadic breast cancer, which most commonly occur in postmenopausal women, the vast majority of patients with germline *TP53* mutations who develop breast cancer do so by age 50, with a mean age of 37.[15] A woman with LFS is thought to have a breast cancer risk of 90%.

Who Should be Tested?

The details of an individual's personal and family history of cancer are very important in determining the likelihood that a germline *TP53* mutation will be detected. An important study by Gonzalez and colleagues[4] examined 525 patients sent for *TP53* testing at the City of Hope clinical genetics laboratory (Philadelphia, PA, USA), among whom 91 mutations were detected. In this series, an individual diagnosed with invasive breast cancer between the ages of 30 and 49 years who had no family history of any of the core Li Fraumeni cancers (except breast cancer) had a 0% (0 out of 15) chance of

Table 2
Li-Fraumeni Syndrome and Li-Fraumeni-Like Syndrome

	Li-Fraumeni Syndrome	Li-Fraumeni-Like Syndrome	
		Birch Criteria	Eeles Criteria
Diagnostic Criteria	Proband with a sarcoma diagnosed before age 45 and A first-degree relative with any cancer <45 and A first- or second-degree relative with any cancer <45, or a sarcoma at any age	Proband with childhood cancer or sarcoma, brain tumor, leukemia or ACC <45 and: First- or second-degree relative with typical Li Fraumeni syndrome cancer and First- or second-degree relative cancer <60	Two different cancers that are part of Li Fraumeni syndrome in first- or second-degree relative at any age
Likelihood of Detecting a TP53 Mutation	80%	7%–22%.[5–7,9]	

a detectable *TP53* mutation. In contrast, a patient with breast cancer under age 30 and family history of one or more core Li Fraumeni cancers (other than breast cancer) in a first- or second-degree relative, had a 100% (five out of five) chance of having a p53 mutation.[4] Probands with adrenal cortical tumors in childhood or choroid plexus tumors had a very high cancer of carrying a *TP53* mutation, with prior probabilities of 67% (14 of 21) and 100% (eight of eight), respectively. Women with breast cancer younger than age 30 without any family history of cancer still had a 7% chance of carrying a *TP53* mutation, a figure consistent with other series.[16] The limitations of this study include small sample size in the individual subgroups and referral bias; however, the data are helpful in the clinic when considering who should undergo genetic testing for this rare syndrome. Because of the very low frequency of germline *TP53* mutations in the general population, women diagnosed with breast cancer after age 30 without a family history suggestive of LFS or Li-Fraumeni-like syndrome (representing the vast majority of breast cancer patients) are very unlikely to have a *TP53* mutation.

Screening, Prevention, and Treatment

Postpubescent females with a family history of LFS should be closely monitored for breast cancer. Although there is a theoretical risk of inducing malignancies in *TP53* mutation carriers through the exposure to radiation, the National Comprehensive Cancer Network (NCCN) Clinical Practice Guidelines in Oncology recommend annual mammograms and magnetic resonance imaging (MRI) scans starting at age 20 to 25 for LFS patients, as the benefits of early detection are believed to be greater than their risks (**Table 3**). Given the high lifetime risk of cancer, prophylactic mastectomy is a reasonable option in *TP53* mutation carriers.[17]

Screening Guidelines for Other Cancers

Individuals with germline *TP53* mutations are at elevated risks for many types of cancer. For this reason, there is great interest in developing effective screening strategies. Garber and colleagues[18] assessed the utility of positron emission tomography/computed tomography (PET/CT) in a small cohort of *TP53* mutation carriers. Cancers were detected in 3 of 15 patients undergoing PET/CT, including two papillary thyroid cancers and a stage 2 esophageal adenocarcinoma. There is significant interest in the potential role of full-body MRI. Individuals with this rare syndrome are encouraged to enroll on clinical studies. Annual comprehensive examinations should be performed with a focus on skin and neurologic examinations. Colonoscopy should be considered starting at age 25 (see **Table 3**).

Therapeutic Implications

Patients who carry a germline *TP53* mutation and are diagnosed with breast cancer should consider mastectomy rather than breast-conserving surgery and radiation. Increased sensitivity to DNA-damaging agents such as ionizing radiation may place individuals with *TP53* mutations at higher risk for developing treatment-induced cancers, particularly sarcomas in the radiation field.[19]

CS

CS, also known as multiple hamartoma syndrome, is a rare cancer predisposition associated with a high rate of breast cancer and mucocutaneous findings, thyroid abnormalities, and endometrial carcinomas (see **Table 1** and **Table 4**). The diagnostic criteria for CS are complex, but are summarized in **Table 4**. Germline mutations in the *PTEN* gene have been found to occur in 80% of strictly defined CS patients.[20,21] The

Table 3
Screening recommendations

	Li-Fraumeni Syndrome	Cowden Syndrome	Hereditary Breast and Ovarian Cancer Syndrome
Breast Self-examination		Monthly, starting at age 18	
Clinical Breast Examination	Semiannually, starting at age 20–25 or 5–10 years before the earliest known breast cancer in the family	Semiannually, starting at age 25 or 5–10 years before the earliest known breast cancer in the family	Semiannually, starting at age 25
Breast Radiographic Screening	Annual mammogram and breast magnetic resonance imaging (MRI) screening starting at age 20–25 or individualized based on earliest age of onset in family	Annual mammography and breast MRI screening starting at age 30–35 or 5–10 years before the earliest known breast cancer in the family (whichever is earlier)	Annual mammogram and breast MRI screening starting at age 25 or individualized based on earliest age of onset in family
Prophylactic Surgery	Discuss option of risk-reducing mastectomy (RRM)	Discuss option of RRM	Discuss option of RRM. Recommend RRSO, ideally between 35 and 40 years of age
Screening for Other Cancers	Colonoscopy every 2–5 years starting at 25. Annual comprehensive examination and neurologic examinations. Ongoing investigations regarding the role of positron emission tomography or MRI	Baseline thyroid ultrasound, consider yearly thyroid ultrasound. Role of yearly endometrial biopsy is debated: not included in current NCCN guidelines	Twice yearly TVUS and CA125 for ovarian cancer screening until the time RRSO. Consider yearly dermatology examination in *BRCA2* mutation carriers. Discussion of prostate cancer screening in male carriers

Abbreviations: NCCN, National Comprehensive Cancer Network; RRSO, risk reducing salpingo-oophorectomy; TVUS, transvaginal ultrasound.

Data from NCCN clinical practice guidelines in oncology – genetic/familial high-risk assessment: breast and ovarian. 2009. Available at: http://www.nccn.org/professionals/physician_gls/PDF/genetics_screening.pdf; and Hobert JA, Eng C. PTEN hamartoma tumor syndrome: an overview. Genet Med 2009;11(10):687–94.

Table 4 Cowden syndrome	
Definition	Any single pathognomonic criterion or ≥2 major criteria or 1 major and ≥3 minor criteria or ≥4 minor criteria[13]
Criteria	
Pathognomonic	Mucocutaneous lesions Facial trichilemnomas Acral keratosis Papillomatous lesions Mucosal lesions Adult Lhermitte Duclos disease
Major	Breast cancer Endometrial cancer Thyroid cancer Macrocephaly
Minor	Fibrocystic breast disease Mental retardation Benign thyroid lesions Hamartomatous polyps Lipomas Fibromas GU tumors Fibroids Renal cell carcinoma

Data from NCCN clinical practice guidelines in oncology - genetic/familial high risk assessment: breast and ovarian. 2009. Available at: http://www.nccn.org/professionals/physician_gls/PDF/genetics_screening.pdf; and Hobert JA, Eng C. PTEN hamartoma tumor syndrome: an overview. Genet Med 2009;11(10):687–94.

PTEN gene encodes the PTEN protein, a lipid phosphatase enzyme involved in the regulation of the cell cycle and apoptosis.[22] *PTEN*, like *TP53*, functions as a tumor suppressor gene.

Inheritance and Penetrance

CS is an autosomal-dominant, highly penetrant genetic disorder. More than 90% of individuals with *PTEN* mutations are believed to manifest some feature of the syndrome (although rarely cancer) by age 20, and by age 30 nearly 100% of carriers are believed to have developed at least some of the mucocutaneous signs.[23]

Women with CS have approximately a 67% to 76% risk for benign breast disease, such as fibroadenomas and fibrocystic breast disease, and a 25% to 50% lifetime risk for breast cancer. The peak incidence of breast cancer in women with CS occurs between the ages of 38 and 46 years, although there is a wide range in age of onset.[23,24] Like LFS, the exact prevalence of CS is unknown, although its prevalence has been estimated to be between 1 case in 200,000 people and 1 case in 250,000 people based on projections from a study of the Dutch national registry.[25] CS, though undoubtedly rare (it is estimated that fewer than 1% of hereditary breast cancer families are caused by CS), may be under-recognized, as women who present with breast cancer and subtle skin findings or common associated features (ie, fibroids or fibrocystic breast disease) may not be recognized as potentially part of the Cowden's spectrum.[26]

Familial data collected by Nelen and colleagues[25] show that there is marked variation in symptom manifestation and age of symptom occurrence in patients with CS. In part because of this phenotypic heterogeneity, and in part because of the occurrence of de novo *PTEN* germline mutations, a family history of breast cancer may not be apparent. For example, in one study of 19 women with breast cancer and CS, only 35% of the women reported a family history of breast cancer.[26]

Screening, Prevention, and Treatment

Women with CS should be monitored closely for breast cancer (see **Table 3**). Breast cancers seen in women with germline *PTEN* mutations show a spectrum of pathology similar to that of sporadic breast cancers in the general population, with the predominant type of breast cancer being ductal carcinoma.[26] Annual screening breast MRI in addition to annual mammograms are recommended for women with *PTEN* mutations starting in their early 30s.[17] Similar to those with *TP53* mutations, screening and prevention information specific to those with *PTEN* mutations are limited because of the rarity of the syndrome. Individuals with *PTEN* mutations are at elevated risk for follicular and papillary carcinoma of the thyroid, and a baseline screening thyroid ultrasound at 18 with consideration of annual ultrasound has been suggested.[17] In addition, because of the increased risk of endometrial cancer (with a potential lifetime risk of 5% to 10%), yearly endometrial biopsy starting at age 35 to 40 years has been recommended by some authors[23] but is not currently part of the NCCN guidelines. The increased risk of developing endometrial cancer with tamoxifen use is of particular concern to those with *PTEN* mutations as such women are already at an increased risk for endometrial cancer. Therefore, if women are interested in primary prevention, raloxifene, with no apparent excess risk of uterine cancer, may be preferred over tamoxifen.[27] As is true for any women at increased risk for the development of breast cancer, prophylactic mastectomy is an option for women with *PTEN* mutations.[17]

HBOC

HBOC has received considerable attention since *BRCA1* and *BRCA2* were cloned in 1994 and 1995, respectively.[28,29] *BRCA1* and *BRCA2*, which function as tumor suppressor genes, are involved in, among other important cellular functions, homologous DNA repair.[30] Germline mutations in *BRCA1* and *BRCA2* are seen in fewer than 5% of unselected breast cancer cases.[31] Features that increase the likelihood that a woman will have a *BRCA1* or *BRCA2* mutation include a family history of ovarian cancer, male breast cancer, or multiple early onset breast cancers. In addition, the presence of Ashkenazi Jewish ancestry increases the likelihood of a *BRCA1* or *BRCA2* mutation. Approximately 1 in 40 Ashkenazi Jewish people is a carrier of one of three founder mutations: 185delAG and 5382insC in *BRCA1* and 6174del T in *BRCA2*.[32,33]

BRCA1 and *BRCA2* mutations are both associated with a high risk of breast and ovarian cancer, but clinical and pathologic differences exist between these two related yet distinct genetic syndromes (see **Table 1**). For example, although the lifetime risk for breast cancer in *BRCA2* mutation carriers is similar to that for *BRCA1* mutation carriers, the mean age of onset of breast cancer is younger in *BRCA1* mutation carriers.[34] *BRCA1* and *BRCA2* mutations are also associated with distinct breast cancer phenotypes; *BRCA1*-associated breast cancers are predominantly estrogen receptor (ER)-negative, whereas most *BRCA2*-associated breast cancers are ER-positive.[35] These differences my have implications in the prevention and treatment of breast cancer in *BRCA1* and *BRCA2* mutation carriers.

Penetrance

Female BRCA1 mutation carriers have a lifetime risk of developing breast cancer of approximately 40% to 80%, while female BRCA2 mutation carriers have a lifetime risk of developing breast cancer of approximately 30% to 60%.[34,36] BRCA mutation carriers are at significant risk of developing ovarian cancer as well as breast cancer, with 36% to 46% of BRCA1 mutation carriers developing ovarian cancer by age 70 years compared with 10% to 20% of BRCA2 mutation carriers.[34,36]

There is good evidence for variation of penetrance of breast and ovarian cancer among BRCA1 and BRCA2 mutation carriers,[37] which is likely due to many factors. Genotype-phenotype correlations exist, with mutations within the ovarian cancer cluster regions associated with higher risks of ovarian cancer.[38,39] Details of the cancer history of the proband and the family clearly matter, which may reflect shared environmental factors or genetic modifiers. Genetic modifiers and the coinheritance of single nucleotide polymorphisms in other genes (such as FGFR2 and MAP3K1) can modify the penetrance of BRCA2, and to a lesser extent, BRCA1.[40] Much of the variability of penetrance remains unexplained, and even the known contributors to this variance are not clinically applicable at this time.

Who Should be Tested?

Guidelines and insurance coverage are variable, but those individuals with a probability of having a BRCA1/2 mutation greater than 5% to 10% are considered candidates for genetic counseling and consideration of testing. Multiple models are available to aid in determining good candidate for genetic testing.[41] Box 1 outlines breast cancer patients who are appropriate candidates for genetic counseling.[17]

Myriad Genetics (Salt Lake City, UT, USA) is currently the only source of commercial testing for BRCA1/2 mutation testing in the United States. Most germline BRCA1/2 mutations are caused by point mutations or small deletions or insertions. However, large genomic rearrangements appear to be the source of a significant minority of BRCA1/2 mutations.[42] The BRACAnalysis Rearrangement Test (BART) is currently available from Myriad as a method of detecting large genomic rearrangements; however, only samples from individuals meeting certain criteria automatically undergo

---

Box 1
Candidates for genetic counseling and testing

Personal history of breast cancer (including ductal carcinoma in situ) plus one or more of the following:

Diagnosis occurred before age 45

Diagnosis occurred before age 50, with at least one close relative diagnosed with breast cancer before age 50 or at least one close relative with ovarian cancer

Two primary breast cancers, with at least one diagnosed before age 50

At least two close relatives with breast or ovarian cancer

Close male relative with breast cancer

Personal history of ovarian cancer

No additional family history may be required for individuals of ethnicities associated with higher mutation frequencies (eg, Ashkenazi Jewish)

Data from NCCN Clinical Practice Guidelines in Oncology—Genetic/Familial High Risk Assessment: Breast and Ovarian. 2009. Available at: http://www.nccn.org/professionals/physician_gls/PDF/genetics_screening.pdf; with permission.

BART testing if testing by full sequencing is negative. For other individuals, BART testing needs to be considered on an individual basis, with the understanding that insurance coverage is variable.

Management

Women who are found to carry a deleterious *BRCA1/2* mutation should begin breast cancer screening at age 25. Current recommendations include a yearly mammogram, yearly MRI, twice-yearly clinical breast examinations, and monthly breast self-examinations (see **Table 3**).[17] MRI has been shown to be significantly more sensitive than mammography in detecting breast cancers in women at high risk.[43–45] Sensitivity of mammography may be particularly poor in *BRCA1* mutation carriers.[45]

Because of the role BRCA1 and BRCA2 play in homologous DNA repair, there have been particular concerns regarding potential risks of screening mammograms with respect to radiation exposure. Although exposure to chest radiographs before age 20 has been associated with an increased risk of breast cancer in *BRCA1/2* mutation carriers,[46] studies have not demonstrated a direct link between mammographic radiation and increased risk of breast cancer. One retrospective case–control study with over 3000 *BRCA1/2* mutation carriers demonstrated no increased risk of breast cancer associated with mammography.[47] A smaller retrospective cohort study of 200 *BRCA1/2* mutation positive women also showed no association between mammogram exposure and risk of breast cancer in the group as a whole, although there was a modest association in *BRCA1* carriers (adjusted OR, 1.08; $P = .03$).[48] Therefore, although theoretical concerns remain,[49] at the current time, the potential benefits of mammogram in this very high-risk population are felt to outweigh any potential risks.

Unlike with breast cancer, no effective screening for ovarian cancer currently exists. Although fewer women develop ovarian cancer compared with breast cancer, the odds of surviving ovarian cancer are far worse than the odds of surviving breast cancer. Between 1999 and 2005, the overall 5-year survival rate for American women with breast cancer was 89.1%, whereas the overall survival rate for American women with ovarian cancer was 45.9%.[50] Consequently, risk-reducing salpingo-oophorectomy (RRSO) is considered the most critical intervention available to *BRCA1/2* mutation carriers. Despite the limited data on the effectiveness of ovarian cancer screening, twice-yearly transvaginal ultrasound and CA-125 levels are recommended beginning at age 30 to 35 years until child-bearing is complete and women are prepared to undergo oophorectomy.[17]

Prevention

The clinical management of healthy *BRCA1/2* carriers depends heavily on individual preferences. Options to be considered include chemoprevention in the form of a selective estrogen receptor modulator (SERM) for breast cancer and oral contraceptives for ovarian cancer, and surgical preventions such as RRSO and risk-reducing mastectomy (RRM).

Chemoprevention

The results of the Breast Cancer Prevention Trial (BCPT) demonstrated that tamoxifen reduced the incidence of invasive breast cancer by 50% among unaffected, high-risk women.[51] Similarly, the study of tamoxifen and raloxifene demonstrated similar efficacy of raloxifene with a different adverse effect profile.[52] Very limited data are available regarding SERMS in women with *BRCA1/2* mutations. An initial study examined data from the BCPT study. Eight *BRCA1* and 11 *BRCA2* mutation carriers with breast cancer were examined. Because of the small numbers, there were insufficient data to draw conclusions about the use of tamoxifen for primary prevention of breast cancer risk in *BRCA1/2* mutation carriers; however, there was a suggestion (which was not statistically significant) that there may be benefit in *BRCA2* versus *BRCA1* mutation carriers.[53] Because *BRCA2*-associated breast cancers are much more likely than *BRCA1*-associated breast cancers to be estrogen receptor positive, this was felt to be plausible. A matched case–control study conducted by the Hereditary Breast Cancer Clinical Study group, however, found tamoxifen to be protective against contralateral breast cancer in both *BRCA1* and *BRCA2* mutation carriers. The study compared self-reported tamoxifen use in *BRCA1/2* mutation-positive women with bilateral breast cancer (n = 285) to those with unilateral breast cancer (n = 751). The results showed a statistically significant reduction in contralateral breast cancer risk among *BRCA1* (odds ratio [OR] 0.50, 95% confidence interval [CI] 0.30–0.85), as well as a reduction among *BRCA2* mutation carriers (OR 0.42, 95% CI 0.17–1.02) who took tamoxifen.[54]

Oral contraceptive pills (OCPs) have been shown to be effective at reducing the risk of ovarian cancer in *BRCA1* and *BRCA2* mutation carriers.[55,56] OCPs, however, also have been associated with a modest excess risk of breast cancer in *BRCA1/2* mutation carriers in some,[57] but not all,[58] studies. Balancing the benefits of OCPs in terms of reduction in ovarian cancer risk and prevention of unintended pregnancy against the potential increase risk of breast cancer needs to be considered on an individual basis.

Surgical Prevention

Risk-reducing surgery is the most effective prevention against breast and ovarian cancer available to *BRCA1/2* mutation carriers. RRSO reduces the risk of ovarian cancer by greater than 85% and reduces the risk of breast cancer by approximately 50%.[59–63] It additionally may improve mortality.[64] The breast cancer risk reduction seen with oophorectomy may be greatest when the surgery is performed before age 40.[61] As is the case with SERMS, hormonal ablation induced by RRSO theoretically would cause a greater reduction in *BRCA2*-associated breast cancers than *BRCA1*-associated cancers because of the differences in estrogen receptor status. A multicenter prospective study involving 1079 *BRCA1/2* mutation carriers found a reduction in breast cancer risk following RRSO in *BRCA2* mutation carriers (hazard ratio [HR] 0.28, 95% CI 0.08–0.92); the risk reduction in *BRCA1* mutation carriers did not reach statistical significance (HR 0.61, 95% CI 0.3–1.22).[65] Further work needs to be done regarding this important topic; however, in a recent meta-analysis, overall RRSO was shown to reduce the risk of breast cancer substantially in both *BRCA1* and *BRCA2* mutation carriers.[63]

A prospective study of the mortality benefit of RRSO found that the procedure was associated with decreased overall mortality (HR 0.26, 95% CI 0.09–0.85), decreased breast-cancer-specific mortality (HR 0.13, 95% CI 0.02–0.81), and decreased ovarian cancer-specific and primary peritoneal cancer-specific mortality (HR 0.05, 95% CI 0.0–0.46).[64] This study was limited by small sample size and limited follow-up; further prospective studies are needed.

RRSO induces surgical menopause years, if not decades, before natural menopause would have occurred. In addition to the menopausal symptoms that young women may experience after undergoing a bilateral oophorectomy, serious long-term consequences of early estrogen deprivation include increased risk of osteoporosis, cardiovascular disease, and stroke. In studies from the general population (reflecting women who do not have the same risk of ovarian and breast cancer as *BRCA1* and *BRCA2* mutation carriers), early oophorectomy also may lead to increased mortality.[66,67] This is in contrast to what has been demonstrated to date in *BRCA1* and *BRCA2* carriers. In premenopausal *BRCA1/2* mutation carriers without prior cancer who undergo RRSO, short-term (2–3 years) hormone replacement therapy (HRT) does not appear to increase breast cancer risk[68,69] and does mitigate menopausal symptoms.[70] Although the overall benefits of RRSO are significant in *BRCA1/2* mutation carriers, careful attention should be paid to noncancer end points, and further studies are needed to help prevent potential adverse outcomes.

Bilateral prophylactic mastectomy, also known as risk-reducing mastectomy (RRM), has been shown to drastically reduce the risk of breast cancer in *BRCA1/2* mutation carriers.[71–73] The option of RRM should be discussed with *BRCA1/2* mutation carriers, with appropriate consideration of breast reconstruction.

Treatment

Women with *BRCA1/2* mutations diagnosed with a first breast cancer have a substantially elevated risk of developing a second primary breast cancer, with a lifetime risk as high as 50%.[74,75] For example, a study involving over 2000 breast cancer patients from families with known *BRCA1* or *BRCA2* mutations demonstrated a cumulative risk for contralateral breast cancer of 47.4% (95% CI 38.8% to 56.0%) at 25 years from the first breast cancer diagnosis.[75] Age at initial breast cancer and type of BRCA mutation (*BRCA1* vs *BRCA2*) impacted the risk of contralateral breast cancer, with younger women and *BRCA1* mutation carriers at higher risk.[75] Although oophorectomy and tamoxifen may decrease the risk of contralateral cancer,[74] the risk is still considerable, and for that reason, some women choose to undergo bilateral mastectomy. It is important, however, to consider the features of the primary tumor in this decision. Women with multiple lymph node-positive tumors are at high risk for systemic recurrence from the primary tumor; prophylactic mastectomy of the contralateral breast, to decrease the risk of a second primary tumor, should be considered in the context of the woman's risk of dying from her primary tumor.

Systemic therapy in breast cancer in *BRCA1/2* mutation carriers is currently managed similarly to sporadic breast cancer, with treatment decisions driven by tumor size, lymph node status, and results of ER, progesterone receptor (PR), and HER2/neu assays. Although initial studies were inconsistent, breast cancers in *BRCA1/2* mutation carriers appear to have a similar prognosis compared with sporadic tumors.[76,77] For *BRCA1* mutation carriers, chemotherapy may be particularly important for comparable outcomes.[76]

In vitro studies have suggested an enhanced sensitivity to platinums and decreased sensitivity to taxanes in *BRCA1/2*-deficient cell lines.[78] Restrospective[79] and small prospective[80] studies have suggested a high response rate to cisplatin in *BRCA1/2* mutation carriers receiving neo-adjuvant chemotherapy for breast cancer. However, results from ongoing studies, including a direct comparison of docetaxel and carboplatin led in the United Kingdom (ISRCTN43372330) in the first-line metastatic setting, are needed before a change in management off of a clinical trial. More recently poly (ADP-ribose) polymerase (PARP) inhibitors have been studied in metastatic breast cancer. In a phase 1 study recently published, olaparib, an oral PARP inhibitor, was found to have low toxicity and demonstrated activity in *BRCA1/2* mutation carriers. In 19 *BRCA1/2* mutation carriers with breast, ovarian, and prostate cancers who were evaluable, 9 had objective responses (response rate 47%), and an additional 3 patients had extended stable disease.[81] Two subsequent phase 2 studies specific to *BRCA1/2* mutation carriers with ovarian cancer and breast cancer have been reported in abstract form with similar response rates at a dose of 400 mg twice daily.[82,83] In parallel to this work, PARP inhibitors have been studied in triple-negative (ER-negative, PR-negative, HER2-negative) metastatic breast cancer. In a study of triple-negative breast cancer patients, the addition of a PARP inhibitor to carboplatin/gemcitabine compared with carboplatin/gemcitabine alone led to an improvement in disease-free survival.[84] A substantial majority of triple-negative breast cancers are of the molecularly classified basal phenotype, similar to *BRCA1* mutation carriers. These parallel lines of investigation demonstrate the ways in which cancers related to inherited syndromes can help inform treatment of sporadic tumors.

SUMMARY

Continued advancements in the field of inherited genetics of breast cancer have not only benefited those individuals with specific gene mutations, but have the potential to impact the management of sporadic breast cancer.

REFERENCES

1. US Preventive Services Task Force. Screening for breast cancer: US Preventive Services Task Force recommendation statement. Ann Intern Med 2009;151(10): 716–26.
2. Li FP, Fraumeni JF, Mulvihill JJ, et al. A cancer family syndrome in twenty-four kindreds. Cancer Res 1988;48(18):5358–62.
3. Malkin D, Li FP, Strong LC, et al. Germ line p53 mutations in a familial syndrome of breast cancer, sarcomas, and other neoplasms. Science 1990;250(4985): 1233–8.
4. Gonzalez KD, Noltner KA, Buzin CH, et al. Beyond Li Fraumeni syndrome: clinical characteristics of families with p53 germline mutations. J Clin Oncol 2009;27(8): 1250–6.
5. Frebourg T, Barbier N, Yan YX, et al. Germ-line p53 mutations in 15 families with Li-Fraumeni syndrome. Am J Hum Genet 1995;56(3):608–15.
6. Varley JM, McGown G, Thorncraft M, et al. Germ-line mutations of TP53 in Li-Fraumeni families: an extended study of 39 families. Cancer Res 1997; 57(15):3245–52.
7. Birch JM, Hartley AL, Tricker KJ, et al. Prevalence and diversity of constitutional mutations in the p53 gene among 21 Li-Fraumeni families. Cancer Res 1994; 54(5):1298–304.
8. Eeles RA. Germline mutations in the TP53 gene. Cancer Surv 1995;25:101–24.
9. Rapakko K, Allinen M, Syrjakoski K, et al. Germline TP53 alterations in Finnish breast cancer families are rare and occur at conserved mutation-prone sites. Br J Cancer 2001;84(1):116–9.
10. Gonzalez KD, Buzin CH, Noltner KA, et al. High frequency of de novo mutations in Li-Fraumeni syndrome. J Med Genet 2009;46(10):689–93.
11. Achatz MI, Hainaut P, Ashton-Prolla P. Highly prevalent TP53 mutation predisposing to many cancers in the Brazilian population: a case for newborn screening? Lancet Oncol 2009;10(9):920–5.
12. Evans DG, Birch JM, Thorneycroft M, et al. Low rate of TP53 germline mutations in breast cancer/sarcoma families not fulfilling classical criteria for Li-Fraumeni syndrome. J Med Genet 2002;39(12):941–4.
13. Borresen AL, Andersen TI, Garber J, et al. Screening for germ line TP53 mutations in breast cancer patients. Cancer Res 1992;52(11):3234–6.
14. Hwang SJ, Lozano G, Amos CI, et al. Germline p53 mutations in a cohort with childhood sarcoma: sex differences in cancer risk. Am J Hum Genet 2003; 72(4):975–83.

15. Kleihues P, Schauble B, zur Hausen A, et al. Tumors associated with p53 germline mutations: a synopsis of 91 families. Am J Pathol 1997;150(1):1–13.
16. Lalloo F, Varley J, Moran A, et al. BRCA1, BRCA2 and TP53 mutations in very early-onset breast cancer with associated risks to relatives. Eur J Cancer 2006; 42(8):1143–50.
17. NCCN clinical practice guidelines in oncology—genetic/familial high-risk assessment: breast and ovarian. 2009. Available at: http://www.nccn.org/professionals/physician_gls/PDF/genetics_screening.pdf. Accessed December 26, 2009.
18. Masciari S, Van den Abbeele AD, Diller LR, et al. F18-fluorodeoxyglucose-positron emission tomography/computed tomography screening in Li-Fraumeni syndrome. JAMA 2008;299(11):1315–9.
19. Salmon A, Amikam D, Sodha N, et al. Rapid development of post-radiotherapy sarcoma and breast cancer in a patient with a novel germline 'de-novo' TP53 mutation. Clin Oncol (R Coll Radiol) 2007;19(7):490–3.
20. Liaw D, Marsh DJ, Li J, et al. Germline mutations of the PTEN gene in Cowden disease, an
   inherited breast and thyroid cancer syndrome. Nat Genet 1997;16(1):64–7.
21. Marsh DJ, Coulon V, Lunetta KL, et al. Mutation spectrum and genotype–phenotype analyses in Cowden disease and Bannayan-Zonana syndrome, two hamartoma syndromes with germline PTEN mutation. Hum Mol Genet 1998;7(3):507–15.
22. Eng C. Will the real Cowden syndrome please stand up: revised diagnostic criteria. J Med Genet 2000;37(11):828–30.
23. Hobert JA, Eng C. PTEN hamartoma tumor syndrome: an overview. Genet Med 2009;11(10):687–94.
24. Brownstein MH, Wolf M, Bikowski JB. Cowden's disease: a cutaneous marker of breast cancer. Cancer 1978;41(6):2393–8.
25. Nelen MR, Kremer H, Konings IB, et al. Novel PTEN mutations in patients with Cowden disease: absence of clear genotype–phenotype correlations. Eur J Hum Genet 1999;7(3):267–73.
26. Schrager CA, Schneider D, Gruener AC, et al. Clinical and pathological features of breast disease in Cowden's syndrome: an under-recognized syndrome with an increased risk of breast cancer. Hum Pathol 1998;29(1):47–53.
27. Nelson HD, Fu R, Griffin JC, et al. Systematic review: comparative effectiveness of medications to reduce risk for primary breast cancer. Ann Intern Med 2009; 151(10):703–15.
28. Miki Y, Swensen J, Shattuck-Eidens D, et al. A strong candidate for the breast and ovarian cancer susceptibility gene BRCA1. Science 1994;266(5182):66–71.
29. Wooster R, Neuhausen SL, Mangion J, et al. Localization of a breast cancer susceptibility gene, BRCA2, to chromosome 13q12-13. Science 1994; 265(5181):2088–90.
30. Gudmundsdottir K, Ashworth A. The roles of BRCA1 and BRCA2 and associated proteins in the maintenance of genomic stability. Oncogene 2006;25(43):5864–74.
31. Malone KE, Daling JR, Doody DR, et al. Prevalence and predictors of BRCA1 and BRCA2 mutations in a population-based study of breast cancer in white and black American women ages 35 to 64 years. Cancer Res 2006;66(16):8297–308.
32. Roa BB, Boyd AA, Volcik K, et al. Ashkenazi Jewish population frequencies for common mutations in BRCA1 and BRCA2. Nat Genet 1996;14(2):185–7.
33. Robson M, Dabney MK, Rosenthal G, et al. Prevalence of recurring BRCA mutations among Ashkenazi Jewish women with breast cancer. Genet Test 1997;1(1):47–51.
34. Antoniou A, Pharoah PD, Narod S, et al. Average risks of breast and ovarian cancer associated with BRCA1 or BRCA2 mutations detected in case series

unselected for family history: a combined analysis of 22 studies. Am J Hum Genet 2003;72(5):1117–30.

35. Lakhani SR, Reis-Filho JS, Fulford L, et al. Prediction of BRCA1 status in patients with breast cancer using estrogen receptor and basal phenotype. Clin Cancer Res 2005;11(14):5175–80.

36. Chen S, Parmigiani G. Meta-analysis of BRCA1 and BRCA2 penetrance. J Clin Oncol 2007;25(11):1329–33.

37. Begg CB, Haile RW, Borg A, et al. Variation of breast cancer risk among BRCA1/2 carriers. JAMA 2008;299(2):194–201.

38. Gayther SA, Warren W, Mazoyer S, et al. Germline mutations of the BRCA1 gene in breast and ovarian cancer families provide evidence for a genotype–phenotype correlation. Nat Genet 1995;11(4):428–33.

39. Gayther SA, Mangion J, Russell P, et al. Variation of risks of breast and ovarian cancer associated with different germline mutations of the BRCA2 gene. Nat Genet 1997;15(1):103–5.

40. Antoniou AC, Spurdle AB, Sinilnikova OM, et al. Common breast cancer-predisposition alleles are associated with breast cancer risk in BRCA1 and BRCA2 mutation carriers. Am J Hum Genet 2008;82(4):937–48.

41. Panchal SM, Ennis M, Canon S, et al. Selecting a BRCA risk assessment model for use in a familial cancer clinic. BMC Med Genet 2008;9:116.

42. Palma MD, Domchek SM, Stopfer J, et al. The relative contribution of point mutations and genomic rearrangements in BRCA1 and BRCA2 in high-risk breast cancer families. Cancer Res 2008;68(17):7006–14.

43. Kriege M, Brekelmans CT, Boetes C, et al. Efficacy of MRI and mammography for breast cancer screening in women with a familial or genetic predisposition. N Engl J Med 2004;351(5):427–37.

44. Kuhl CK, Schrading S, Leutner CC, et al. Mammography, breast ultrasound, and magnetic resonance imaging for surveillance of women at high familial risk for breast cancer. J Clin Oncol 2005;23(33):8469–76.

45. Leach MO, Boggis CR, Dixon AK, et al. Screening with magnetic resonance imaging and mammography of a UK population at high familial risk of breast cancer: a prospective multicentre cohort study (MARIBS). Lancet 2005; 365(9473):1769–78.

46. Andrieu N, Easron DF, Chang-Claude J, et al. Effect of chest X-rays on the risk of breast cancer among BRCA1/2 mutation carriers in the international BRCA1/2 carrier cohort study: a report from the EMBRACE, GENEPSO, GEO-HEBON, and IBCCS Collaborators' Group. J Clin Oncol 2006;24(21):3361–6.

47. Narod SA, Lubinshi J, Ghadirian P, et al. Screening mammography and risk of breast cancer in BRCA1 and BRCA2 mutation carriers: a case-control study. Lancet Oncol 2006;7(5):402–6.

48. Goldfrank D, Chuai S, Bernstein JL, et al. Effect of mammography on breast cancer risk in women with mutations in BRCA1 or BRCA2. Cancer Epidemiol Biomarkers Prev 2006;15(11):2311–3.

49. Berrington de Gonzalez A, Berg CD, Visvanathan K, et al. Estimated risk of radiation-induced breast cancer from mammographic screening for young BRCA mutation carriers. J Natl Cancer Inst 2009;101(3):205–9.

50. Jemal A, Siegel R, Ward E, et al. Cancer statistics, 2009. CA Cancer J Clin 2009; 59(4):225–49.

51. Fisher B, Costantino JP, Wickerham DL, et al. Tamoxifen for the prevention of breast cancer: current status of the National Surgical Adjuvant Breast and Bowel Project P-1 study. J Natl Cancer Inst 2005;97(22):1652–62.

52. Vogel VG, Constantino JP, Wickerham DL, et al. Effects of tamoxifen vs raloxifene on the risk of developing invasive breast cancer and other disease outcomes: the NSABP Study of Tamoxifen and Raloxifene (STAR) P-2 trial. JAMA 2006;295(23): 2727–41.

53. King MC, Wieand S, Hale K, et al. Tamoxifen and breast cancer incidence among women with inherited mutations in BRCA1 and BRCA2: National Surgical Adjuvant Breast and Bowel Project (NSABP-P1) Breast Cancer Prevention Trial. JAMA 2001;286(18):2251–6.

54. Gronwald J, Tung N, Foulkes WD, et al. Tamoxifen and contralateral breast cancer in BRCA1 and BRCA2 carriers: an update. Int J Cancer 2006;118(9): 2281–4.

55. Narod SA, Dube MP, Klijn J, et al. Oral contraceptives and the risk of breast cancer in BRCA1 and BRCA2 mutation carriers. J Natl Cancer Inst 2002; 94(23):1773–9.

56. Whittemore AS, Balise RR, Pharoah PD, et al. Oral contraceptive use and ovarian cancer risk among carriers of BRCA1 or BRCA2 mutations. Br J Cancer 2004; 91(11):1911–5.

57. Brohet RM, Goldgar DE, Easton DF, et al. Oral contraceptives and breast cancer risk in the international BRCA1/2 carrier cohort study: a report from EMBRACE, GENEPSO, GEO-HEBON, and the IBCCS Collaborating Group. J Clin Oncol 2007;25(25): 3831–6.

58. Haile RW, Thomas DC, McGuire V, et al. BRCA1 and BRCA2 mutation carriers, oral contraceptive use, and breast cancer before age 50. Cancer Epidemiol Biomarkers Prev 2006;15(10):1863–70.

59. Rebbeck TR, Lynch HT, Neuhausen SL, et al. Prophylactic oophorectomy in carriers of BRCA1 or BRCA2 mutations. N Engl J Med 2002;346(21):1616–22.

60. Kauff ND, Satagopan JM, Robson ME, et al. Risk-reducing salpingo-oophorectomy in women with a BRCA1 or BRCA2 mutation. N Engl J Med 2002;346(21):1609–15.

61. Eisen A, Lubinski J, Klijn J, et al. Breast cancer risk following bilateral oophorectomy in BRCA1 and BRCA2 mutation carriers: an international case-control study. J Clin Oncol 2005;23(30):7491–6.

62. Finch A, Beiner M, Lubinski J, et al. Salpingo-oophorectomy and the risk of ovarian, fallopian tube, and peritoneal cancers in women with a BRCA1 or BRCA2 Mutation. JAMA 2006;296(2):185–92.

63. Rebbeck TR, Kauff ND, Domchek SM. Meta-analysis of risk reduction estimates associated with risk-reducing salpingo-oophorectomy in BRCA1 or BRCA2 mutation carriers. J Natl Cancer Inst 2009;101(2):80–7.

64. Domchek SM, Friebel TM, Neuhausen SL, et al. Mortality after bilateral salpingo-oophorectomy in BRCA1 and BRCA2 mutation carriers: a prospective cohort study. Lancet Oncol 2006;7(3):223–9.

65. Kauff ND, Domchek SM, Friebel TM, et al. Risk-reducing salpingo-oophorectomy for the prevention of BRCA1- and BRCA2-associated breast and gynecologic cancer: a multicenter, prospective study. J Clin Oncol 2008;26(8):1331–7.

66. Parker WH, Broder MS, Chang E, et al. Ovarian conservation at the time of hysterectomy and long-term health outcomes in the nurses' health study. Obstet Gynecol 2009;113(5):1027–37.

67. Rocca WA, Grossardt BR, de Andrade M, et al. Survival patterns after oophorectomy in premenopausal women: a population-based cohort study. Lancet Oncol 2006;7(10):821–8.

68. Rebbeck TR, Friebel T, Wagner T, et al. Effect of short-term hormone replacement therapy on breast cancer risk reduction after bilateral prophylactic oophorectomy in BRCA1 and BRCA2 mutation carriers: the PROSE Study Group. J Clin Oncol 2005;23(31):7804–10.
69. Eisen A, Lubinski J, Gronwald J, et al. Hormone therapy and the risk of breast cancer in BRCA1 mutation carriers. J Natl Cancer Inst 2008;100(19):1361–7.
70. Madalinska JB, van Beurden M, Bleiker EM, et al. The impact of hormone replacement therapy on menopausal symptoms in younger high-risk women after prophylactic salpingo-oophorectomy. J Clin Oncol 2006;24(22):3576–82.
71. Hartmann LC, Sellers TA, Schaid DJ, et al. Efficacy of bilateral prophylactic mastectomy in BRCA1 and BRCA2 gene mutation carriers. J Natl Cancer Inst 2001;93(21):1633–7.
72. Meijers-Heijboer H, van Geel B, van Putten WL, et al. Breast cancer after prophylactic bilateral mastectomy in women with a BRCA1 or BRCA2 mutation. N Engl J Med 2001;345(3):159–64.
73. Rebbeck TR, Friebel T, Lynch HT, et al. Bilateral prophylactic mastectomy reduces breast cancer risk in BRCA1 and BRCA2 mutation carriers: the PROSE Study Group. J Clin Oncol 2004;22(6):1055–62.
74. Metcalfe K, Lynch HT, Ghadirian P, et al. Contralateral breast cancer in BRCA1 and BRCA2 mutation carriers. J Clin Oncol 2004;22(12):2328–35.
75. Graeser MK, Engel C, Rhiem K, et al. Contralateral breast cancer risk in BRCA1 and BRCA2 mutation carriers. J Clin Oncol 2009;27(35):5887–92.
76. Rennert G, Bisland-Naggan S, Bernett-Griness O, et al. Clinical outcomes of breast cancer in carriers of BRCA1 and BRCA2 mutations. N Engl J Med 2007; 357(2):115–23.
77. Bordeleau L, Panchal S, Goodwin P. Prognosis of BRCA-associated breast cancer: a summary of evidence. Breast Cancer Res Treat 2010;119(1):13–24.
78. Tutt A, Ashworth A. Can genetic testing guide treatment in breast cancer? Eur J Cancer 2008;44(18):2774–80.
79. Byrski T, Gronwald J, Huzarski T, et al. Response to neo-adjuvant chemotherapy in women with BRCA1-positive breast cancers. Breast Cancer Res Treat 2008; 108(2):289–96.
80. Byrski T, Huzarski T, Dent R, et al. Response to neoadjuvant therapy with cisplatin in BRCA1-positive breast cancer patients. Breast Cancer Res Treat 2009;115(2): 359–63.
81. Fong PC, Boss DS, Yap TA, et al. Inhibition of poly(ADP-ribose) polymerase in tumors from BRCA mutation carriers. N Engl J Med 2009;361(2):123–34.
82. Audeh MW, Penson RT, Friedlander M, et al. Phase II trial of the oral PARP inhibitor olaparib in BRCA-deficient advanced ovarian cancer. J Clin Oncol 2009; 27(15S):277s.
83. Tutt A, Robson M, Garber JE, et al. Phase II trial of the oral PARP inhibitor olaparib in BRCA-deficient advanced breast cancer. J Clin Oncol 2009;27(15S):7s.
84. O'Shaughnessy OC, Pippen J, Yoffe M, et al. Efficacy of BSI-201, a poly (ADP-ribose) polymerase-1 (PARP1) inhibitor, in combination with gemcitabine/carboplatin (G/C) in patients with metastatic triple-negative breast cancer: results of a randomized trial. J Clin Oncol 2009;27(15s):6s.
85. Howlett NG, Taniguchi T, Olson S, et al. Biallelic inactivation of BRCA2 in Fanconi anemia. Science 2002;297(5581):606–9.

Upper Gastrointestinal Cancer Predisposition Syndromes

Manish A. Shah, MD[a,b,]*, Robert C. Kurtz, MD[b,c]

KEYWORDS

- Gastrointestinal • Cancer • Malignancy
- Genetic predisposition • Hereditary

Upper gastrointestinal malignancies encompass a heterogenous group of cancers that carry the worst prognosis of solid tumor malignancies of the entire gastrointestinal tract. Cancers of the esophagus, stomach, pancreas, and gastrointestinal stroma are commonly diagnosed in an advanced stage, when treatment goals are for disease control rather than cure. Although they have varying epidemiology and biology, there are several genetic predisposition syndromes that carry an increased risk for these malignancies, many of which are overlapping.

This review highlights the known genetic predisposition syndromes associated with upper gastrointestinal malignancies. Genetic risk may be grouped by family history, high-penetrance alleles, and low-penetrance polymorphisms. Low-penetrance polymorphisms for upper gastrointestinal malignancies are often associated with gene/environment interactions. This article highlights the known genetic risks for developing the each of these individual diseases in the context of these broad categories to provide a clinically relevant, comprehensive review of upper gastrointestinal genetic predisposition syndromes.

CANCER OF THE ESOPHAGUS

During the past 50 years, the epidemiology of esophageal cancer has changed considerably.[1,2] Historically, squamous cell carcinoma (SCC) of the esophagus

---

[a] Gastrointestinal Oncology Service, Department of Medicine, Memorial Sloan-Kettering Cancer Center, 1275 York Avenue, H910, New York, NY 10065, USA
[b] Department of Medicine, Weill Medical College of Cornell University, 1300 York Avenue, New York, NY 10065, USA
[c] Gastroenterology and Nutrition Service, Department of Medicine, Memorial Sloan-Kettering Cancer Center, 410 East 68th Street, H374, New York, NY 10065, USA
* Corresponding author. Gastrointestinal Oncology Service, Department of Medicine, Memorial Sloan-Kettering Cancer Center, 1275 York Avenue, H910, New York, NY 10065.
E-mail address: shah1@mskcc.org

Hematol Oncol Clin N Am 24 (2010) 815–835
doi:10.1016/j.hoc.2010.06.007
0889-8588/10/$ – see front matter © 2010 Elsevier Inc. All rights reserved.

hemonc.theclinics.com

accounted for more than 90% of the newly diagnosed cases, with common risk factors including heavy tobacco and alcohol use. Since the 1970s, the incidence of adenocarcinoma of the distal esophagus has increased by 4% to 10%/y, and has recently eclipsed the SCC of the esophagus.[3] The risk factors for esophageal adenocarcinoma are obesity, gastroesophageal reflux disease, and the associated pathologic changes characteristic of Barrett esophagus.[4] Annually, approximately 14,000 new cases of esophageal adenocarcinoma and SCC are diagnosed in the United States, with a high ratio of fatalities to cases (0.89).[5] This article reviews the limited knowledge of genetic predisposition syndromes associated with esophageal cancer, highlighting tylosis, *BRCA2* kindreds, familial Barrett esophagus, and low-penetrance genetic polymorphisms linked with the development of esophageal carcinoma.

Tylosis: Association with Esophageal SCC

Tylosis is a rare autosomal dominant skin disorder characterized by hyperkeratosis of the palms and soles. This condition has also been associated with the development of esophageal SCC,[6–10] initially observed in large pedigrees from the United Kingdom[9] and from the United States[7] that demonstrate an autosomal dominant inheritance pattern with complete penetrance of the skin changes by the age of 20 years. The estimated lifetime risk of developing esophageal cancer ranges from 40% (United States pedigree) to 92% (United Kingdom pedigree) by the age of 70 years.[10]

Linkage analysis identifies a 42.5 kb region on chromosome 17q25 that is strongly linked with the disease.[11,12] Recently, downregulation of cytoglobin gene expression has been associated with the development of tylosis.[13] The proposed mechanism of a germline mutation causing disease is novel: impaired cytoglobin gene transcription and the altered expression of an associated, but as yet unidentified, target gene may be caused by the production of aberrant RNA that is capable of reduced transcription but also by interaction with the cytoglobin gene product.[13]

BRCA2: A Linkage with Esophageal SCC?

BRCA2 was identified in families with breast cancer who did not have a mutation in *BRCA1* and had a high incidence of male breast cancer.[14] *BRCA2*, located on chromosome 13q12 to 13, encodes a large 3418–amino-acid protein and is believed to be important in facilitating repair of double-stranded breaks by binding directly to the Rad51 protein[15] and recruiting this recombinase protein to sites of DNA damage.[16] This protein has been associated with familial kindreds of SCC of the esophagus in high-risk areas in the Shanxi Province in China[17] and among the Turkmen population of Iran.[18] In the study from the Shanxi Province, investigators identified 5 germline mutations (4 missense and 1 deletion) among 44 patients with esophageal cancer all with a family history, whereas no germline *BRCA2* mutations were identified among the cases without a family history ($P = .078$).[17] In the Turkmen study from Iran, a single nonsense variation (K3326X) was identified in 9 patients with squamous cell cancer of the esophagus versus 2/254 controls (odds ratio [OR] 6.0, 95% confidence interval [CI] 1.3–28),[18] thus further implicating this gene in the development of some familial kindreds of esophageal cancer. However, neither the Chinese missense mutations nor the K3266X alteration are clearly associated with loss of BRCA2 function, raising the possibility that these associations may not be causative. In support of this, in these esophageal squamous cell cancer kindreds with *BRCA2* variation, no cases of breast or ovarian cancer were identified.[17]

Familial Barrett Esophagus: Association with Esophageal Adenocarcinoma

Barrett esophagus describes the replacement of the normal squamous lining of the esophagus with metaplastic columnar epithelium as a result of chronic gastric acid reflux. Barrett esophagus associated with high-grade dysplasia is considered a premalignant condition with the annual risk for transformation estimated at 1% to 2%.[19] Although traditionally believed to be an acquired condition, there is increasing evidence that a subset of patients with Barrett esophagus may have a genetic predisposition to developing the disease.[20–22] The risk of developing adenocarcinoma in patients with familial Barrett esophagus seems to be variable, but may be as much as twice that of malignant transformation from sporadic Barrett esophagus.[22]

The familial clustering of Barrett esophagus may be multifactorial, including from shared genes and environmental influences. Twin studies can minimize the confounding of shared environments, and have been examined to identify concordance of Barrett esophagus among monozygotic and dizygotic twins. In 3 separate studies, although the concordance for Barrett esophagus was significantly higher for monozygotic twins than dizygotic twins,[23–25] the concordance ranged from 19% to 42%, suggesting the presence of additional environmental factors that may modify the penetrance of the disease phenotype.

Low-penetrance Polymorphisms Linked to Esophageal Cancer: Gene-Environment Interaction

Genetic polymorphisms linked to esophageal cancer have been examined for both squamous cell and esophageal adenocarcinoma, evaluating polymorphisms in metabolic pathway proteins or in proteins involved in DNA repair, cell cycle, and apoptosis (reviewed by Cheung and Liu[26]). Although susceptibility studies across various populations have rarely been consistent, thereby dampening enthusiasm for identification of a true linkage with disease, several studies demonstrate gene-environmental interactions that are highly suggestive of modulation of risk of developing esophageal cancer. For example, 1 polymorphism associated with squamous cell esophageal cancer risk involves the aldehyde dehydrogenase gene, *ALDH2*, which is involved in the metabolism of alcohol.[27,28] Heterozygous individuals, *ALDH ∗1/∗2*, particularly those who have high alcohol consumption, are at a significant risk of developing squamous cell cancer of the esophagus, with an estimated OR of 3.2.[28] Heterozygous individuals who do not drink alcohol, or homozygous (∗2/∗2) individuals (typically associated with alcohol intolerance) are at reduced risk of SCC.[28] As another example, homozygous carriers of a DNA repair protein, O(6)-methylguanine-DNA methyltransferase (MGMT) polymorphism (rs12268840) who suffer from acid reflux are at significantly higher risk for developing esophageal adenocarcinoma, with an OR of 15.5.[29] These studies suggest that evaluation of at least some low-penetrance polymorphisms must be taken in the appropriate clinical and environmental context for an association to be identified and, potentially, validated.

CANCER OF THE STOMACH

Gastric cancer represents an enormous global health burden. Gastric cancer is the second most common cause of cancer-related deaths worldwide, with 700,349 deaths annually,[30] and is the third most common malignancy worldwide, with 974,000 new cases in the year 2000. Although the incidence of gastric cancer in the United States has declined in the past several decades, it remains a significant health problem throughout southeast Asia, eastern Europe, and Central America. Nearly two-thirds of cases occur in eastern Europe, South America, and Asia, with 42% in China alone. In the United States, an estimated 21,500 new cases (14th most common) of gastric cancer were diagnosed in 2008 with 10,880 deaths (13th most common).[31]

Gastric cancers are often grouped together, although there are considerable clinical and pathologic differences in disease, distinguished by disease location, histology, and molecular characteristics. Virtually all stomach cancers are adenocarcinomas that can be pathologically distinguished according to the Lauren classification as intestinal or diffuse subtypes.[32] Intestinal gastric cancers are generally well differentiated with a glandular appearance, and tend to expand through the stomach wall, whereas diffuse gastric cancers are more commonly poorly differentiated and spread as single discohesive cells that infiltrate throughout the stomach wall. Intestinal gastric cancers are more prevalent in high-incidence areas and are responsible for much of the observed global ethnic variation.[33] In contrast, the incidence of diffuse gastric cancer is approximately the same, independent of geography or race. It is more infrequent than intestinal gastric cancer, occurring at an incidence of 0.3 to 1.8 per 100,000 people. When reviewing the genetics of gastric cancer, it is important to place this information in context with disease biology. As understanding of the biology of this heterogeneous disease improves, the ability to screen for early stage disease and treat more advanced disease should also improve.

Familial Gastric Cancer

A family history of gastric cancer confers an OR of 2.1 to 6 for developing gastric cancer.[34–36] The risk of developing gastric cancer increases with increasing numbers of family members with the disease, up to an OR of 8.5 when 2 or more siblings are affected,[35] and, in a study of twin siblings, the sibling of a male monozygotic twin who had stomach cancer has an OR of 9.9 for developing gastric cancer, compared with an individual without a twin without gastric cancer.[37] The cause for the high risk of gastric cancer conferred by a familial history is largely unknown. Approximately 15% of all new gastric cancer diagnoses are heritable, whereas the remaining 85% are sporadic.

Hereditary Diffuse Gastric Cancer

Hereditary diffuse gastric cancer (HDGC) is a genetic predisposition syndrome that was defined in 1999 by the International Gastric Cancer Linkage Consortium (IGCLC) as any family that fulfills 1 of the following criteria: (1) 2 or more documented cases of diffuse gastric cancer in first- or second-degree relatives, with at least 1 diagnosed before the age of 50 years; or (2) 3 or more cases of diffuse gastric cancer in first- or second-degree relatives, independent of age.[38] HDGC (Online Mendelian Inheritance in Man [OMIM] # gastric cancer 137215) is an autosomal dominant syndrome characterized by a 60% to 80% penetrance for the development of diffuse-type gastric cancer. Families with HDGC also have a higher prevalence of developing lobular breast cancer and signet ring cell colon cancer. Thus, modified HDGC criteria now also include a family history of 1 of these cancers in addition to early-onset diffuse gastric cancer as sufficient criteria for the syndrome.

HDGC is caused by functional mutations or deletions in the E-cadherin (CDH1) gene on chromosome 16q22.[39–41] E-cadherin is a calcium-dependent cell-to-cell adhesion molecule on epithelial cells that maintains intercellular adhesion and epithelial cell architecture. Loss of E-cadherin expression has been demonstrated in many sporadic human cancers and is associated with malignancy, invasion, and metastasis. CDH1 is believed to have both tumor suppressor and invasion suppressor functions. A CDH1 mutation was first identified in several Maori kindreds with familial gastric cancer in 1998.[39] To date, more than 70 families with CDH1 mutations have been identified, each with a predominance of early-onset diffuse gastric adenocarcinoma. Many different mutations, rather than a few recurring alterations, have been identified.[42] More recently, *CDH1* allelic expression imbalance was seen in 70% of patients with diffuse gastric cancer meeting HDGC criteria who were mutation or deletion negative, suggesting that additional mechanisms of allelic loss of *CDH1* are likely present in those familial kindreds without *CDH1* mutation or deletion.[43] E-cadherin loss is observed by immunohistochemistry in approximately 50% of patients with sporadic diffuse gastric cancer, suggesting that this pathway may present a possible molecular target to exploit.

There are preliminary clues to a potential racial variance with regard to the occurrence of CDH1 mutations. *CDH1* is a highly polymorphic gene with significant variance throughout each of its 16 exons and coding regions, and no regions considered as mutational hot spots. Germline mutations in CDH1 occur in as many as 20% of patients with sporadic diffuse gastric cancer who developed the disease before the age of 50 years. However, in high-incidence areas (ie, Asia/Central America), germline CDH1 mutations in sporadic diffuse gastric cancer are found less often, at about 1% to 2%.[32] Recently, a large registry-based cohort study reported that the incidence of germline CDH1 mutations occurred in 30% of families with a family history of gastric cancer, and in 20% of isolated early-onset diffuse gastric cancer cases.[11] However, this study included only 3 African Americans, and 4 Asian/Pacific Islander families, out of a total of 31 tested, again highlighting the lack of racial/minority representation in this type of registry research. This study was not powered to determine whether the incidence of CDH1 mutations in familial and early-onset gastric cancer differed based on race or ethnicity. The current recommendations for therapy for patients harboring a *CDH1* mutation is prophylactic gastrectomy, which is felt to greatly reduce the risk of developing gastric cancer.[44]

Other Germline Genetic Causes of Heritable Gastric Cancer

HDGC represents approximately 30% of all familial gastric cancers. The genetic cause of the remainder is yet to be identified.[42,45] There has been 1 reported gastric cancer familial kindred having a germline mutation in *MET*, the genet that encodes for cMET, a transmembrane receptor tyrosine kinase responsible for cellular proliferation, migration, invasion in embryogenesis, and wound healing. This has prompted significant research in cMET signaling as a potential target for gastric cancer, and has led to multiple (ie, >6) novel cMET inhibitors in clinical evaluation, several of which are specifically for gastric cancer. Other rare genetic causes of familial gastric cancer include hereditary nonpolyposis colon cancer syndrome (HNPCC), FAP, Li-Fraumeni syndrome (p53 mutations), and Peutz-Jeghers syndrome (PJS).[45]

Lynch[46] syndrome (also known as HNPCC) is an autosomal dominant condition caused by germline mutations in one of the mismatch repair genes *MLH1*, *MSH2*, *MSH6*, *PMS1*, and *PMS2*. Microsatellite instability characterizes all of the tumors that arise in association with Lynch syndrome. Endometrial and colorectal cancers are the most commonly described cancers in this syndrome. Lynch[47] syndrome accounts for about 3% of the more than 1 million cases of colorectal cancer that will occur worldwide this year. Stomach cancers arise in approximately 11% of Lynch syndrome families carrying germline mutations in *MLH1*, *MSH2*, or *MSH6*. Most malignancies are Laurens intestinal histology, and have the same natural history as sporadic intestinal gastric cancer.[48,49]

Familial adenomatous polyposis (FAP) is a condition associated with significant increased development of foregut as well as hindgut adenomatous polyps. Patients with FAP carry a germline mutation in adenomatous polyposis coli (*APC*), a tumor suppressor gene located on chromosome 5q21.[50,51] Loss of heterozygosity (ie, a second hit) inactivates the second allele and begins the cascade to polyp formation.

Subsequent somatic mutations are required, including *KRAS* and *p53*, that in turn lead to progression from an adenoma to a carcinoma.[52] Upper gastrointestinal polyps commonly occur in the gastric antrum (fundic gland polyps) and duodenum.[53] In the stomach, the development of fundic gland polyps does not seem to increase the rate of antral adenocarcinoma in North American or European patients,[54] but may in Japanese or Korean families that carry a germline *APC* mutation.[45]

Li-Fraumeni syndrome, carrying a germline *p53* mutation, is associated with a variety of malignancies, most notably soft tissue sarcoma, leukemia, brain cancer, adrenal cortical cancer, and breast cancer. Oliveira and colleagues[55] describe one family with a *p53* germline mutation (R158G, G → C471) with a cluster of predominant gastric cancers. PJS is an autosomal dominant hereditary disease characterized by hamartomatous polyps of the gastrointestinal tract, described more fully later.

Genetics of Intestinal Gastric Cancer: Low-penetrance Polymorphisms and Helicobacter pylori Infection

The development of intestinal gastric cancer, particularly of the body and fundus, is closely related to infection with *Helicobacter pylori*,[56,57] a gram-negative bacillus discovered in 1983 to be the pathogen responsible for gastric ulcers and peptic ulcer disease. In 1994, the World Health Organization and the International Agency for Research on Cancer consensus group classified *H pylori* as a class I carcinogen.[58] However, although *H pylori* is a common worldwide pathogen, less than 2% of infected patients develop gastric cancer during their lifetime. *H pylori* is an endemic pathogen with high prevalence rates in both developing and industrialized countries. The bacterium is present in the stomachs of at least half of the world's population, is usually acquired in childhood, and, when left untreated, generally persists for the host's lifetime. As such, exposure to this pathogen is chronic and long standing. The rate of *H pylori* infection is highest amongst the elderly minority population, with a rate of 73% in non-Hispanic blacks, and 74% in Hispanic individuals.[59] In approximately 10% of cases, the pathogen is associated with diverse clinical outcomes, including nonulcer dyspepsia, peptic ulcer disease, and distal gastric cancer.[57,60]

Several studies have examined low-penetrance polymorphisms and their association with *H pylori* associated gastric cancer. Although *H pylori* is a common worldwide pathogen, less than 5% of infected patients develop gastric cancer during their lifetime. The host's immune response to this pathogen has been implicated in determining the risk of developing gastric cancer, and, in particular, cytokines interleukin (IL)-1 and IL-8, which mediate the inflammatory response to the bacterial infection (**Table 1**). The IL-1 gene cluster is on chromosome 2q, and contains 3 related genes within a 430-kb region, *IL-1A*, *IL-1B*, and *IL-1RN*, which encode for IL-1α, IL-1β and their receptor antagonist, IL-1ra.[61] IL-1β is a potent proinflammatory cytokine and powerful inhibitor of gastric acid secretion that plays an important primary role in the initiation and amplification of the inflammatory response to *H pylori* infection.[62] Polymorphisms in the 3' regulatory region of *IL-1B* (*IL-1B* C-T -551 and -31) and *IL-1RN* (*IL-1RN*∗2) are associated with an increased risk of hypochlorhydria, decreased acid secretion, and are also associated with a significantly higher risk of gastric cancer following *H pylori* infection.[63] The estimated OR for developing gastric cancer with the *IL-1B-31T* allele was 1.6 (95% CI 1.2–2.2) and for the *IL-1RN*∗2/∗2 allele was 2.9 (95% CI 1.9–4.4).[63] These IL-1–related polymorphisms and the association with gastric cancer have now been reported in several other populations.[64,65]

IL-8 is a member of the CXC chemokine family that functions as a potent chemoattractant for neutrophils and lymphocytes. IL-8 levels are increased tenfold in gastric cancer specimens compared with normal gastric tissues.[66] Activation of *IL-8* gene

Table 1
Immune system genetic polymorphisms and gastric cancer risk

Gene	Function of Gene Product	Polymorphism	Gastric CA OR
IL-1β	Induces expression of inflammatory cytokines, inhibits gastric acid production	−31 C-T −511 C-T	2.5 (1.6–3.8) 2.6 (1.7–3.9)
IL-1Rβ	Receptor for IL-1β	Penta-allelic 86-bp tandem repeat (IN 2)	2.9 (1.9–4.4)
TNF-α	Activates inflammation and apoptosis signaling pathways; inhibits acid secretion	−308 A/A	1.9 (1.2–2.8)
IL-10	Inhibits production of proinflammatory cytokines	−591 ATA/ATA −819 ATA/ATA −1082 ATA/ATA	3.4 (1.4–8.1)
IL-8	T allele increases IL-8 promoter activity	−251 A/T	2.1–2.52

Data from Peek RMJ, Blaser MJ. Helicobacter pylori and gastrointestinal tract adenocarcinomas. Nat Rev Cancer 2002;2:28–37.

expression is mediated by *H pylori* activation of nuclear factor-κB,[67] a nuclear transcription factor also implicated in the pathogenesis of gastric cancer[68,69] and a negative prognostic factor for patients with the disease.[69] The A→T promoter polymorphism at -251 (*IL-8 -251T*) has two- to fivefold higher promoter activity than the *IL-8 -251A* allele, because of high-affinity binding of the -251A allele to a nuclear protein that acts as a negative regulator of promoter function.[70] In a Chinese cohort study, the *IL-8* AT or TT genotype (associated with increased IL-8 expression) was significantly associated with an increased risk of gastric cancer. Importantly, this association was identified specifically in patients with diffuse gastric cancer in the setting of prior or current *H pylori* infection (*IL-8 -251A/T* OR 2.12, 95% CI 1.17–3.86; *IL-8 -251T/T* OR 2.52, 95% CI 1.3–4.9), whereas those patients without *H pylori* infection had no increased risk of gastric cancer associated with *IL-8 -251T* * genotype.[70]

Recently, investigators examined 12 meta-analyses and 1 meta-analysis and pooled analysis that were published from 2005 to 2008, focusing on genes involved in inflammation, detoxification of carcinogens (*GSTM1*, *GSTT1*, *CYP2E1*), folate metabolism (*MTHFR*), adhesion (*CDH1*), and cell cycle regulation (*p53*).[71] Most of the polymorphisms have a small effect in increasing gastric cancer risk, and are of borderline significance or are not significant (**Table 2**).[71]

CANCER OF THE PANCREAS

Pancreatic cancer is the second most common gastrointestinal cancer in the United States, with an annual incidence of more than 37,000 cases and a mortality that approaches the annual incidence. The strikingly high mortality has not improved in the past 20 years, with 1-year survival for newly diagnosed patients approximately 19% and the 5-year survival less than 5%.[72] This high mortality is believed to be related to the almost universal advanced stage of pancreatic cancer at the time of

Table 2
Summary of low-penetrance genes possibly associated with gastric cancer

Gene	Meta-OR	Confidence Limits
CYP2E1 Pst1/Rsa1 c2c2	1.36	0.82–2.25
GSTM1 null	1.24	1.00–1.54
GSTTf null	1.09	0.97–1.21
	1.06	0.94–1.18
MTHFR 677TT	1.68	1.29–2.19
	1.59	1.28–1.98
	1.52	1.31–1.77
MTHFR 1298CC	0.90	0.44–1.57
	0.94	0.65–1.35
p53 codon 72 Arg/Arg	0.96	0.78–1.24
CDH1 -160A	0.98	0.78–1.24

Data from Gianfagna F, et al. A systematic review of meta-analyses on gene polymorphisms and gastric cancer risk. Curr Genomics 2008;9:361–74.

clinical presentation. Strategies to improve this dismal survival rate include identifying patients who have early, localized disease at presentation, and developing a greater understanding of environmental susceptibility and inherited risk. Only a small number of patients with pancreatic cancer have a definable genetic predisposition. About 10% of pancreatic cancers are believed to have a hereditary predisposition.[73] Two broad categories of hereditary pancreatic cancer can be defined. Familial pancreatic cancer is an inherited predisposition based on family clustering in families in which there are multiple first- and second-degree relatives with ductal pancreatic adenocarcinoma in the absence of a known genetic syndrome. As pancreatic cancer is common, several family members may be affected by chance alone. There also may be common environmental factors, an unidentified common genetic factor, or low-penetrance polymorphisms responsible for the familial clustering. Pancreatic cancer also occurs in certain well-defined cancer syndromes in which an identifiable germline mutation may lead to the development of pancreatic adenocarcinoma.[74,75]

Germline Mutations and Pancreatic Cancer

BRCA1 and BRCA2
One of the best known of the cancer predisposition syndromes is the hereditary breast and ovarian cancer syndrome. This syndrome is caused by mutation in the BRCA1 or BRCA2 tumor suppressor genes. Women who carry gene mutations of BRCA1 or BRCA2 have high lifetime risks for breast and ovarian cancers. Mutations in BRCA1 or BRCA2 are commonly the reason for families having multiple individuals with breast cancer diagnosed before the age of 60 years.[76] In a multi-institutional study, the risk of non–breast or ovarian cancer was investigated in 173 families with BRCA2 mutations identified from 20 centers in Europe and North America. Several cancers were found to have a statistically significant increased risk. These cancers included prostate, gallbladder, bile duct, stomach, and pancreas. For pancreatic cancer, the relative risk was 3.51; (95% CI 1.87–6.58).[77]

Other studies have demonstrated that BRCA2 mutations are associated with pancreatic adenocarcinoma, especially in Ashkenazi Jews. Using direct sequencing of constitutional DNA, Murphy and colleagues[78] at Johns Hopkins analyzed samples from patients with pancreatic cancer for mutations in 4 tumor suppressor candidate genes including BRCA2. Samples were taken from highly informative families in which 3 or more family members were affected with pancreatic cancer, with at least 2 first-degree relatives. BRCA2 gene sequencing identified 5 mutations believed to be deleterious (17.2%). Three patients harbored the 6174delT frameshift mutation. Two of the 5 carriers reported a family history of breast cancer, but none reported a family history of ovarian cancer. These findings confirm the increased risk of pancreatic cancer (approximately 10-fold) in individuals with BRCA2 mutations. The investigators also concluded that germline BRCA2 mutations are the most common inherited genetic alteration in familial pancreatic cancer.

BRCA1 mutations were initially not believed to have the same association with pancreatic adenocarcinoma as BRCA2; however, in a study by Lynch and colleagues,[79] pancreatic cancer was seen in 9 of 15 families in which the BRCA1 mutations was either confirmed or inferred as probable obligate BRCA1 mutation carriers. Thompson and colleagues[80] analyzed data on 11,847 individuals from 699 families with a BRCA1 mutation. They found that the relative risk of developing pancreatic cancer in BRCA1 mutation carriers was statistically significant (about two-fold).

Lynch syndrome: HNPCC

Pancreatic cancer was first reported in a family with Lynch syndrome in 1985.[81] Studies of the risk of pancreatic carcinoma in patients with Lynch syndrome compared with the general population have been variable. Pancreatic cancer has been included as an HNPCC-associated tumor in the revised Bethesda guidelines.[82] Geary and colleagues[83] reviewed the family histories of 130 individuals with documented mismatch repair gene mutations. They found 22 cases of pancreatic cancer. Half were in proven or obligate carriers. The risk as define by their study was about 7 times expected. Young age of onset was also characteristic, with 14 of 20 with a known age less than 60 years. Three of 7 families with small bowel cancer also had pancreatic cancer. There have also been case reports of individuals with Lynch syndrome who have developed medullary carcinoma of the pancreas. The link between Lynch syndrome and medullary carcinomas of the pancreas was suggested by Wilentz and colleagues.[84] Three of their 18 patients with medullary cancer of the pancreas had a first-degree relative with colon cancer. One patient in this study had both a medullary carcinoma of the pancreas and a colorectal cancer. Both tumors were found to be positive for microsatellite instability. A report was recently published of a patient with a medullary carcinoma of the pancreas in which a germline mutation in the MSH2 gene was identified, further supporting an association between medullary carcinoma of the pancreas and Lynch syndrome.[85] Individuals with medullary carcinoma of the pancreas should be considered for evaluation of a mutated mismatch repair gene, especially if their pancreatic cancer is tested and found to be positive for microsatellite instability. In a study from Italy,[86] a series of 135 consecutive patients with pancreatic cancer were examined for suspected Lynch syndrome by reviewing their historical data. Nineteen patients with pancreatic cancer were characterized as suspected cases of Lynch syndrome. DNA was available for study in 11 cases, and 4 were found to have a novel variant of either MLH1 or MSH2 not known to cause a mismatch repair defect. The investigators concluded that only a small percentage of patients with pancreatic cancer would be expected to carry a mismatch repair gene mutation. Kastrinos and colleagues[87] found 31 of 147 families with mismatch repair gene mutations where there was at least 1 reported case of pancreatic cancer. The cumulative risk of pancreatic cancer in their families with gene mutations was calculated to be 1.31% (0.31%–2.32%) in young individuals up to age 50 years.

This rose to 3.68% (1.45%–5.88%) up to age 70 years, an 8.6-fold increase. Yamamoto and colleagues[88] described 3 patients with Lynch syndrome with high levels of microsatellite instability in their pancreatic cancers. These individuals had a significantly longer overall survival than patients with pancreatic cancer with low tumor levels of microsatellite instability or patients who were microsatellite stable.

Familial atypical multiple mole melanoma syndrome

The familial atypical multiple mole melanoma (FAMMM) syndrome is caused by a germline mutation in the tumor suppressor gene CDKN2A (p16) on chromosome 9. Mutations in CDKN2A occur in about 20% of familial melanoma families in North America, Asia, Australia, and Europe.[89] Several studies have demonstrated an increased risk of pancreatic cancer among CDKN2A melanoma–prone families.[90–93] In the Dutch FAMMM registry, pancreatic cancer was found to be the second most common cancer after melanoma in mutation carriers.[93]

Lynch and colleagues[94] described the pedigrees of 8 families with FAMMM with CDKN2A mutations and pancreatic cancer. The investigators suggested that the FAMMM phenotype could be a potential benefit in identifying individuals at high risk for the development of pancreatic cancer and allow for selective use of screening strategies.

PJS

PJS is an autosomal dominant disease characterized by hamartomatous polyps of the gastrointestinal tract and by mucocutaneous melanin deposits, and caused by germline mutations of STK11 (serine threonine kinase 11). These mutations can be found in most (66%–94%) of patients with PJS.[95] In 1987, Giardiello and colleagues[96] described the increased risk of both gastrointestinal and nongastrointestinal cancers in patients with PJS. Cancer developed in 15 of the 31 patients (48%). Relative-risk analysis showed that the development of cancer in patients with PJS was 18 times greater than expected in the general population, and the cumulative lifetime risk for pancreatic cancer from age 15 to 64 years was 36%. Ninety-six cancers were found in 419 individuals with PJS, of which 297 had documented STK11/LKB1 mutations. The most frequent cancers represented in this analysis were gastroesophageal, small bowel, colorectal, and pancreatic.[97] An individual patient meta-analysis comparing the risk of cancer in PJS with the general population, based on 210 individuals described in 6 publications, found similar results.[98] Lim and colleagues[99] found 54 cancers in 240 individuals with PJS, with germline mutations in STK11. Multiple sites of gastrointestinal cancers were seen, which included pancreatic cancer. The issue of ascertainment bias inflating the overall cancer risk was raised by Giardeillo and colleagues.[95]

FAP

FAP is an autosomal dominantly inherited disorder caused by germline mutation of the APC gene on chromosome 5q. Although colorectal cancer is the major cancer risk in affected individuals, the relative risk of other cancers, such as thyroid and pancreas, has also been described.[100] These investigators looked at the Johns Hopkins Polyposis Registry and found 4 patients with pancreatic cancer in their cohort of 1391 patients with FAP. Patients with FAP are now surviving longer because of early identification and management of their colorectal cancer risk. As a result, more-frequent diagnoses of extracolonic cancers, such as pancreatic cancer, can be expected.[101] Horii and colleagues[102] looked for somatic mutations in the APC gene in sporadic pancreatic cancer tissue and found 4 mutations in 10 pancreatic cancers. Each of these mutations would lead to a truncated protein, suggesting that somatic mutations in the APC gene might play a role in the development of sporadic pancreatic cancer. Gupta and Mazzara[103] described a woman with FAP and a precancerous pancreatic lesion, high-grade pancreatic intraepithelial neoplasia (PanIN)-3.

Hereditary pancreatitis

Hereditary pancreatitis is an autosomal dominant disease. Acute pancreatitis begins early and can lead to chronic pancreatitis. The disease has variable expression and penetrance is estimated to be about 80%.[104] In 1996, Whitcomb and colleagues[105] reported that an arginine-histidine substitution at residue 117 of the cationic trypsinogen gene was likely the cause of hereditary pancreatitis. They found this mutation in affected individuals and obligate carriers in 5 kindreds, but not in spousal controls. The gene for hereditary pancreatitis was found to map to chromosome 7q35.[105] Pancreatitis has been linked to pancreatic cancer, and an international multi-institutional study estimated the risk of pancreatic cancer in affected individuals in hereditary pancreatitis cohorts to be about 40% by age 70 years.[104]

Familial Pancreatic Cancer

The inherited susceptibility to pancreatic cancer has been well described for several decades in multiple case reports. Reimer and colleagues[106] reported a father and son who were both affected by pancreatic cancer and who also had occupational exposure to vinyl chloride. Another early report of the familial occurrence of pancreatic cancer described 3 women in successive generations who, over 11 years, each developed pancreatic cancer at a younger age. The investigators speculated that inheritance may play a role in some pancreatic cancers.[107] A similar report described pancreatic cancer in 2 brothers and a sister, all in their 70s with pancreatic cancer.[108] Lynch and colleagues,[109] in a clinicopathologic study, described 47 individuals with pancreatic cancer from 18 families recruited to the Hereditary Cancer Institute at Creighton University in Omaha. A family history of pancreatic cancer is found in up to 10% of patients with pancreatic cancer.[110] A population-based case-control study conducted in Montreal, found that 7.2% of patients with pancreatic cancer had a family history of pancreatic cancer, compared with only 0.6% in the control group.[108] Lal and colleagues[111] define patients with pancreatic cancer by likelihood of familial risk by constructing 3 generation pedigrees. They analyzed 38 out of their cohort of 102 patients with pancreatic cancer with high or intermediate risk for germline mutations. Germline mutations were found in 5 patients, 1 with a p16 (CDKN2A) mutation and 4 Ashkenazi Jews with either BRCA 1 or 2 mutations. The investigators concluded that, in most of their patients at high and intermediate risk for pancreatic cancer, an unidentified gene or genes were causing a susceptibility to this disease. A hospital-based segregation analysis also concluded that there is a rare major gene responsible for the increased susceptibility to this disease.[112] The group at Johns Hopkins using the National Familial Pancreas Tumor Registry found that, when at least 1 pair of first-degree relatives were affected with pancreatic cancer, the risk of developing pancreatic cancer was 18 times that for relatives of an individual with sporadic pancreatic cancer. In those pancreatic cancer kindreds with 3 or more affected family members, there was a 57-fold (95% CI 12.4–175) increased risk of pancreatic cancer.[113] In these families with familial pancreatic cancer, the risk of developing pancreatic cancer is closely related to the number of first-degree relatives in the family with the disease. Klein and colleagues[114] noted that environmental factors can also have an effect on pancreatic risk, because this risk was higher in smokers than in nonsmokers.

The group at the University of Washington described a susceptibility locus for familial pancreatic cancer in one of their familial pancreatic cancer cohorts (family X) that mapped to chromosome location 4q32 to 34. Further work by this group revealed a germline missense mutation in the gene Palladin (PALLD). This gene encodes for a component of the cytoskeleton that controls cell shape and motility. They demonstrated that paladin RNA was overexpressed in tissue from both dysplasia and pancreatic adenocarcinoma in both familial and sporadic pancreatic cancer.[115] Subsequent studies have not confirmed the link of Palladin to familial pancreatic cancer.[116–118] Klein and colleagues[119] performed DNA sequence analysis of the Palladin gene in 48 individuals with familial pancreatic cancer and failed to find any deleterious mutations that would identify Palladin as a susceptibility gene in familial pancreatic cancer.

Management of high-risk individuals from families with pancreatic cancer remains an important issue. Several familial pancreatic cancer registries have been developed in the United States and worldwide.[120] Pancreatic cancer precursor lesions, such as intraductal papillary mucinous neoplasms (IPMNs) and PanINs have been well described.[121] Screening programs to identify these pancreatic lesions in at-risk healthy family members are underway and several have begun to report their preliminary findings. Brentnall and colleagues,[122] at the University of Washington, studied 14 individuals from 3 unrelated pancreatic cancer kindreds (families X, Y, and Z) that had 2 or more affected members in at least 2 generations. Fourteen patients were evaluated for evidence of pancreatic abnormalities with multiple diagnostic imaging laboratory studies. Seven of these patients had endoscopic retrograde cholangiopancreatography (ERCP) findings of ectatic branch ducts and abnormalities of the main pancreatic duct. Because of these findings, these 7 patients were referred for pancreatectomy. Six of these patients were from 1 family (family X). All 7 patients were found to have pancreatic duct epithelial dysplasia ranging from low to high grade. No invasive cancer was found. Canto and colleagues[123] at Johns Hopkins, using endoscopic ultrasound and ERCP, initially reported a diagnostic yield of 5.3% in a pilot study of 38 patients. One invasive cancer was detected.[123] In a second report from Johns Hopkins, Canto and colleagues[124] identified 7 high-risk individuals with pathologically confirmed IPMNs, and 1 patient had a PanIN for a diagnostic yield of 10%. Our group at Memorial Sloan-Kettering Cancer Center, in a similar screening program using cross-sectional imaging (magnetic resonance cholangiopancreatography and computed tomography) based on our Memorial Sloan-Kettering Cancer Center Familial Pancreatic Tumor Registry, found IMPNs in 8 of 113 healthy at-risk individuals (unpublished data). Langer and colleagues[125] recently published their results of screening 76 individuals from 34 familial pancreatic cancer families culled from the German National Collection for Familial Pancreatic Cancer. Ten individuals were found to have solitary pancreatic lesions, and 7 of these underwent surgery. No cancers were identified and only 1 IPMN was found, for a low diagnostic yield of 1.3%.

The Fourth International Symposium of Inherited Diseases of the Pancreas recommends that screening of familial pancreatic cancer family members is appropriate in the context of a clinical trial.[126] They recommend screening for healthy individuals with at least 3 affected first-degree relatives and in individuals with a known BRCA2 mutation, at least 1 family member with pancreatic cancer. The age when screening should begin follows the colon cancer model, which is starting at age 50 years, or 10 years younger than the youngest affected family member. The frequency of screening remains an unanswered question, but genetic counseling was strongly recommended.

GASTROINTESTINAL STROMAL TUMOR

Gastrointestinal stromal tumors (GISTs) were originally believed to be of smooth muscle origin but have been shown to be related to the interstitial cells of Cajal (ICC)[127,128] whose function is to enable physiologic movement throughout the gastrointestinal tract. Many GISTs were initially noted to have a positive immunohistochemical stain for CD34.[129] This positive immunohistochemical staining was the initial tumor marker for GIST and led to the possibility that the cell of origin of GIST was the ICC. CD34 was dropped as a marker for GIST when it was noted that Schwann cells and other tumors of smooth muscle origin expressed CD34. GIST represents the most common gastrointestinal connective tissue malignancy. Incidence is estimated to be 10 to 13 cases per million annually.[130] Both genders are equally affected and there are no known specific risk factors. Most GISTs occur in the stomach (60%–70%). The small intestine is less frequently involved (20%–30%). The esophagus, colon, and rectum represent uncommon sites of primary GIST (<10%). Extraintestinal intraabdominal sites of involvement of primary GIST include omentum, mesentery, and retroperitoneum.[131] Hirota and colleagues[132] were the first to described the molecular genetic event that is responsible for the development of GIST; in gain-of-function mutations of c-KIT in 49 GIST tissue specimens, 94% expressed c-KIT. c-KIT mutations are seen in more than 90% of sporadic GIST. c-KIT encodes for a transmembrane tyrosine kinase inhibitor. GIST and its associated c-KIT mutations has become one of the important oncologic models for the application of kinase-targeted treatment. Initial treatment of GIST is primarily surgical, but advanced disease has been found to be dramatically responsive to tyrosine kinase inhibitors such as imatinib and sunitinib.[133] Imatinib prevents substrate phosphorylation by occupying the ATP-binding pocket of KIT, and prevents downstream signaling leading to impaired cellular proliferation. Additionally, studies of imatinib used in the adjuvant setting after surgery have demonstrated an increase in recurrence-free survival.[134]

Familial GIST

In 1998, Nishida and colleagues[135] described a Japanese family with multiple GISTs who had c-KIT mutations in their tumors as well as their leukocytes, indicating a germline mutation. This mutation was found in exon 11 of c-KIT. They also noted that the perineal and hand hyperpigmentation and mast cell hyperplasia seen in this familial aggregation of GIST are related to the c-KIT mutation. Several families with GISTs have subsequently been described with either c-KIT mutations or mutations in platelet-derived growth factor A.[136] Most familial GISTs express CD 34 and KIT protein (CD117). Familial GIST is believed to follow an autosomal dominant pattern of inheritance with high penetrance.[137]

Clinical differences have been noted between sporadic and familial GIST. Age at diagnosis seems to be approximately 1 decade earlier in familial GIST but with an equal distribution between genders.[137,138] Familial GIST is likely autosomal dominant with high penetrance. Unlike sporadic GIST, in which the stomach is the most common site of origin, in familial GIST the small bowel seems to be most commonly affected. One GIST family was described as having associated dysphagia caused by esophageal leiomyomatosis and achalasia.[139] Familial GIST should be treated in a fashion similar to sporadic GIST, and although there are no specific clinical trials for patients with familial GIST, the general belief is that these individuals do at least as well with surgical resection and the treatment of advanced disease as do their sporadic counterparts. Other uncommon forms of hereditary GIST include Carney triad and Carney-Stratakis syndrome. GIST in patients with Carney triad do not overexpress c-KIT or have somatic mutations of platelet-derived growth factor receptor α (PDGFRA).[140,141] Although neurofibromatosis type 1 is not a hereditary GIST syndrome, GIST has been described in patients with NF-1.[142] There is no clear understanding yet as to whether GISTs in these patients are caused by c-KIT or PDGFRA mutations.

REFERENCES

1. Blot WJ, DeVesa SS, Kneller RW, et al. Rising incidence of adenocarcinoma of the esophagus and gastric cardia. JAMA 1991;265:1287–9.
2. Blot WJ, McLaughlin JK. The changing epidemiology of esophageal cancer. Semin Oncol 1999;26:2–13.
3. Brown LM, Devesa SS, Chow WH. Incidence of adenocarcinoma of the esophagus among white Americans by sex, stage, and age. J Natl Cancer Inst 2008; 100:1184–7.
4. Crew KD, Neugut AI. Epidemiology of gastric cancer. World J Gastroenterol 2006;12(3):354–62.
5. Jemal A, Siegel R, Ward E, et al. Cancer statistics, 2009. CA Cancer J Clin 2009; 59(4):225–49.
6. Clarke CA, McConnell RB. Six cases of carcinoma of the oesophagus occurring in one family. Br Med J 1954;2:1137–8.
7. Stevens HP, Kelsell DP, Bryant SP, et al. Linkage of an American pedigree with palmo-plantar keratoderma and malignancy (palmoplantar ectodermal dysplasia type III) to 17q24. Literature survey and proposed updated classification of the keratodermas. Arch Dermatol 1996;132:640–51.
8. Hennies HC, Hagedorn M, Reis A. Palmoplantar keratoderma in association with carcinoma of the oesophagus maps to chromosome 17q distal to the keratin gene cluster. Genomics 1995;29:537–40.
9. Ellis A, Field JK, Field AE, et al. Tylosis associated with carcinoma of the oesophagus and oral leukoplakia in a large Liverpool family – a review of six generations. Eur J Cancer B Oral Oncol 1994;30:102–11.
10. Robertson EV, Jankowski JA. Genetics of gastroesophageal cancer: paradigms, paradoxes, and prognostic utility. Am J Gastroenterol 2008;103:443–9.
11. Risk JM, Evans KE, Jones J, et al. Characterization of a 500kb region on 17q25 and the exclusion of candidate genes as the familial tylosis oesophageal cancer (TOC) locus. Oncogene 2002;21:6395–402.
12. Langan JE, Cole CG, Huckle EJ, et al. Novel microsatellite markers and single nucleotide polymorphisms refine the tylosis with oesophageal cancer (TOC) minimal region on 17q25 to 42.5kb: sequencing does not identify causative gene. Hum Genet 2004;114:534–40.
13. McRonald FE, Liloglou T, Xinarianos G, et al. Down-regulation of the cytoglobin gene, located on 17q25, in tylosis with oesophageal cancer (TOC): evidence for transallele repression. Hum Mol Genet 2006;15:1271–7.
14. Stratton MR, Ford D, Neuhasen S, et al. Familial male breast cancer is not linked to the BRCA1 locus on chromosome 17q. Nat Genet 1994;7(1):103–7.
15. Chen PL, Chen CF, Chen Y, et al. The BRC repeats in BRCA2 are critical for Rad51 binding and resistance to methyl methanesulfonate treatment. Proc Natl Acad Sci U S A 1998;95(9):5287–92.
16. Boulton SJ. Cellular functions of the BRCA tumour-suppressor proteins. Biochem Soc Trans 2006;34(5):633–45.
17. Nan H, Wang C, Han X-Y, et al. Evaluation of BRCA2 in the genetic susceptibility of familial esophageal cancer. Oncogene 2004;23:852–8.

18. Akbari MR, Malekzadeh R, Nasrollahzadeh D, et al. Germline BRCA2 mutations and the risk of esophageal squamous cell carcinoma. Oncogene 2008;27(9): 1290–6.
19. Cameron AJ, Romero Y. Symptomatic gastro-oesophageal reflux as a risk factor for oesophageal adenocarcinoma. Gut 2000;46(6):754–5.
20. Chak A, Faulx A, Kinnard M, et al. Identification of Barrett's esophagus in relatives by endoscopic screening. Am J Gastroenterol 2004;99:2107–14.
21. Drovdlik CM, Goddard KAB, Chak A, et al. Demographic and phenotypic features of 70 families segregating Barrett's esophagus and esophageal adenocarcinoma. J Med Genet 2003;40:651–6.
22. Sappati Biyyani RS, Chessler L, McCain E, et al. Familial trends of inheritance in gastro-esophageal reflux disease, Barrett's esophagus and Barrett's adenocarcinoma: 20 families. Dis Esophagus 2007;20:53–7.
23. Cameron AJ, Lagergren J, Henriksson C, et al. Gastroesophageal reflux disease in monozygotic and dizygotic twins. Gastroenterology 2002;122:55–9.
24. Mohammed I, Cherkas LF, Riley SA, et al. Genetic influences in gastro-esophageal reflux disease: a twin study. Gut 2003;52:1085–9.
25. Zaman MS, Hur C, Jones MP, et al. Concordance of reflux among monozygotic and dizygotic twins. Gastroenterology 2001;120(Suppl 5):A418.
26. Cheung WY, Liu G. Genetic variations in esophageal cancer risk and prognosis. Gastroenterol Clin North Am 2009;38:75–91.
27. Lee CH, Lee JM, Wu DC, et al. Carcinogenetic impact of ADH1B and ALDH2 genes on squamous cell carcinoma risk of the esophagus with regard to the consumption of alcohol, tobacco, and betel quid. Int J Cancer 2008;122(6): 1347–56.
28. Lewis SJ, Smith GD. Alcohol, ALDH2, and esophageal cancer: a meta-analysis which illustrates the potentials and limitations of a Mendelian randomization approach. Cancer Epidemiol Biomarkers Prev 2005;14:1967–71.
29. Doecke J, Zhao ZZ, Pandeya N, et al. Polymorphisms in MGMT and DNA repair genes and the risk of esophageal adenocarcinoma. Int J Cancer 2008;123: 174–80.
30. Parkin DM, Bray FI, Ferlay J, et al. Global cancer statistics: 2002. CA Cancer J Clin 2005;55:74–108.
31. American Cancer Society. Cancer facts and figures. Atlanta: American Cancer Society; 2008. p. 4–17.
32. Lauren T. The two histologic main types of gastric carcinoma. Acta Pathol Microbiol Scand 1965;64:34.
33. Munoz N, Correa P, Cuello C, et al. Histologic types of gastric carcinoma in high- and low-risk areas. Int J Cancer 1968;3:809–18.
34. Nagase H, Ogino K, Yoshida I, et al. Family history-related risk of gastric cancer in Japan: a hospital-based case-control study. Jpn J Cancer Res 1996;87(10): 1025–8.
35. Palli D, Galli M, Caporaso NE, et al. Family history and risk of stomach cancer in Italy. Cancer Epidemiol Biomarkers Prev 1994;3(1):15–8.
36. Zanghieri G, Di Gregorio C, Sacchetti C, et al. Familial occurrence of gastric cancer in the 2-year experience of a population-based registry. Cancer 1990; 66:2047–51.
37. Lichtenstein P, Holm NV, Verkasalo PK, et al. Environmental and heritable factors in the causation of cancer. N Engl J Med 2000;343(2):78–85.
38. Caldas C, Carniero F, Lynch HT, et al. Familial gastric cancer: overview and guidelines for management. J Med Genet 1999;36:873–80.

39. Guilford P, Hopkins J, Harraway J, et al. E-cadherin germline mutations in familial gastric cancer. Nature 1998;392:402–5.
40. Guilford PJ, Hopkins JB, Grady WM, et al. E-cadherin germline mutations define an inherited cancer syndrome dominated by diffuse gastric cancer. Hum Mutat 1999;14(3):249–55.
41. Oliveira C, Senz J, Kaurah P, et al. Germline CDH1 deletions in hereditary diffuse gastric cancer families. Hum Mol Genet 2009;18(9):1545–55.
42. Kaurah P, MacMillan A, Boyd N, et al. Founder and recurrent CDH1 mutations in families with hereditary diffuse gastric cancer. JAMA 2007; 297(21):2360–72.
43. Pinheiro H, Bordeira-Carrico R, Seixas S, et al. Allele-specific CDH1 downregulation and hereditary diffuse gastric cancer. Hum Mol Genet 2010; 19(5):943–52.
44. Huntsman DG, Carneiro F, Lewis FR, et al. Early gastric cancer in young, asymptomatic carriers of germ-line E-cadherin mutations. N Engl J Med 2001; 344(25):1904–9.
45. Lynch HT, Grady W, Suriano G, et al. Gastric cancer: new genetic developments. J Surg Oncol 2005;90(3):114–33.
46. Lynch HT, Lanspa SJ, Boman BM, et al. Hereditary nonpolyposis colorectal cancer–Lynch syndromes I and II. Gastroenterol Clin North Am 1988;17(4):679–712.
47. Lynch HT, Lynch PM, Lanspa SJ, et al. Review of the Lynch syndrome: history, molecular genetics, screening, differential diagnosis, and medicolegal ramifications. Clin Genet 2009;76(1):1–18.
48. Aarnio M, Salovaara R, Aaltonen L, et al. Features of gastric cancer in hereditary non-polyposis colorectal cancer syndrome. Int J Cancer 1997;74(5):551–5.
49. Vasen HF, Wijnen JT, Menko FH, et al. Cancer risk in families with hereditary non-polyposis colorectal cancer diagnosed by mutation analysis. Gastroenterology 1996;110(4):1020–7.
50. Bodmer WF, Bailey CJ, Bodmer J, et al. Localization of the gene for familial adenomatous polyposis on chromosome 5. Nature 1987;328:614–6.
51. Groden J, Thliveris A, Samowitz W, et al. Identification and characterization of the familial adenomatous polyposis gene. Cell 1991;66:589–600.
52. Vogelstein B, Kinzler KW. The multistep nature of cancer. Trends Genet 1993;9: 138–41.
53. Gallagher MC, Phillips RK, Bulow S. Surveillance and management of upper gastrointestinal disease in familial adenomatous polyposis. Fam Cancer 2006; 5:263–73.
54. Offerhaus GJ, Giardiello FM, Krush AJ, et al. The risk of upper gastrointestinal cancer in familial adenomatous polyposis. Gastroenterology 1992;102: 1980–2.
55. Oliveira C, Ferreira P, Nabais S, et al. E-cadherin, CDH1, and p53 rather than SMAD4 and Caspase-10 germline mutations contribute to genetic predisposition in Portuguese gastric cancer patients. Eur J Cancer 2004; 40:1897–903.
56. Peek RM, Blaser MJ. Helicobacter pylori and gastrointestinal tract adenocarcinomas. Nat Rev Cancer 2002;2:28–37.
57. Uemura N, Okamoto S, Yamamoto S, et al. Helicobacter pylori infection and the development of gastric cancer. N Engl J Med 2001;345(11):784–9.
58. Schistosomes, liver flukes and Helicobacter pylori. IARC Working Group on the Evaluation of Carcinogenic Risks to Humans. Lyon, 7–14 June 1994. IARC Monogr Eval Carcinog Risks Hum 1994;61:1–241.

59. Everhart JE, Kruszon-Moron D, Perez-Perez GI, et al. Seroprevalence and ethnic differences in *Helicobacter pylori* infection among adults in the United States. J Infect Dis 2000;181:1359–63.

60. Dunn BE, Cohen H, Blazer MJ. *Helicobacter pylori*. Clin Microbiol Rev 1997;10: 720–41.

61. Dinarello CA. Biologic basis for interleukin-1 in disease. Blood 1996;87(6): 2095–147.

62. Basso D, Scrigner M, Toma A, et al. *Helicobacter pylori* infection enhances mucosal interleukin-1 beta, interleukin-6, and the soluble receptor of interleukin-2. Int J Clin Lab Res 1996;26:207–10.

63. El Omar EM, Carrington M, Chow WH, et al. Interleukin-1 polymorphisms associated with increased risk of gastric cancer. Nature 2000;404:398–402.

64. Figueiredo C, Machado JC, Pharoah P, et al. *Helicobacter pylori* and interleukin-1 genotyping: an opportunity to identify high-risk individuals for gastric adenocarcinoma. J Natl Cancer Inst 2002;94(22):1680–7.

65. Li C, Xia HH, Xie W, et al. Association between interleukin-1 gene populations and *Helicobacter pylori* infection in gastric carcinogenesis in a Chinese population. J Gastroenterol Hepatol 2007;22(2):234–9.

66. Taguchi A, Ohmiya N, Shirai K, et al. Interleukin-8 promoter polymorphism increases the risk of atrophic gastritis and gastric cancer in Japan. Cancer Epidemiol Biomarkers Prev 2005;15:2487–93.

67. Sharma SA, Tummuru MK, Blaser MJ, et al. Activation of IL-8 gene expression by *Helicobacter pylori* is regulated by transcription factor nuclear factor-B in gastric epithelial cells. J Immunol 1998;160:2401–7.

68. Karin M, Cao Y, Greten FR, et al. NF-kB in cancer: from innocent bystander to major culprit. Nat Rev Cancer 2002;2:301–10.

69. Sasaki N, Morisaki T, Hashizume K, et al. Nuclear factor-kB p65 (RelA) transcription factor is constitutively activated in human gastric carcinoma tissue. Clin Cancer Res 2001;7:4136–42.

70. Lee WP, Tai DI, Lan KH, et al. The -251T allele of the interleukin-8 promoter is associated with increased risk of gastric carcinoma featuring diffuse-type histopathology in Chinese population. Clin Cancer Res 2005;11(18): 6431–41.

71. Gianfagna F, De Feo E, Van Duijn CM, et al. A systematic review of meta-analyses on gene polymorphisms and gastric cancer risk. Curr Genomics 2008;9:361–74.

72. Greenlee RT, Hill-Harmon MB, Murray T, et al. Cancer statistics, 2001. CA Cancer J Clin 2001;51(1):15–36.

73. Klein AP, Hruban RH, Brune KA, et al. Familial pancreatic cancer. Cancer J 2001;7(4):266–73.

74. Brand RE, Lynch HT. Hereditary pancreatic adenocarcinoma. A clinical perspective. Med Clin North Am 2000;84(3):665–75.

75. Lynch HT, Brand RE, Deters CA, et al. Hereditary pancreatic cancer. Pancreatology 2001;1(5):466–71.

76. Bishop DT. BRCA1 and BRCA2 and breast cancer incidence: a review. Ann Oncol 1999;10(Suppl 6):113–9.

77. Cancer risks in BRCA2 mutation carriers. The Breast Cancer Linkage Consortium. J Natl Cancer Inst 1999;91(15):1310–6.

78. Murphy KM, Brune KA, Griffin C, et al. Evaluation of candidate genes MAP2K4, MADH4, ACVR1B, and BRCA2 in familial pancreatic cancer: deleterious BRCA2 mutations in 17%. Cancer Res 2002;62(13):3789–93.

79. Lynch HT, Detres CA, Snyder CL, et al. BRCA1 and pancreatic cancer: pedigree findings and their causal relationships. Cancer Genet Cytogenet 2005;158(2):119–25.

80. Thompson D, Easton DF. Breast Cancer Linkage Consortium. Cancer incidence in BRCA1 mutation carriers. J Natl Cancer Inst 2002;94(18):1358–65.

81. Lynch HT, Voorhees GJ, Lanspa SJ, et al. Pancreatic carcinoma and hereditary nonpolyposis colorectal cancer: a family study. Br J Cancer 1985; 52(2):271–3.

82. Umar A, Boland CR, Terdiman JP, et al. Revised Bethesda guidelines for hereditary nonpolyposis colorectal cancer (Lynch syndrome) and microsatellite instability. J Natl Cancer Inst 2004;96(4):261–8.

83. Geary J, Sasieni P, Houlston R, et al. Gene-related cancer spectrum in families with hereditary non-polyposis colorectal cancer (HNPCC). Fam Cancer 2008; 7(2):163–72.

84. Wilentz RE, Goggins M, Redston M, et al. Genetic, immunohistochemical, and clinical features of medullary carcinoma of the pancreas: a newly described and characterized entity. Am J Pathol 2000;156(5):1641–51.

85. Banville N, Geraghty R, Fox E, et al. Medullary carcinoma of the pancreas in a man with hereditary nonpolyposis colorectal cancer due to a mutation of the MSH2 mismatch repair gene. Hum Pathol 2006;37(11):1498–502.

86. Gargiulo S, Torrini M, Ollila S, et al. Germline MLH1 and MSH2 mutations in Italian pancreatic cancer patients with suspected Lynch syndrome. Fam Cancer 2009;8(4):547–53.

87. Kastrinos F, Mukherjee B, Tayob N, et al. Risk of pancreatic cancer in families with Lynch syndrome. JAMA 2009;302(16):1790–5.

88. Yamamoto H, Itoh F, Nakamura H, et al. Genetic and clinical features of human pancreatic ductal adenocarcinomas with widespread microsatellite instability. Cancer Res 2001;61(7):3139–44.

89. Goldstein AM. Familial melanoma, pancreatic cancer and germline CDKN2A mutations. Hum Mutat 2004;23(6):630.

90. Bergman W, Gruis N. Familial melanoma and pancreatic cancer. N Engl J Med 1996;334(7):471–2.

91. Bergman W, Watson P, de Jong J, et al. Systemic cancer and the FAMMM syndrome. Br J Cancer 1990;61(6):932–6.

92. Borg A, Sandberg T, Nilsson K, et al. High frequency of multiple melanomas and breast and pancreas carcinomas in CDKN2A mutation-positive melanoma families. J Natl Cancer Inst 2000;92(15):1260–6.

93. Vasen HF, Gruis NA, Frants RR, et al. Risk of developing pancreatic cancer in families with familial atypical multiple mole melanoma associated with a specific 19 deletion of p16 (p16-Leiden). Int J Cancer 2000;87(6):809–11.

94. Lynch HT, Brand RE, Hogg D, et al. Phenotypic variation in eight extended CDKN2A germline mutation familial atypical multiple mole melanoma-pancreatic carcinoma-prone families: the familial atypical mole melanoma-pancreatic carcinoma syndrome. Cancer 2002;94(1):84–96.

95. Giardiello FM, Trimbath JD. Peutz–Jeghers syndrome and management recommendations. Clin Gastroenterol Hepatol 2006;4(4):408–15.

96. Giardiello FM, Welsh SB, Hamilton SR, et al. Increased risk of cancer in the Peutz–Jeghers syndrome. N Engl J Med 1987;316(24):1511–4.

97. Hearle N, Schumacher V, Menko FH, et al. Frequency and spectrum of cancers in the Peutz–Jeghers syndrome. Clin Cancer Res 2006;12(10):3209–15.

98. Giardiello FM, Brensinger JD, Tersmette AC, et al. Very high risk of cancer in familial Peutz–Jeghers syndrome. Gastroenterology 2000;119(6):1447–53.

99. Lim W, Olschwang S, Keller JJ, et al. Relative frequency and morphology of cancers in STK11 mutation carriers. Gastroenterology 2004;126(7):1788–94.

100. Giardiello FM, Offerhaus GJ, Lee DH, et al. Increased risk of thyroid and pancreatic carcinoma in familial adenomatous polyposis. Gut 1993;34(10):1394–6.

101. Groen EJ, Roos A, Muntinghe FL, et al. Extra-intestinal manifestations of familial adenomatous polyposis. Ann Surg Oncol 2008;15(9):2439–50.

102. Horii A, Nakatsuru S, Miyoshi Y, et al. Frequent somatic mutations of the APC gene in human pancreatic cancer. Cancer Res 1992;52(23):6696–8.

103. Gupta C, Mazzara PF. High-grade pancreatic intraepithelial neoplasia in a patient with familial adenomatous polyposis. Arch Pathol Lab Med 2005; 129(11):1398–400.

104. Lowenfels AB, Maisonneuve P, DiMagno EP, et al. Hereditary pancreatitis and the risk of pancreatic cancer. International Hereditary Pancreatitis Study Group. J Natl Cancer Inst 1997;89(6):442–6.

105. Whitcomb DC, Gorry MC, Preston RA, et al. Hereditary pancreatitis is caused by a mutation in the cationic trypsinogen gene. Nat Genet 1996;14(2):141–5.

106. Reimer RR, Fraumeni JF, Ozols RF, et al. Pancreatic cancer in father and son. Lancet 1977;1(8017):911.

107. Ehrenthal D, Haeger L, Griffin T, et al. Familial pancreatic adenocarcinoma in three generations. A case report and a review of the literature. Cancer 1987; 59(9):1661–4.

108. Ghadirian P, Boyle P, Simard A, et al. Reported family aggregation of pancreatic cancer within a population-based case-control study in the Francophone community in Montreal, Canada. Int J Pancreatol 1991;10(3–4):183–96.

109. Lynch HT, Fitzsimmons ML, Smyrk TC, et al. Familial pancreatic cancer: clinicopathologic study of 18 nuclear families. Am J Gastroenterol 1990;85(1):54–60.

110. Hruban RH, Petersen GM, Goggins M, et al. Familial pancreatic cancer. Ann Oncol 1999;10(Suppl 4):69–73.

111. Lal G, Liu G, Schmocker B, et al. Inherited predisposition to pancreatic adenocarcinoma: role of family history and germ-line p16, BRCA1, and BRCA2 mutations. Cancer Res 2000;60(2):409–16.

112. Klein AP, Beaty TH, Bailey-Wilson JE, et al. Evidence for a major gene influencing risk of pancreatic cancer. Genet Epidemiol 2002;23(2):133–49.

113. Tersmette AC, Petersen GM, Offerhaus GJ, et al. Increased risk of incident pancreatic cancer among first-degree relatives of patients with familial pancreatic cancer. Clin Cancer Res 2001;7(3):738–44.

114. Klein AP, Brune KA, Petersen GM, et al. Prospective risk of pancreatic cancer in familial pancreatic cancer kindreds. Cancer Res 2004;64(7):2634–8.

115. Pogue-Geile KL, Chen R, Bonner MP, et al. Palladin mutation causes familial pancreatic cancer and suggests a new cancer mechanism. PLoS Med 2006; 3(12):e516.

116. Klein AP, de Andrade M, Hruban RH, et al. Linkage analysis of chromosome 4 in families with familial pancreatic cancer. Cancer Biol Ther 2007;6(3):320–3.

117. Slater E, Amrillaeva V, Fendrich V, et al. Palladin mutation causes familial pancreatic cancer: absence in European families. PLoS Med 2007;4(4):e164.

118. Zogopoulos G, Rothenmund H, Eppel A, et al. The P239S palladin variant does not account for a significant fraction of hereditary or early onset pancreas cancer. Hum Genet 2007;121(5):635–7.

119. Klein AP, Borges M, Griffith M, et al. Absence of deleterious palladin mutations in patients with familial pancreatic cancer. Cancer Epidemiol Biomarkers Prev 2009;18(4):1328–30.

120. Greenhalf W, Malats N, Nilsson M, et al. International registries of families at high risk of pancreatic cancer. Pancreatology 2008;8(6):558–65.
121. Singh M, Maitra A. Precursor lesions of pancreatic cancer: molecular pathology and clinical implications. Pancreatology 2007;7(1):9–19.
122. Brentnall TA, Bronner MP, Byrd DR, et al. Early diagnosis and treatment of pancreatic dysplasia in patients with a family history of pancreatic cancer. Ann Intern Med 1999;131(4):247–55.
123. Canto MI, Goggins M, Yeo CJ, et al. Screening for pancreatic neoplasia in high-risk individuals: an EUS-based approach. Clin Gastroenterol Hepatol 2004;2(7): 606–21.
124. Canto MI, Goggins M, Hruban RH, et al. Screening for early pancreatic neoplasia in high-risk individuals: a prospective controlled study. Clin Gastroenterol Hepatol 2006;4(6):766–81 [quiz 665].
125. Langer P, Kann PH, Fendrich V, et al. Five years of prospective screening of high-risk individuals from families with familial pancreatic cancer. Gut 2009; 58(10):1410–8.
126. Brand RE, Lerch MM, Rubinstein WS, et al. Advances in counselling and surveillance of patients at risk for pancreatic cancer. Gut 2007;56(10):1460–9.
127. Kindblom LG, Remotti HE, Aldenborg F, et al. Gastrointestinal pacemaker cell tumor (GIPACT): gastrointestinal stromal tumors show phenotypic characteristics of the interstitial cells of Cajal. Am J Pathol 1998;152(5):1259–69.
128. Mazur MT, Clark HB. Gastric stromal tumors. Reappraisal of histogenesis. Am J Surg Pathol 1983;7(6):507–19.
129. Miettinen M, Majidi M, Lasota J. Pathology and diagnostic criteria of gastrointestinal stromal tumors (GISTs): a review. Eur J Cancer 2002;38(Suppl 5): S39–51.
130. Reichardt P, Hogendoorn PC, Tamborini E, et al. Gastrointestinal stromal tumors I: pathology, pathobiology, primary therapy, and surgical issues. Semin Oncol 2009;36(4):290–301.
131. Stamatakos M, Douzinas E, Stefanaki C, et al. Gastrointestinal stromal tumor. World J Surg Oncol 2009;7:61.
132. Hirota S, et al. Gain-of-function mutations of c-kit in human gastrointestinal stromal tumors. Science 1998;279(5350):577–80.
133. Kingham TP, DeMatteo RP. Multidisciplinary treatment of gastrointestinal stromal tumors. Surg Clin North Am 2009;89(1):217–33, x.
134. DeMatteo RP. Nanoneoadjuvant therapy of gastrointestinal stromal tumor (GIST). Ann Surg Oncol 2009;16(4):799–800.
135. Nishida T, Hirota S, Taniguchi M, et al. Familial gastrointestinal stromal tumours with germline mutation of the KIT gene. Nat Genet 1998;19(4):323–4.
136. Agarwal R, Robson M. Inherited predisposition to gastrointestinal stromal tumor. Hematol Oncol Clin North Am 2009;23(1):1–13, vii.
137. Robson ME, Glogowski E, Sommer G, et al. Pleomorphic characteristics of a germ-line KIT mutation in a large kindred with gastrointestinal stromal tumors, hyperpigmentation, and dysphagia. Clin Cancer Res 2004;10(4): 1250–4.
138. Kleinbaum EP, Lazar AJ, Tamborini E, et al. Clinical, histopathologic, molecular and therapeutic findings in a large kindred with gastrointestinal stromal tumor. Int J Cancer 2008;122(3):711–8.
139. Marshall JB, Diaz-Arias AA, Bochna GS, et al. Achalasia due to diffuse esophageal eiomyomatosis and inherited as an autosomal dominant disorder. Report of a family study. Gastroenterology 1990;98(5 pt 1):1358–65.

140. Agaimy A, Pelz AF, Corless CL, et al. Epithelioid gastric stromal tumours of the antrum in young females with the Carney triad: a report of three new cases with mutational analysis and comparative genomic hybridization. Oncol Rep 2007; 18(1):9–15.
141. Knop S, Schupp M, Warderlmann E, et al. A new case of Carney triad: gastrointestinal tumours and leiomyoma of the oesophagus do not show activating mutations of KIT and platelet-derived growth factor receptor alpha. J Clin Pathol 2006;59(10): 1097–9.
142. Fuller CE, Williams GT. Gastrointestinal manifestations of type 1 neurofibromatosis (von Recklinghausen's disease). Histopathology 1991;19(1):1–11.

Clinical Genetics of Hereditary Colorectal Cancer

Derek G. Power, MD[a], Emily Gloglowski, MS, MSc[a],
Steven M. Lipkin, MD, PhD[b],*

KEYWORDS

- Colorectal cancer • Genetics • Hereditary • Germline
- Lynch syndrome • Mismatch repair

Colorectal cancer (CRC) is a significant worldwide health care problem. Global cancer statistics from 2002 report CRC as the third most common cancer with around a million cases and the third and fourth most common cause of cancer-related mortality in men and women, respectively, accounting for approximately 508,000 deaths.[1] In the United States, in 2009 there were an estimated 149,000 new cases of CRC with 49,000 deaths (second most common).[2] Most (70%–80%) CRCs are sporadic. Around 20% to 30% of cases have a familial component, that is, one or more affected first- or second-degree relatives (or both), and a potentially definable genetic basis **(Fig. 1)**.[3,4] In the United States, around 10% to 15% of adults have a history of CRC in a first-degree relative.[5] Because early diagnosis of CRC is directly related to prognosis, there has been much interest in screening for this disease. Compelling evidence supports screening in average-risk individuals older than 50 years to reduce CRC mortality by detecting cancer at an early stage and by detecting and removing clinically significant adenomas. Early detection is especially important in high-risk groups (those with a CRC-positive family history) because CRC in this setting tends to occur at an earlier age compared with the average-risk population and may result in a disproportionate loss of years of life.

Over the last 10 to 15 years, molecular genetics has made a significant impact by identifying germline and somatic mutations associated with the development of CRC.[6] Single-gene germline mutations conferring a hereditary susceptibility to CRC account for around 6% to 7% of all CRCs.[4] Mutations in DNA repair genes (*MLH1*, *MSH2*, *MSH6*, *PMS2*, *MYH*) as well as in genes involved in signal transduction (*APC*, *SMAD4*) are associated with true hereditary syndromes. Much of the inherited

No finding support was received for the compilation of this work.
[a] Clinical Genetics, Department of Medicine, Memorial Sloan-Kettering Cancer Center, 1275 York Avenue, New York, NY 10065, USA
[b] Gastroenterology, Department of Medicine, Weill Cornell College of Medicine, Caspary Research Building, 541 East 71st Street, New York, NY 10021, USA
* Corresponding author.
E-mail address: stl2012@med.cornell.edu

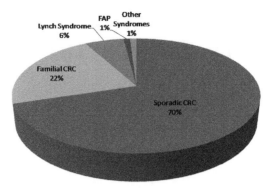

Fig. 1. Contribution of familial and hereditary factors to CRC.

components in the remaining familial cases of CRC is likely polygenic, and many of the genetic changes involved are as yet unidentified. This article addresses the most important CRC genetic syndromes.

LYNCH SYNDROME, DNA MISMATCH REPAIR, AND MICROSATELLITE INSTABILITY

Lynch syndrome (LS; previously known as hereditary nonpolyposis CRC, HNPCC) is the most common form of hereditary CRC.[4] In the early 1990s, linkage analysis discovered the genetic basis of LS with the identification of germline mutations in the DNA mismatch repair (MMR) genes *MLH1* and *MSH2*. Mutations in these genes explained more than 90% of LS cases. Subsequently, germline mutations in the *MSH6* and *PMS2* MMR genes were also shown to result in LS and may be more common than initially thought.[7–9] Rare atypical LS pedigrees with identifiable *MLH3* mutations have also been described.[10,11] The phenotypic spectrum of LS includes cancers of the colorectum (right-sided colon in up to two-thirds of cases), endometrium, stomach, upper urinary tract, small bowel, ovary, bile ducts, brain, and skin (sebaceous tumors and keratoacanthomas in the Muir-Torre variant [frequently caused by *MSH2* mutations]). Clinical criteria based on family history, the Amsterdam I and II criteria (**Table 1**), were originally devised to identify patients with an inherited form of CRC, that is, HNPCC.[12,13] However, problems were encountered with these criteria because these identified a heterogeneous group of patients with some cancers caused by MMR gene mutations and others caused by MMR gene inactivation or unknown etiology.[14] Recently, it has been proposed to use the term LS to specifically refer to those patients with HNPCC who carry a pathogenic mutation in DNA MMR genes.[15] An earlier-onset syndrome, known as constitutional MMR deficiency syndrome, occurs in the presence of homozygous or heterozygous mutations in MMR genes, especially *PMS2*.[16]

LS-associated CRC has a higher incidence of several recognizable histopathologic features, such as poorly differentiated mucinous appearance, characteristic lymphocytic infiltrate, histologic heterogeneity, and signet-ring cell features.[17] An identifiable molecular feature of LS-associated CRC is microsatellite instability (MSI). Because the MMR system is responsible for surveillance and correction of errors in DNA replication, it was discovered that sequences of DNA that are prone to accumulation of mutations, such as microsatellite repetitive sequences consisting of mononucleotide, dinucleotide, or higher-order nucleotide repeats, are not repaired if MMR genes are dysfunctional. This MSI phenotype (also known as the mutator phenotype), despite

Table 1
Clinical criteria for identifying hereditary nonpolyposis CRC

Classic ICG-HNPCC (Amsterdam I) Criteria[12]	Revised ICG-HNPCC (Amsterdam II) Criteria[13]	Revised Bethesda Guidelines (for MSI Testing)[19]
Three relatives (or more) with CRC (at least 1 of whom is a first-degree relative of the other 2)	Three relatives (or more) with an HNPCC-associated cancer[a] (at least 1 of whom is a first-degree relative of the other 2)	CRC diagnosed at age <50 y
Two successive generations (or more) with CRC	Two successive generations (or more) with an HNPCC-associated cancer	Presence of synchronous, metachronous colorectal, or other HNPCC-related tumors[a] regardless of age
One family member with CRC diagnosed before age 50 y	One family member with an HNPCC-associated cancer diagnosed before age 50 y	CRC diagnosed in 1 or more first-degree relatives with an HNPCC-related tumor with 1 of the cancers being diagnosed under age 50 y
FAP should be excluded	FAP should be excluded in the CRC cases, if any	CRC diagnosed in 2 or more first- or second-degree relatives with HNPCC-related tumors, regardless of age
Tumors should be verified by pathologic examination	Tumors should be verified by pathologic examination	CRC with MSI-H histology[b] diagnosed in a patient who is younger than 60 y

Abbreviations: FAP, familial adenomatous polyposis; ICG-HNPCC, International Collaborative Group on Hereditary Nonpolyposis CRC; MSI, microsatellite instability.

[a] Colorectal, endometrial, stomach, ovarian, pancreas, ureter and renal pelvis, biliary tract, and brain (usually glioblastoma as seen in Turcot syndrome) tumors, sebaceous gland adenomas and keratoacanthomas in Muir-Torre syndrome, and carcinoma of the small bowel.

[b] Presence of tumor-infiltrating lymphocytes, Crohn's-like lymphocytic reaction, mucinous/signet-ring differentiation, or medullary growth pattern.

being a hallmark of LS, is also observed in 10% to 15% of sporadic CRCs. Many genes, such as *TGF-β*, *BAX*, and *HDAC2*, develop mutations in microsatellite repeats in MMR-deficient CRCs. MSI is now routinely detected in tumor blocks, and a consensus conference in Bethesda established a panel of microsatellite markers (initially 5 markers, now expanded to 10) to identify MSI CRC.[18,19] Based on these markers, MSI is judged to be high (MSI-H), low (MSI-L), or stable (MSS). The Bethesda criteria and later-revised Bethesda criteria (see **Table 1**) were developed to identify those patients whose CRC warrants molecular testing for MSI. However, there has been much debate as to the utility of these criteria to identify patients suitable for MMR germline testing. Recently, it has been shown that immunohistochemical (IHC) analysis of MMR protein expression can help guide further genetic testing (see the following sections).

EPIGENETICS

Epigenetics refers to stable changes in gene expression resulting from changes in a chromosome without alteration of the actual gene sequence.[20] For example, on a somatic level, methylation of GC- and CpG-rich areas (usually located near the promoter regions of widely expressed genes) that are known as CpG islands contributes to gene inactivation in most cases (up to 84%) of *MLH1* loss in MSI-H CRCs.[21] It also appears that MSI CRC has more endogenous CpG methylation than MSS CRCs and this, in turn, is responsible for a greater rate of genetic change in these tumors. Tumor suppressor genes inactivated by hypermethylation include *APC*, *BRAF*, and *MRE11A*. Thus, detected loss of *MLH1* on IHC analysis may be caused by spontaneous hypermethylation of the promoter region, resulting in *MLH1* inactivation, even in a suspected LS tumor. Germline sequencing may not be required in such cases, although the challenge lies in separating these from the actual LS tumors.

Recent work on the *RAF/MEK/ERK/MAPK* kinase signaling pathway has shown that somatic changes in *KRAS* and *BRAF* are important in CRC tumorigenesis and therapeutics. Activating mutations in the *KRAS* gene are seen in 30% to 40% of CRCs, and mutually exclusive activating mutations in *BRAF* are present in 10% of CRCs. These mutations predict resistance to anti-epidermal growth factor receptor antibodies (eg, cetuximab).[6,22,23] *BRAF* mutations are almost exclusively seen in sporadic MSI CRCs and result from somatic hypermethylation of *MLH1*.[24] Testing CRCs for somatic *BRAF* mutations (the most common being V600E) has therefore been suggested to rule out LS, in cases in which the tumor is MSI-H or family history suggests a genetic predisposition.[25] *KRAS* mutations are more common in MSS tumors.[22] Some recent studies have focused on genetic and epigenetic classifications, defining clinical phenotype, and determining patient outcomes in CRC.[26] Sanchez and colleagues[26] analyzed tumors from 391 unselected patients with CRC for MSI, CpG island methylator phenotype (CIMP), and *BRAF* and *KRAS* mutations. The investigators concluded that the population was heterogeneous. CIMP-H and MSI-H tumors were not interchangeable and both molecular subtypes had a high frequency of *BRAF* mutation and a low rate of *KRAS* mutation. Most tumors were MSS/CIMP-negative (70%). Divergent survival was seen amongst the different groups, with MSI-H/CIMP-negative tumors showing the best survival for stages I to III (stage IV was the strongest determinant of survival and was removed from the analysis). Others have confirmed these findings and have highlighted the molecular complexity of CRCs based on genetic and epigenetic profiles.[27]

Adding further complexity to the identification of potential patients with LS, there are reports that the LS phenotype can be inherited via germline epigenetic changes affecting *MLH1* or *MSH2*. A heritable somatic mutation in *MSH2* has been reported, resulting from germline deletions in the *TACSTD1* gene, which lies directly upstream of *MSH2* and encodes Ep-CAM. Such deletions result in the silencing of *MSH2* by hypermethylation.[28] It has been proposed that clinical genetics workup should include deletion analysis of the 3' region of the *TACSTD1* gene in those cases in which IHC analysis shows *MSH2/MSH6* protein loss, and no mutation is found in the coding regions of the *MSH2/MSH6* genes.[29] A recent report of 331 LS-suspected patients, who had no germline *MLH1*, *MSH2*, or *MSH6* mutation and whose tumors showed MSI-H or loss of *MLH1* or *MSH2*, revealed 2 patients with germline *MLH1* promoter hypermethylation and 3 patients with somatic *MSH2* promoter hypermethylation in their tumors caused by a germline *TACSTD1* deletion.[30] Thus germline epigenetic changes can mimic hereditary cancer syndromes. More recent data suggest that somatic methylation of *MSH2* in patients with LS is common (24% of cases of LS patients with *MSH2* mutations) and may serve as the second hit at the wild-type *MSH2* allele.[31]

MISSENSE MMR MUTATIONS

There is, as yet, no consensus as to what level of evidence is sufficient to classify germline MMR mutations as deleterious. Yet unclassified mutations are referred to as variants of uncertain significance. There is significant variation with regard to age of onset, clinical phenotypes, and tumor spectrum among individuals and families with MMR gene mutations. The clinical phenotype ranges from families satisfying the highly restrictive Amsterdam criteria[19] to familial CRC, isolated early-onset disease, and even sporadic CRC.[32] Part of the large variation is attributable to the frequent occurrence of missense mutations that can account for up to 24% of all LS mutations (typical mutations are truncating genomic deletions, duplications, and rearrangements).[32] Missense mutations can cause a loss of protein function and result in a phenotype similar to mutations that truncate the protein prematurely; others create proteins that retain partial function or result in non-functional proteins that are still expressed and scored as wild type on IHC analysis.[33] There is widespread agreement that correct interpretation of the clinical significance of specific missense mutations (even with bioinformatic algorithms) is extremely challenging and complicates the genetic counseling and medical management of the families involved.[34] A pervasive weakness of risk-prediction models for LS is that they cannot distinguish to what extent a variant is a causative deleterious mutation. Approaches to combine mutation risk prediction and missense variant classification have been developed for the *BRCA1/BRCA2* genes, and it is hoped that a similar approach in CRC, such as missense variants with multivariate analysis of protein polymorphisms mismatch repair (MAPP-MMR) or align–Grantham variation-Grantham deviation (A-GVGD) combined with risk-prediction models, can help to more accurately define missense variants.

IDENTIFYING PATIENTS WITH LS

As the clinical management and prognosis of MMR mutation versus non mutation carriers differs significantly, it is imperative to identify those patients with LS. It is not practical to perform germline testing on all patients. The Amsterdam and broader Bethesda criteria help define a high-risk population in whom germline testing should be considered. However, these criteria have low sensitivities (40%–80%, respectively) among selected (CRC patients referred to a genetics clinic) and unselected patients.[35]

Molecular pre-screening using MSI testing or IHC analysis of tumor tissue for MMR protein loss has been proposed as a primary screening tool for all patients with CRC. The rationale for using IHC analysis is that loss of MMR protein expression identifies the relevant deficient MMR gene in a quick, inexpensive, and reproducible manner. When a mismatch is detected, *MSH2* associates with *MSH6* (predominantly) and *MLH1* couples with *PMS2*. It follows that absence of *MLH1* and *PMS2* on IHC most likely represents *MLH1* expression loss (*PMS2* loss is secondary). In that case, the germline workup should therefore initially focus on *MLH1*. Given the accessibility of immunohistochemistry, many institutions now routinely test colon cancers (especially those patients younger than 60 years) for MMR proteins. An algorithm for the proposed institution-wide clinical evaluation for LS is summarized in **Fig. 2**. If no tumor tissue is available and the suspicion for LS is strong, it is reasonable to proceed directly to MMR germline sequencing.

IHC analysis and MSI testing have limitations as screening tools. As discussed earlier, MSI tumors are seen in 10% to 15% of sporadic CRCs and most *MLH1* protein loss on IHC analysis is caused by hypermethylation of the promoter in the absence of a germline mutation. A recent report from the Evaluation of Genomic Applications in Practice and Prevention Working Groups has reviewed the clinical validity of IHC analysis and MSI testing before MMR germline sequencing. For MSI, the clinical sensitivity (ability to identify LS) was 85% for *MLH1* mutations, 85% for *MSH2* mutations, and 69% for *MSH6* mutations. The overall clinical specificity was 90% (95% confidence interval [CI], 87%–93%).[14] The overall clinical sensitivity of IHC testing to identify LS was 83% for *MLH1*, *MSH2*, and *MSH6* (95% CI, 65%–93%).[14] Clinical specificity was 89% (95% CI, 68%–95%). Recent data from the United States have shown that the use of IHC analysis and MSI testing as preliminary tests for all CRCs is cost-effective (<$75,000 per life year saved compared with age-targeted testing),[36] and universal testing using MSI or IHC detected nearly twice as many cases of LS as targeting younger patients.

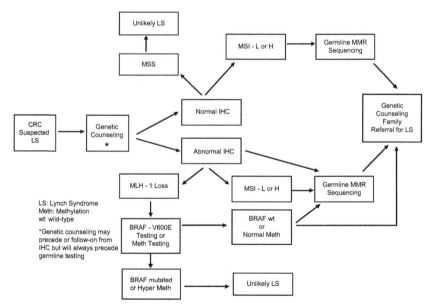

Fig. 2. Algorithm for molecular diagnosis of LS.

In a cohort of 1566 unselected patients with CRC form the Columbus metropolitan area, IHC analysis for the 4 MMR proteins and MSI were both performed. If either preliminary test was abnormal, complete sequencing for germline mutations was performed.[35] The overall prevalence of LS was at least 2.8% (44 out of 1566 patients). Of the 44 patients diagnosed with LS, 249 relatives of 33 probands were tested for germline mutations in MMR genes and 109 relatives tested positive, amounting to more than 3 relatives per proband with mutations. The strongest predictors of germline mutations were absence of *MSH2* with or without absence of *MSH6* on IHC analysis (66.7%), absence of *MSH6* or *PMS2* alone on IHC analysis (23.5% and 55.6%), and absence of *MLH1* without *MLH1* promoter hypermethylation (33.3%). Patients whose tumors had abnormal IHC results were just as likely to have LS as those patients whose tumors were MSI-H (21.4% vs 20.8%, $P = .9847$, χ^2 test). Younger (age <50 years) patients were more likely to have LS than patients who were older than 50 years. In this study, if tumor analysis had been limited to those patients who fulfilled the Bethesda criteria, 1 in 4 cases of LS would not have been identified.

The optimal diagnostic strategy for LS is still under debate. Researchers have recently hypothesized that *BRAF* testing on tumor tissue with absent *MLH1* staining could identify sporadic CRC cases that would not benefit from *MLH1* sequencing. Several studies have reported sensitivity and specificity of *BRAF* testing for sporadic CRC in patients with absent *MLH1* expression on IHC analysis.[14,25,37,38] Overall sensitivity was 69% (95% CI, 57%–79%) and specificity was 100% (95% CI, 93%–100%). Thus evidence suggests that *BRAF* V600E mutation testing and *MLH1* promoter hypermethylation testing in those CRC cases with absent *MLH1* protein on IHC analysis may avoid unnecessary *MLH1* sequencing without a loss in LS detection.[14]

Molecular prescreening using MSI or IHC testing assumes that tumor tissue is readily available. Also, these patients already have CRC, yet the major aim of any screening strategy is to identify LS prior to the development of cancer. In recent years, several models have been developed to predict the likelihood of carrying a germline mutation.[39–43] Tumor tissue is not required for these models (except for MMRPro[42]) and information from personal and/or family history is an input to predict the probability of carrying a mutation. The models, using either logistic regression or Bayesian analytical approaches, can also be applied to those individuals in whom germline testing has found no mutation. To date, all of these models have been shown to outperform the revised Bethesda guidelines in terms of MMR mutation risk. Comparison of 4 models[39–42] in high-risk patients and also in patients with CRC found that all 4 models could discriminate between carriers and noncarriers.[15] As the penetrance of mutations in *MSH6* and *PMS2* is lower than that of *MLH1* and *MSH2*, it was not surprising that *MSH6* mutation carriers had lower risk scores from all 4 models ($P<.015$) (no model took into account mutations in *PMS2*).[9,44] The investigators found that all 4 models had diagnostic utility in identifying patients with CRC from the general population who should receive further evaluation. When corrections were made for family size, the MMR predict model[40] performed the best, achieving a sensitivity of 94% (95% CI, 73%–99%) and a specificity of 91% (95% CI, 88%–93%). This model could better identify a subset (11%) of all patients who should have additional molecular or IHC testing compared with the revised Bethesda criteria (sensitivity = 94% and specificity = 51%), which suggested additional testing for 50% of patients. As per the investigators, another advantage of all 4 models is the identification of at-risk family members who should be offered screening for colonic and extracolonic tumors while awaiting the probands' molecular test results. All risk-prediction models are freely available on the Internet and can be easily used in the clinic to guide germline mutation testing.

MANAGEMENT AND SURVEILLANCE OF PATIENTS WITH LS

Data on future cancer risk (penetrance) in MMR germline mutation carriers are varied and inconsistent amongst published series. One reason for this is the heterogeneity of populations studied; earlier studies focused on families with many affected members, whereas more recent studies tend to be population based. Results in both groups may be confounded by other genetic and environmental influences. Because of these inconsistencies, it is impossible to give a single summary statistic for CRC risk in MMR mutation carriers. The risk of CRC with *MLH1/MSH2* mutations by age 70 years is 80% (men) and the overall risk is 10% lower for *MSH6* and *PMS2* mutations.[45] Earlier studies suggested similar risks for women, but in recent studies, women have a lower risk (20%–40% lower) of developing CRC. In studies that are population based (and so avoid high-risk family bias), estimates for penetrance by age 70 years are 45% for men and 35% for women. Of note, the risk for other LS-associated cancers varies greatly depending on the gene studied; for example, endometrial cancer risk may be preferentially increased in *MSH6* mutation carriers.[46]

Based on the risk of CRC in MMR mutation carriers, surveillance guidelines have been proposed.[47–49] Individuals with a known or suspected MMR mutation, or who are at risk based on a documented family mutation, should undergo colonoscopy at least every 1 to 2 years, starting at age 20 to 25 years (some have suggested starting at age 30 years in families with *MSH6* mutations).[48] Such frequent screening is advised based on the rapid transformation of polyp to carcinoma observed in the syndrome. Recent data from the Netherlands further support the efficacy of surveillance. In a cohort study of 2788 members from 146 families with LS, the standardized mortality ratio for CRC was decreased by 70% when compared with the subjects who did (n = 897) or did not (n = 1073) have surveillance colonoscopies (P<.001).[50] In those families without detectable MMR mutations, enhanced screening is also recommended based on data on the efficacy of colonoscopy in average- and high-risk populations.[51] Joint guidelines from the American Cancer Society, the US Multi-Society Task Force on Colorectal Cancer, the American College of Radiology, and the American Gastroenterology Association (AGA) recommend that individuals with a family history of CRC or adenomatous polyps in a first-degree relative before age 60 years or in 2 or more first-degree relatives of any age (no genetic cause found) should have a colonoscopy at age 40 years or 10 years before the youngest case in the immediate family, whichever comes first. If normal, colonoscopy should be repeated every 5 years.[51] Similar recommendations have been put forward by the AGA for individuals with a first-degree relative with CRC or advanced adenomatous polyps.

Surgery

Prophylactic colectomy is typically not performed in patients with MMR germline mutations.[52] However, in patients with LS diagnosed with CRC, there is an increased risk of metachronous CRC (16% after 10-year follow-up[53]), and surgeons are faced with the decision to perform a segmental colectomy (SEG) or total abdominal colectomy (TAC) with ileorectal anastomosis (IRA). The latter has been proposed as the standard operation to decrease the risk of metachronous tumors, although this is largely based on expert opinion rather than empirical data.[54] Quality-of-life issues can be significant after TAC.[55] Maeda and colleagues[56] used mathematical modeling to compare SEG and TAC in patients with LS. Predicted mean survival for young (30 years) patients was slightly better with TAC than with SEG (35.5 years vs 34.8 years.) However, when quality-adjusted life-years (QALYs) were considered, both the strategies were essentially equivalent. With advancing years, SEG became a more favorable strategy. Previous studies reported a better survival for TAC but did not account for QALYs.[57] Thus the decision to perform SEG or TAC should be individualized based on patient factors, patient preferences, and ability of the patient to follow surveillance guidelines if SEG is chosen.

Surgical management and surveillance of other LS-associated cancers are dealt with elsewhere in this issue.

Chemotherapy

There is level I evidence supporting the efficacy of systemic chemotherapy in the treatment of stage II (high-risk only, ie, tumors causing bowel perforation or obstruction, large tumors with diffuse lymphovascular space and perineural invasion), III, and IV CRC.[58,59] It is accepted that MSI-H tumors have a more favorable prognosis and are less likely to present with lymph node positive or metastatic disease.[60,61] Recent data from large adjuvant clinical trials reported that MSI had more prognostic value in stage II than in stage III tumors.[62] Until recently, MSI or MMR protein loss by IHC analysis has not routinely been used to inform decision making regarding chemotherapy treatment. Conflicting data, in retrospective studies, exist on the effect of 5-fluorouracil/leucovorin in MSI-H tumors.[63–65] Irinotecan is a commonly used drug in metastatic CRC. Irinotecan binds to topoisomerase and generates double-strand DNA breaks. Homologous recombination helps to repair this DNA damage, and important in this process is the *MRE11A/hRAD50/NBS1* (*MRN*) gene complex. Up to 85% of MSI CRCs tend to accumulate mutations in mononucleotide-repeat coding sequences in *MRE11A* and *RAD50*. Cell line work has shown that such mutations render cells that are highly sensitive to irinotecan because double-stranded breaks cannot be repaired by homologous recombination.[22] MSI subset analyses of irinotecan-based chemotherapy given in the adjuvant and metastatic setting have reported conflicting results. Some trials report an increased benefit in MSI-H tumors treated with irinotecan, and others report no difference between MSI-H and MSS cancers.[62,66] The question of increased sensitivity of MSI CRC to irinotecan-based chemotherapy is not yet fully answered. Of note, there does not appear to be any difference in response or outcome to oxaliplatin-based treatment in MSI CRC.[67] Poly(ADP)ribose polymerase (PARP) enzymes are critical components of the base excision repair (BER) pathway effecting single-strand break repair. Background endogenous single-strand breaks, if not repaired by the BER (nucleotide excision or MMR) pathways, can progress to double-strand breaks. MSI cell lines deficient in homologous repair pathways have been shown to be highly sensitive to *PARP* inhibitors compared with MSS cell lines.[68] Studies are now underway in CRCs, stratified by microsatellite status, to study the efficacy of *PARP* inhibitors alone and in combination with chemotherapy that induces double-strand breaks (NCT00912743; www.clinicaltrials.gov). Mammalian target of rapamycin inhibitors are also likely to be evaluated. As most MSI-H tumors do not occur in individuals with LS, these studies may or may not ultimately prove to be relevant to LS tumors.

Chemoprevention

The role of nonsteroidal anti-inflammatory drugs (NSAIDs) and cyclooxygenase-2 (*COX-2*) inhibitors has been well studied in patients with familial adenomatous polyposis (FAP; discussed in the following sections).[48] In patients with LS, chemoprevention is less well studied. However, a recent randomized study of 1071 patients with LS reported no significant difference in the detection of one or more colorectal adenomas or CRC in those who took aspirin, resistant starch (undigested portion of starch that can suppress the proliferation of colonic cells), or both every day for up to 4 years.[69]

Phase I/II multicenter trials of celecoxib in patients with LS have been completed and are yet to be reported (www.clinicaltrials.gov; NCT00001693). Recent concern regarding the cardiovascular safety of COX-2 inhibitors has cast doubt on the future role of NSAIDs in adenoma and CRC prevention.[70]

FAP

The second most common, but most easily recognizable, form of hereditary CRC is FAP (see **Fig. 1**). The prevalence of FAP is around 1 in 8000 individuals. This syndrome is characterized by hundreds or thousands of adenomatous polyps in the colon and rectum, beginning in the late teens or early 20s (median age of adenomas is 16 years) and progressing to CRC by 40 to 50 years of age in virtually every case.[4] A minimum of 100 polyps are generally necessary to diagnose the classic form of FAP, whereas LS mutation carriers rarely have more than 12 polyps. Benign hamartomas are seen in the gastric fundus and body in about half of the patients and duodenal polyps in about 90% (4%–12% resulting in duodenal/ampullary carcinoma). There is also an increased risk for thyroid cancer (especially papillary), mostly in women, and young children are at risk for hepatoblastoma.[71] CNS tumors (medulloblastomas) can be seen in the Turcot variant of FAP.[72] The Gardner syndrome variant of FAP is characterized by cutaneous soft tissue lipomas, fibromas, epidermoid/sebaceous cysts on legs, face, scalp, and arms, osteomas (skull and mandible), supernumerary teeth, congenital hypertrophy of the retinal pigment epithelium (CHRPE), and desmoid tumors and mesenteric fibromatosis.[73]

The gene responsible for FAP is the APC gene, a large gene with 15 exons, located at chromosome 5q21. Somatic mutations and deletions that inactivate both copies of APC are present in 60% to 80% of sporadic CRCs and adenomatous polyps.[66] This gene encodes a large protein that acts in the Wnt pathway via several domains to regulate the cell cycle and apoptosis, stabilize the cytoskeleton, and mediate intercellular adhesion.[74] The protein product of the APC gene has been shown to associate with proteins (catenins) that bind to the cell surface molecules (cadherins) essential for cellular adhesion. Activation of the Wnt signaling pathway via mutations in the APC gene is regarded as the initiating event in sporadic CRC.[75] Germline mutations in genes that produce scaffold proteins, for example, AXIN1 and CTNNB1, can lead to multiple polyps, which suggests that all elements of the Wnt signaling pathway can be considered putative CRC-causing genes because mutations in these genes may impact degradation of the key effector molecule of the pathway, β-catenin.[76] Most mutations in the APC gene (98%) lead to protein truncation. Germline mutations in APC are inherited in an autosomal dominant fashion and are 100% penetrant. Approximately 30% occur de novo.[77]

Variable genotype or phenotype correlations have been demonstrated in large kindred series.[78] Severe polyposis is associated with APC mutations in codons 1250 to 1464, sparser polyps with mutations in codons 213 to 1249 and 1465 to 1597, CHRPE with mutations in codons 311 to 1444, and Gardner syndrome with mutations in codons 1395 to 1578.[79] Two hotspots, codon 1061 and 1309 mutations, account for 11% and 13% of all germline mutations, respectively, with codon 1309 mutation being associated with a younger age of onset of CRC.[80] Variable expressivity, for example, age of onset of CRC, has also been noted even within families with identical APC mutations, suggesting that modifier genes play a role.[81,82]

Genetic Testing and Management

Gastroenterologists and surgeons may consider genetic testing unnecessary in patients with presumed FAP because diagnosis by sigmoidoscopy is clear and the prognosis remains unchanged (100% penetrance). However, determination of family members at risk through genetic testing can reduce unnecessary screening from a young age.[83] Given the 100% penetrance for colon cancer, prophylactic colectomy is standard.[84] Guidelines for the management of patient with FAP have been promulgated by the AGA and the National Comprehensive Cancer Network (NCCN) and should be consulted as they are updated regularly.[85,86] In general, patients with *APC* mutations should undergo flexible sigmoidoscopy annually, starting at age 10 to 12 years or during the midteen years, with colonoscopy once polyps are detected and colectomy for dense polyposis (>approximately 20–30). Surgical options include colectomy and IRA, proctocolectomy with ileostomy, and proctocolectomy with ileal pouch–anal anastomosis (IPAA). The goal of colectomy and IRA is to preserve rectal function,[87] and postsurgical flexible sigmoidoscopy surveillance of the rectum with endoscopic snare polypectomy and argon coagulation endoscopy ablation are suggested at 6-month intervals.[88] A large analysis of the Danish, Swedish, Finnish, and Dutch polyposis registries revealed 47 rectal carcinoma diagnoses among 659 patients who had IRA surgery. The cumulative risk according to chronologic age was 30% at 60 years and higher in patients undergoing surgery after 25 years ($P = .0016$). Of 167 individuals harboring known *APC* mutations, 7 had rectal cancer diagnoses. The 5-year median survival rate after rectal carcinoma diagnosis was 60%.[87] In patients with FAP, regression of rectal polyps has been noted after IRA, suggesting possible environmental modulators of the phenotype. Upper gastrointestinal (GI) endoscopy should be performed in patients with FAP every 1 to 4 years with baseline examination by age 25 to 30 years, and their thyroid glands should also be palpated. At-risk infants may be considered for screening for hepatoblastoma (age 0–5 years). Presymptomatic individuals with a family history of FAP, but for whom mutation status is unknown, should have annual flexible sigmoidoscopy beginning at age 10 to 12 years until age 24 years, every 2 years until age 34 years, every 3 years until age 44 years, and every 3 to 5 years thereafter; colonoscopy should be considered at 10-year intervals starting at age 20 years.

Because the progression from initiation of adenoma to carcinoma can take several years, there is a window of opportunity to potentially intervene. NSAIDs and the more selective *COX-2* inhibitors have demonstrated significant chemopreventive benefits in FAP (reduction in the size and number of rectal adenomas) as evidenced by at least 4 randomized trials.[89] NSAIDs, however, have not been shown to prevent colorectal neoplasia in patients with FAP.[90] The response to NSAIDs may be genetically determined.[91] Despite these data, surgery is still the primary treatment of FAP. NSAID chemoprevention is an adjunct to surgery to address remaining rectal tissue, or may permit surgery to be delayed. Postmenopausal hormone replacement therapy has been suggested as a chemoprevention for colon cancer.[92] Case reports of polyp regression after cytotoxic chemotherapy have been published. Further studies are required to determine whether cytotoxic chemotherapy may be an alternative for patients with FAP for whom colectomy is not an option or for duodenal or ampullary polyps that may be less amenable to surgery or treatment with NSAIDs.[93]

ATTENUATED FAP

An attenuated form of FAP (AFAP) has been described in adult patients with greater than 10 but less than 100 cumulative colorectal adenomas. This entity arises from *APC* mutations at the 5′ or 3′ ends of the *APC* gene or in certain areas of exon 9,[94] giving rise to hypomorphic alleles that do not completely inactivate the protein product. This syndrome is characterized by later onset of polyposis, average age of

44 years, and CRC by average age of 56 years.[95] In general, AFAP has fewer colonic adenomas (<100), without associated CHRPE, but patients can have upper GI and other extracolonic features similar to classic FAP. Genotype-phenotype correlations have been reported. Mutations upstream of codon 169 are thought to be mild because downstream, at codon 184, there is an in-frame ATG amino acid sequence that can reinitiate protein translation. A Canadian study of 11 kindreds with AFAP found that those with mutations in the 5′ region had more severe upper GI manifestations. Mutations in the 3′ and exon 9 regions resulted in fewer more distally located adenomas.[96] Another report of a large kindred with an exon 9 mutation noted marked variable expressivity, ranging from a complete lack of clinical or endoscopic findings in 4 individuals to classic FAP findings or CRC in 16 of 22 members. The mutation was an 11–base-pair insertion that causes truncation of exon 9 with possible alternative splicing or unknown modifying factors.[97] The phenotypic features of adenomas may also vary in AFAP because both serrated polyps and flat adenomas (of the LS type) have been reported.[88,98]

A hypermutable region exists at codon 1307 in the *APC* gene. This mutation does not lead to classic FAP with 100 to 1000 polyps but causes an increased risk of colon cancer.[99] About 6% to 8% of Ashkenazi Jews (AJ) have the *I1307K* mutation resulting in approximately 10% to 20% lifetime risk of colon cancer.[100] Of AJs with CRC, 8% to 15% have this mutation.

Genetic Testing and Management

NCCN guidelines recommend *APC* testing in the affected proband to confirm the diagnosis of AFAP and allow for mutation-specific testing in other family members.[85] If no *APC* mutation is found, *MYH* testing should be considered (discussed later). For patients with AFAP, it is generally recommended that colonoscopy should be performed every 2 to 3 years from the late teens and every 1 to 2 years once adenomas are found, while the burden is low (<20 adenomatous polyps, all <1 cm in size with no advanced histology). Upper GI screening should also begin at age 25 to 30 years, and surveillance for skin, soft tissue, eye, and other manifestations of FAP is also appropriate. The role of prophylactic colectomy is less well established, but strong consideration should be given to this procedure around age 40 years or when polyposis load becomes unmanageable with polypectomy. Annual rectal endoscopy should be done postcolectomy.

MYH-ASSOCIATED POLYPOSIS (MAP)

A proportion of probands with FAP who test negative for germline *APC* mutations may harbor bi-allelic truncations or missense mutations in the BER gene *MYH*, the human homologue of the *Escherichia coli mutY* gene. Patients with multiple (>15) adenomas and without *APC* mutations are more likely to have homozygous or bi-allelic *MYH* mutations than controls.[101] The phenotype is often indistinguishable from either FAP or AFAP. Microadenomas in the background colorectal mucosa in bi-allelic *MYH* mutation carriers were once considered pathognomonic of FAP.[102] MAP is considered to display recessive inheritance because parents of affected homozygote or compound heterozygote mutation carriers are typically unaffected.[103] However, both mono-allelic and bi-allelic germline mutations in *MYH* have been associated with multiple adenomas and a CRC risk (the CRC risk being much more pronounced in bi-allelic than in monoallelic mutation carriers, 50-fold vs 1- to 3-fold, respectively).[103–105]

The *MYH* gene is located on chromosome 1p35 and is a BER gene involved in repairing DNA damage induced by ionizing radiation and reactive oxygen species. Genetic testing for FAP that includes *MYH* sequencing in addition to *APC* sequencing mutations increased the positive yield from 34% to 41% in patients referred for testing.[106] Loss of *MYH* activity leads to a high frequency of G:C to T:A transversions, resulting in nonsense or splice-site mutations in *APC*. In one series, bi-allelic *MYH* mutations were found in 8 of 107 patients with polyposis (7%) and 6 of 152 patients with multiple adenoma (4%). All *MYH* positive patients had family histories consistent with autosomal recessive inheritance patterns and all tumors had somatic *APC* G:C to T:A transversions. No cases with germline *MYH* mutations had severe expression of more than 100 adenomas in this series, but 3 cases exhibited extracolonic manifestations, including 2 patients with duodenal polyps and 1 patient with CHPRE.[102] The mutations *Y165C* and *G382D* appear to be mutational hotspots, especially in Caucasian Europeans, compromising 86% of bi-allelic mutations in large series,[102,103] with an estimated carrier frequency of about 2%. Bi-allelic inheritance of the *Y165C* and *G382D* mutations was associated with the presence of 20 or more colonic polyps and age of CRC onset before age 51 years among 984 subjects.[107,108]

MYH mutations have been studied worldwide and there is a large population genetics literature suggesting discrepancies in mutation carrier frequencies based on ethnicity. For example, in a series of 219 North Americans with CRC in whom no *APC* mutations were identified, 13 patients biallelic for *Y165C* and *G382D* were found. Of 15 Y165C or G382D heterozygotes identified in this series, sequencing revealed additional mutations in 9 individuals. Moreover, 2 patients harbored homozygous mutations other than *Y165C* and *G382D* (*466delE* and *1395delGGA*), suggesting that *MYH* sequencing may uncover additional deleterious mutations.[106] The largest series screened 2239 patients with CRC and 1845 controls for germline *MYH* mutations and found that biallelic *MYH* defects accounted for a 93-fold increased risk of CRC (0.54% of the cohort and 0.8% of cases >age 55 years).[109] Other population-based studies have confirmed this.[105]

Genetic Testing and Management

Genetic testing of *MYH* should be performed in those individuals who present with classic features of FAP or AFAP and in whom a germline mutation in the *APC* gene has not been found (10%–30% of FAP cases and 70%–90% of AFAP cases).[3] Partners of known bi-allelic mutation carriers may also be considered for genetic testing because the offspring can be affected if the partner is a monoallelic carrier.

In general, management of bi-allelic *MYH* mutation carriers is identical to that of those with FAP. Prophylactic colectomy is considered according to the phenotype, whether it be closer to FAP or AFAP. Given that more than a third of bi-allelic *MYH* mutation carriers may not develop multiple polyps but remain at elevated risk for CRC, it has been suggested that colonoscopy with polypectomies may not be sufficiently preventative for this population.[110] Further study is needed. Surgical options for mutant gene carriers include IRA for younger patients with few rectal adenomas, attenuated polyposis, and/or a milder family history or total proctocolectomy with the creation of an IPAA for more aggressive polyposis. NCCN guidelines are regularly updated and are essential reading for the management of these patients, including individuals with unknown or negative *APC* and *MYH* mutation status and a personal or family history of polyposis.

HAMARTOMATOUS POLYPOSIS SYNDROMES
Peutz-Jeghers Syndrome

Peutz-Jeghers Syndrome (PJS) is a rare autosomal dominant syndrome characterized by hamartomatous polyposis of the GI tract (virtually pathognomonic) and melanin pigmentation (oral and anal mucous membranes, palms of the hands and feet), and has variable expression within families.[111,112] The average age of diagnosis is in the early 20s. The most common associated cancers are small intestine, stomach, pancreatic adenocarcinomas, and CRC. An increased risk of breast and uterine cancer, testicular and ovarian sex cord tumors, and lung cancer is also reported. The cumulative risk for all cancer types has been reported in a meta-analysis of 6 publications and was 93% from age 15 to 64 years.[113] Risks of breast cancer were 54%, CRC 39%, pancreas cancer 36%, stomach cancer 29%, and ovarian cancer 21%. A more recent large series recorded lower cancer risks, although the overall cancer risk for age 70 years was still 85%.[114] PJS occurs because of germline mutations in the *STK11* gene (also known as the *LKB1* gene) on chromosome 19p13.3.[115] *STK11* mutations are inactivating and the wild-type alleles are lost in hamartomas, suggesting a 2-hit mechanism.[115] Because of the distinctive histopathologic phenotype, molecular studies are often unnecessary to make the diagnosis.[115] Mutations are detected in 70% of those with a family history of the disease and in 20% to 30% of those without a family history.[116] Some groups[117] found evidence suggestive of locus heterogeneity, and families with PJS unlinked to 19p13.3 have been reported.[118] In one study of patients with unexplained hamartomatous polyps, a mutation in *PTEN* was found in a patient who was misclassified as having PJS.[119]

Genetic testing and management

Genetic testing of *STK11/LKB1* should be offered to individuals with clinical signs of PJS and to unaffected family members of known mutation carriers.[120] The age of genetic testing is generally at age 8 to 10 years because small bowel obstruction secondary to polyps or massive bleeding polyps occurs in 30% of patients with PJS by 10 years of age. The stomach, large bowel, and small bowel are generally screened with upper and lower endoscopy, with removal of polyps when possible. Data on the optimal age and interval for screening are limited, so the specifics are based largely on expert opinion. The NCCN suggests that endoscopy should start at age 10 years and colonoscopy in the late teens, and that both be repeated at 2- to 3-year intervals. Recent advances to visualize the small bowel include wireless capsule endoscopy with push enteroscopy.[121] Screening for extracolonic cancers is as per NCCN guidelines.[85]

Juvenile Polyposis Syndrome

Juvenile polyposis syndrome (JPS) is a rare autosomal dominant disorder (1 in 100,000 live births) characterized by multiple juvenile polyps (10 or more) in the GI tract. The phenotypic manifestations are found in childhood to adolescence and the term 'juvenile' refers to the type of polyp seen. The cumulative risk of CRC is around 40% to 50%, and the risk of gastric cancer is 20%. Germline mutations in *BMPR1A* (bone morphogenic protein receptor 1A), *SMAD4*, and rarely *ENG* (endoglin, an accessory receptor for *TGF-β*) have been reported in JPS; however, a large subset of patients with JPS does not harbor these mutations.[122] The NCCN recommends that colonoscopic screening and upper endoscopy start at 15 years, and are repeated every 2 to 3 years if normal and annually once polyps are found.[85] A combined syndrome of JPS and hereditary hemorrhagic telangiectasia is present in 15% to 22% of individuals with an *SMAD4* mutation and requires special management.

Cowden Syndrome

Cowden syndrome is an autosomal dominant disorder affecting 1 in 200,000 live births. Hamartomatous polyps (juvenile, lipomas, lymphoid, ganglioneuromas, and inflammatory) may be found throughout the GI tract. CRC may be associated, although this has not yet been systemically studied. The lifetime risk for thyroid (follicular and papillary) cancer is 3% to 10%, and for endometrial cancer 5% to 10%. The lifetime risk of (early onset) breast cancer is far in excess of this and can approach 50%.[123] Cutaneous changes, for example, trichilemmomas of the face as well as a large head circumference, are classic findings. Lhermitte-Duclos disease can also be associated. Germline mutations in the tumor suppressor gene *PTEN* (a negative regulator of the PI3 kinase and MAP kinase pathways) located on chromosome 10 are responsible for Cowden syndrome. Somatic mutations in, and epigenetic silencing of, *PTEN* have been reported with greater frequency in MSI-H than in MSS tumors.[124]

Individuals with *PTEN* mutations should be monitored carefully for thyroid and breast lesions as well as GI (mostly colonic) polyps. Germline PTEN mutations are seen in the broader PTEN hamartoma tumor syndrome, which includes the allelic Cowden syndrome, Bannayan-Ruvalcha-Riley syndrome, and Proteus syndrome. The risk of malignancy in these rarer *PTEN*-associated syndromes is unclear.[123]

Others

Mixed polyposis syndrome was diagnosed by the investigation of large kindreds with mixed hamartomatous and hyperplastic polyps (especially of the GI tract) and genetic linkage to chromosome 6q, 15q13-14. and 10q23.[122] Neurofibromatosis type 1, multiple endocrine neoplasia type 2b, and Gorlin syndrome are associated with GI tract hamartomas, although colonic polyposis is not a major feature of these syndromes. The risk of CRC with these syndromes is largely unreported. The genetic change responsible for Gorlin syndrome is a germline mutation in the *PTCH* gene on chromosome 9q22.3. This gene is critical in sonic hedgehog signaling.[122] Approximately 70% to 80% of probands have inherited the condition from a parent and approximately 20% to 30% of probands have a de novo mutation. There is considerable overlap in the phenotypic features of Gorlin syndrome, FAP and its Turcot variant (medulloblastoma and germline *APC* mutations), and Muir-Torre variant of LS (sebaceous cancers with MSI), raising the possibility of *Wnt* signaling and sonic hedgehog signaling interactions.[122]

HYPERPLASTIC POLYPOSIS

Hyperplastic polyps, of which there are many different types, for example, sessile serrated, traditional serrated adenoma, and mixed, can lead to CRC. The molecular pathway for the progression of hyperplastic polyps to CRC is different from the well known chromosomal instability pathway seen in the progression of adenomatous polyps to CRC. MSI (hypermethylation of the *MLH1* MMR gene promoter), hypermethylation of CpG islands, and *BRAF* mutations may all play a role.[125] Criteria have been developed for the clinical recognition of hyperplastic polyposis syndrome, but it remains a poorly defined entity with unclear inheritance.

FAMILIAL CANCER TYPE X

In recent years, families who satisfy the Amsterdam I criteria but do not have identifiable mutations in known susceptibility genes have been investigated. In 2003, Renkonen and colleagues[127] described 15 families (all with MSS CRCs, median age of onset 54 years) that met Amsterdam I criteria. Tumors occurred in the distal colon and rectum in these patients more commonly than in those with LS and were less poorly differentiated, more often aneuploid, and had less mucinous pathology compared with the tumors in families that demonstrated MSI.[126] These families were followed by Abdel-Rahman and colleagues,[128] and no molecular features (apart from microsatellite status) to distinguish these families from those with LS or sporadic CRCs were identified. However, comparing the original Renkonen families (known as Finnish familial CRC syndrome X) to *MLH1/MSH2/MSH6* gene mutation–positive families, the former had significantly more CRCs with aberrant *CTNNB1* localization, p53 mutations, and other features associated with sporadic MSS colorectal tumors.

There is unlikely to be one answer that universally addresses the question of how to define familial CRC type X. Phenotypic and molecular characteristics have been studied in several series, but apart from a later mean age of onset of CRC and possibly a lack of increased extracolonic cancer risks, there was no one clinical or molecular feature common to all families that met MSS Amsterdam I criteria (with no identifiable mutations in known genes).[129–132] An interesting hypothesis is that familial CRC type X is caused by an aggregation of low-penetrance CRC susceptibility alleles. The *APC* gene was not sequenced in these studies, so low-penetrance alleles analogous to *APC* I1307K are difficult to exclude.[133] RNA microarray studies have not solved this problem as of yet, and more precise molecular and histopathologic studies of CRC are required.[126] The advent of genome-wide association studies (GWAS) has made the identification of these low-penetrant susceptibilities possible.

GWAS

As only approximately 6% of CRCs occur in the setting of a known high-penetrance cancer predisposition syndrome, such as FAP or LS, some of the genetic risk in the remaining 24% of CRCs with an apparent inherited susceptibility may be accounted for by other forms of genetic variation. Single nucleotide polymorphisms (SNPs) represent the most common form of such variation, and growing evidence suggests that the cumulative effects of SNPs across the genome confer a small-to-modest risk for CRC. GWAS provide a systematic hypotheses-free search for SNPs across the genome to identify associations with a disease. To date, GWASs have identified at least 10 independent susceptibility loci associated with CRC risk.[134] The effect size for each individual risk SNPs is modest, resulting in a 10% to 30% increase in the relative risk of CRC. A detailed discussion on recent developments in GWAS is provided elsewhere in this issue.

REFERENCES

1. Parkin DM, Bray F, Ferlay J, et al. Global cancer statistics, 2002. CA Cancer J Clin 2005;55:74–108.
2. Jemal A, Siegel R, Ward E, et al. Cancer statistics, 2009. CA Cancer J Clin 2009; 59:225–49.
3. Kastrinos F, Syngal S. Recently identified colon cancer predispositions: MYH and MSH6 mutations. Semin Oncol 2007;34:418–24.
4. Lynch HT, de la Chapelle A. Hereditary colorectal cancer. N Engl J Med 2003; 348:919–32.
5. Fuchs CS, Giovannucci EL, Colditz GA, et al. A prospective study of family history and the risk of colorectal cancer. N Engl J Med 1994;331:1669–74.
6. Markowitz SD, Bertagnolli MM. Molecular origins of cancer: molecular basis of colorectal cancer. N Engl J Med 2009;361:2449–60.
7. Offit K. MSH6 mutations in hereditary nonpolyposis colon cancer: another slice of the pie. J Clin Oncol 2004;22:4449–51.
8. Plaschke J, Engel C, Kruger S, et al. Lower incidence of colorectal cancer and later age of disease onset in 27 families with pathogenic MSH6 germline

mutations compared with families with MLH1 or MSH2 mutations: the German Hereditary Nonpolyposis Colorectal Cancer Consortium. J Clin Oncol 2004;22: 4486–94.

9. Senter L, Clendenning M, Sotamaa K, et al. The clinical phenotype of Lynch syndrome due to germ-line PMS2 mutations. Gastroenterology 2008;135:419–28.

10. Liu HX, Zhou XL, Liu T, et al. The role of hMLH3 in familial colorectal cancer. Cancer Res 2003;63:1894–9.

11. Nicolaides NC, Papadopoulos N, Liu B, et al. Mutations of two PMS homologues in hereditary nonpolyposis colon cancer. Nature 1994;371:75–80.

12. Vasen HF, Mecklin JP, Khan PM, et al. The International Collaborative Group on Hereditary Non-Polyposis Colorectal Cancer (ICG-HNPCC). Dis Colon Rectum 1991;34:424–5.

13. Vasen HF, Watson P, Mecklin JP, et al. New clinical criteria for hereditary nonpolyposis colorectal cancer (HNPCC, Lynch syndrome) proposed by the International Collaborative group on HNPCC. Gastroenterology 1999;116:1453–6.

14. Palomaki GE, McClain MR, Melillo S, et al. EGAPP supplementary evidence review: DNA testing strategies aimed at reducing morbidity and mortality from Lynch syndrome. Genet Med 2009;11:42–65.

15. Green RC, Parfrey PS, Woods MO, et al. Prediction of Lynch syndrome in consecutive patients with colorectal cancer. J Natl Cancer Inst 2009;101:331–40.

16. Kratz CP, Holter S, Etzler J, et al. Rhabdomyosarcoma in patients with constitutional mismatch-repair-deficiency syndrome. J Med Genet 2009;46:418–20.

17. Jass JR. Familial colorectal cancer: pathology and molecular characteristics. Lancet Oncol 2000;1:220–6.

18. Boland CR, Thibodeau SN, Hamilton SR, et al. A National Cancer Institute Workshop on microsatellite instability for cancer detection and familial predisposition: development of international criteria for the determination of microsatellite instability in colorectal cancer. Cancer Res 1998;58:5248–57.

19. Umar A, Boland CR, Terdiman JP, et al. Revised Bethesda guidelines for hereditary nonpolyposis colorectal cancer (Lynch syndrome) and microsatellite instability. J Natl Cancer Inst 2004;96:261–8.

20. Hesson LB, Hitchins MP, Ward RL. Epimutations and cancer predisposition: importance and mechanisms. Curr Opin Genet Dev 2010;31:31.

21. Cunningham JM, Christensen ER, Tester DJ, et al. Hypermethylation of the hMLH1 promoter in colon cancer with microsatellite instability. Cancer Res 1998;58:3455–60.

22. Vilar E, Gruber SB. Microsatellite instability in colorectal cancer—the stable evidence. Nat Rev Clin Oncol 2010;7:153–62.

23. Lievre A, Laurent-Puig P. Genetics: predictive value of KRAS mutations in chemoresistant CRC. Nat Rev Clin Oncol 2009;6:306–7.

24. Rajagopalan H, Bardelli A, Lengauer C, et al. Tumorigenesis: RAF/RAS oncogenes and mismatch-repair status. Nature 2002;418:934.

25. Loughrey MB, Waring PM, Tan A, et al. Incorporation of somatic BRAF mutation testing into an algorithm for the investigation of hereditary non-polyposis colorectal cancer. Fam Cancer 2007;6:301–10.

26. Sanchez JA, Krumroy L, Plummer S, et al. Genetic and epigenetic classifications define clinical phenotypes and determine patient outcomes in colorectal cancer. Br J Surg 2009;96:1196–204.

27. Ogino S, Nosho K, Kirkner GJ, et al. CpG island methylator phenotype, microsatellite instability, BRAF mutation and clinical outcome in colon cancer. Gut 2009;58:90–6.

28. Ligtenberg MJ, Kuiper RP, Chan TL, et al. Heritable somatic methylation and inactivation of MSH2 in families with Lynch syndrome due to deletion of the 3' exons of TACSTD1. Nat Genet 2009;41:112–7.

29. Kovacs ME, Papp J, Szentirmay Z, et al. Deletions removing the last exon of TACSTD1 constitute a distinct class of mutations predisposing to Lynch syndrome. Hum Mutat 2009;30:197–203.

30. Niessen RC, Hofstra RM, Westers H, et al. Germline hypermethylation of MLH1 and EPCAM deletions are a frequent cause of Lynch syndrome. Genes Chromosomes Cancer 2009;48:737–44.

31. Nagasaka T, Rhees J, Kloor M, et al. Somatic hypermethylation of MSH2 is a frequent event in lynch syndrome colorectal cancers. Cancer Res 2010;70: 3098–108.

32. Peltomaki P, Vasen H. Mutations associated with HNPCC predisposition—update of ICG-HNPCC/INSiGHT mutation database. Dis Markers 2004;20:269–76.

33. Wahlberg SS, Schmeits J, Thomas G, et al. Evaluation of microsatellite instability and immunohistochemistry for the prediction of germ-line MSH2 and MLH1 mutations in hereditary nonpolyposis colon cancer families. Cancer Res 2002; 62:3485–92.

34. Chao EC, Velasquez JL, Witherspoon MS, et al. Accurate classification of MLH1/MSH2 missense variants with multivariate analysis of protein polymorphisms-mismatch repair (MAPP-MMR). Hum Mutat 2008;29:852–60.

35. Hampel H, Frankel WL, Martin E, et al. Feasibility of screening for Lynch syndrome among patients with colorectal cancer. J Clin Oncol 2008;26:5783–8.

36. Mvundura M, Grosse SD, Hampel H, et al. The cost-effectiveness of genetic testing strategies for Lynch syndrome among newly diagnosed patients with colorectal cancer. Genet Med 2010;12:93–104.

37. Kambara T, Simms LA, Whitehall VL, et al. BRAF mutation is associated with DNA methylation in serrated polyps and cancers of the colorectum. Gut 2004; 53:1137–44.

38. Jensen LH, Lindebjerg J, Byriel L, et al. Strategy in clinical practice for classification of unselected colorectal tumours based on mismatch repair deficiency. Colorectal Dis 2008;10:490–7.

39. Wijnen JT, Vasen HF, Khan PM, et al. Clinical findings with implications for genetic testing in families with clustering of colorectal cancer. N Engl J Med 1998;339:511–8.

40. Barnetson RA, Tenesa A, Farrington SM, et al. Identification and survival of carriers of mutations in DNA mismatch-repair genes in colon cancer. N Engl J Med 2006;354:2751–63.

41. Balmana J, Stockwell DH, Steyerberg EW, et al. Prediction of MLH1 and MSH2 mutations in Lynch syndrome. JAMA 2006;296:1469–78.

42. Chen S, Wang W, Lee S, et al. Prediction of germline mutations and cancer risk in the Lynch syndrome. JAMA 2006;296:1479–87.

43. Marroni F, Pastrello C, Benatti P, et al. A genetic model for determining MSH2 and MLH1 carrier probabilities based on family history and tumor microsatellite instability. Clin Genet 2006;69:254–62.

44. Hendriks YM, Wagner A, Morreau H, et al. Cancer risk in hereditary nonpolyposis colorectal cancer due to MSH6 mutations: impact on counseling and surveillance. Gastroenterology 2004;127:17–25.

45. Wagner A, Hendriks Y, Meijers-Heijboer EJ, et al. Atypical HNPCC owing to MSH6 germline mutations: analysis of a large Dutch pedigree. J Med Genet 2001;38:318–22.

46. Buttin BM, Powell MA, Mutch DG, et al. Penetrance and expressivity of MSH6 germline mutations in seven kindreds not ascertained by family history. Am J Hum Genet 2004;74:1262–9.
47. Vasen HF, Moslein G, Alonso A, et al. Guidelines for the clinical management of Lynch syndrome (hereditary non-polyposis cancer). J Med Genet 2007;44: 353–62.
48. Lindor NM, Petersen GM, Hadley DW, et al. Recommendations for the care of individuals with an inherited predisposition to Lynch syndrome: a systematic review. JAMA 2006;296:1507–17.
49. Levin B, Lieberman DA, McFarland B, et al. Screening and surveillance for the early detection of colorectal cancer and adenomatous polyps, 2008: a joint guideline from the American Cancer Society, the US Multi-Society Task Force on Colorectal Cancer, and the American College of Radiology. Gastroenterology 2008;134:1570–95.
50. de Jong AE, Hendriks YM, Kleibeuker JH, et al. Decrease in mortality in Lynch syndrome families because of surveillance. Gastroenterology 2006;130: 665–71.
51. Levin B, Lieberman DA, McFarland B, et al. Screening and surveillance for the early detection of colorectal cancer and adenomatous polyps, 2008: a joint guideline from the American Cancer Society, the US Multi-Society Task Force on Colorectal Cancer, and the American College of Radiology. CA Cancer J Clin 2008;58:130–60.
52. Guillem JG, Wood WC, Moley JF, et al. ASCO/SSO review of current role of risk-reducing surgery in common hereditary cancer syndromes. J Clin Oncol 2006; 24:4642–60.
53. de Vos tot Nederveen Cappel WH, Nagengast FM, Griffioen G, et al. Surveillance for hereditary nonpolyposis colorectal cancer: a long-term study on 114 families. Dis Colon Rectum 2002;45:1588–94.
54. Van Dalen R, Church J, McGannon E, et al. Patterns of surgery in patients belonging to Amsterdam-positive families. Dis Colon Rectum 2003;46:617–20.
55. You YN, Chua HK, Nelson H, et al. Segmental vs. extended colectomy: measurable differences in morbidity, function, and quality of life. Dis Colon Rectum 2008;51:1036–43.
56. Maeda T, Cannom RR, Beart RW Jr, et al. Decision model of segmental compared with total abdominal colectomy for colon cancer in hereditary nonpolyposis colorectal cancer. J Clin Oncol 2010;28:1175–80.
57. de Vos tot Nederveen Cappel WH, Buskens E, van Duijvendijk P, et al. Decision analysis in the surgical treatment of colorectal cancer due to a mismatch repair gene defect. Gut 2003;52:1752–5.
58. Andre T, Boni C, Mounedji-Boudiaf L, et al. Oxaliplatin, fluorouracil, and leucovorin as adjuvant treatment for colon cancer. N Engl J Med 2004;350:2343–51.
59. Tournigand C, Andre T, Achille E, et al. FOLFIRI followed by FOLFOX6 or the reverse sequence in advanced colorectal cancer: a randomized GERCOR study. J Clin Oncol 2004;22:229–37.
60. Malesci A, Laghi L, Bianchi P, et al. Reduced likelihood of metastases in patients with microsatellite-unstable colorectal cancer. Clin Cancer Res 2007;13:3831–9.
61. Popat S, Hubner R, Houlston RS. Systematic review of microsatellite instability and colorectal cancer prognosis. J Clin Oncol 2005;23:609–18.
62. Roth AD, Tejpar S, Delorenzi M, et al. Prognostic role of KRAS and BRAF in stage II and III resected colon cancer: results of the translational study on the PETACC-3, EORTC 40993, SAKK 60-00 trial. J Clin Oncol 2010;28:466–74.

63. Ribic CM, Sargent DJ, Moore MJ, et al. Tumor microsatellite-instability status as a predictor of benefit from fluorouracil-based adjuvant chemotherapy for colon cancer. N Engl J Med 2003;349:247–57.

64. Liang JT, Huang KC, Lai HS, et al. High-frequency microsatellite instability predicts better chemosensitivity to high-dose 5-fluorouracil plus leucovorin chemotherapy for stage IV sporadic colorectal cancer after palliative bowel resection. Int J Cancer 2002;101:519–25.

65. Sargent DJ, Marsoni S, Thibodeau SN, et al. Confirmation of deficient mismatch repair (dMMR) as a predictive marker for lack of benefit from 5-FU based chemotherapy in stage II and III colon cancer (CC): a pooled molecular reanalysis of randomized chemotherapy trials [abstract #4008]. American Society of Clinical Oncology Annual Meeting 2008.

66. Bertagnolli MM, Niedzwiecki D, Compton CC, et al. Microsatellite instability predicts improved response to adjuvant therapy with irinotecan, fluorouracil, and leucovorin in stage III colon cancer: cancer and leukemia Group B Protocol 89803. J Clin Oncol 2009;27:1814–21.

67. Kim ST, Lee J, Park SH, et al. Clinical impact of microsatellite instability in colon cancer following adjuvant FOLFOX therapy. Cancer Chemother Pharmacol 2009;24:24.

68. Vilar Sanchez E, Chow A, Raskin L, et al. Preclinical testing of the PARP inhibitor ABT-888 in microsatellite instable colorectal cancer [abstract #11028]. American Society of Clinical Oncology Annual Meeting 2009.

69. Burn J, Bishop DT, Mecklin JP, et al. Effect of aspirin or resistant starch on colorectal neoplasia in the Lynch syndrome. N Engl J Med 2008;359:2567–78.

70. Solomon SD, Pfeffer MA, McMurray JJ, et al. Effect of celecoxib on cardiovascular events and blood pressure in two trials for the prevention of colorectal adenomas. Circulation 2006;114:1028–35.

71. Lee S, Hong SW, Shin SJ, et al. Papillary thyroid carcinoma associated with familial adenomatous polyposis: molecular analysis of pathogenesis in a family and review of the literature. Endocr J 2004;51:317–23.

72. Giardiello FM, Offerhaus GJ, Krush AJ, et al. Risk of hepatoblastoma in familial adenomatous polyposis. J Pediatr 1991;119:766–8.

73. Bisgaard ML, Bulow S. Familial adenomatous polyposis (FAP): genotype correlation to FAP phenotype with osteomas and sebaceous cysts. Am J Med Genet A 2006;140:200–4.

74. Fearnhead NS, Britton MP, Bodmer WF. The ABC of APC. Hum Mol Genet 2001; 10:721–33.

75. Goss KH, Groden J. Biology of the adenomatous polyposis coli tumor suppressor. J Clin Oncol 2000;18:1967–79.

76. Salahshor S, Woodgett JR. The links between axin and carcinogenesis. J Clin Pathol 2005;58:225–36.

77. Laurent-Puig P, Beroud C, Soussi T. APC gene: database of germline and somatic mutations in human tumors and cell lines. Nucleic Acids Res 1998; 26:269–70.

78. Al-Sukhni W, Aronson M, Gallinger S. Hereditary colorectal cancer syndromes: familial adenomatous polyposis and lynch syndrome. Surg Clin North Am 2008; 88:819–44, vii.

79. Wallis YL, Morton DG, McKeown CM, et al. Molecular analysis of the APC gene in 205 families: extended genotype–phenotype correlations in FAP and evidence for the role of APC amino acid changes in colorectal cancer predisposition. J Med Genet 1999;36:14–20.

80. Caspari R, Friedl W, Mandl M, et al. Familial adenomatous polyposis: mutation at codon 1309 and early onset of colon cancer. Lancet 1994;343:629–32.
81. Houlston R, Crabtree M, Phillips R, et al. Explaining differences in the severity of familial adenomatous polyposis and the search for modifier genes. Gut 2001; 48:1–5.
82. Crabtree MD, Tomlinson IP, Hodgson SV, et al. Explaining variation in familial adenomatous polyposis: relationship between genotype and phenotype and evidence for modifier genes. Gut 2002;51:420–3.
83. de la Chapelle A. Genetic predisposition to colorectal cancer. Nat Rev Cancer 2004;4:769–80.
84. Merg A, Lynch HT, Lynch JF, et al. Hereditary colorectal cancer—part II. Curr Probl Surg 2005;42:267–333.
85. National Comprehensive Cancer Network. National Comprehensive Cancer Network - guidelines for detection, prevention, risk reduction: colorectal cancer screening; 2010.
86. Vasen HF, Moslein G, Alonso A, et al. Guidelines for the clinical management of familial adenomatous polyposis (FAP). Gut 2008;57:704–13.
87. Bulow C, Vasen H, Jarvinen H, et al. Ileorectal anastomosis is appropriate for a subset of patients with familial adenomatous polyposis. Gastroenterology 2000;119:1454–60.
88. Gallagher MC, Phillips RK. Serrated adenomas in FAP. Familial adenomatous polyposis. Gut 2002;51:895–6 author reply 896.
89. Keller JJ, Giardiello FM. Chemoprevention strategies using NSAIDs and COX-2 inhibitors. Cancer Biol Ther 2003;2:S140–9.
90. Utech M, Bruwer M, Buerger H, et al. [Rectal carcinoma in a patient with familial adenomatous polyposis coli after colectomy with ileorectal anastomosis and consecutive chemoprevention with sulindac suppositories]. Chirurg 2002;73: 855–8 [in German].
91. Hisamuddin IM, Wehbi MA, Schmotzer B, et al. Genetic polymorphisms of flavin monooxygenase 3 in sulindac-induced regression of colorectal adenomas in familial adenomatous polyposis. Cancer Epidemiol Biomarkers Prev 2005;14: 2366–9.
92. Giardiello FM, Hylind LM, Trimbath JD, et al. Oral contraceptives and polyp regression in familial adenomatous polyposis. Gastroenterology 2005;128: 1077–80.
93. Jones DH, Silberstein PT, Lynch H, et al. Regression of colorectal adenomas with intravenous cytotoxic chemotherapy in a patient with familial adenomatous polyposis. J Clin Oncol 2005;23:6278–80.
94. Knudsen AL, Bisgaard ML, Bulow S. Attenuated familial adenomatous polyposis (AFAP). A review of the literature. Fam Cancer 2003;2:43–55.
95. Hernegger GS, Moore HG, Guillem JG. Attenuated familial adenomatous polyposis: an evolving and poorly understood entity. Dis Colon Rectum 2002;45: 127–34 [discussion: 134–26].
96. Soravia C, Berk T, Madlensky L, et al. Genotype–phenotype correlations in attenuated adenomatous polyposis coli. Am J Hum Genet 1998;62:1290–301.
97. Rozen P, Samuel Z, Shomrat R, et al. Notable intrafamilial phenotypic variability in a kindred with familial adenomatous polyposis and an APC mutation in exon 9. Gut 1999;45:829–33.
98. Lynch HT, Smyrk T, McGinn T, et al. Attenuated familial adenomatous polyposis (AFAP). A phenotypically and genotypically distinctive variant of FAP. Cancer 1995;76:2427–33.

99. Laken SJ, Petersen GM, Gruber SB, et al. Familial colorectal cancer in Ashkenazim due to a hypermutable tract in APC. Nat Genet 1997;17:79–83.

100. Gryfe R, Di Nicola N, Lal G, et al. Inherited colorectal polyposis and cancer risk of the APC I1307K polymorphism. Am J Hum Genet 1999;64:378–84.

101. Jo WS, Bandipalliam P, Shannon KM, et al. Correlation of polyp number and family history of colon cancer with germline MYH mutations. Clin Gastroenterol Hepatol 2005;3:1022–8.

102. Sieber OM, Lipton L, Crabtree M, et al. Multiple colorectal adenomas, classic adenomatous polyposis, and germ-line mutations in MYH. N Engl J Med 2003;348:791–9.

103. Jones S, Emmerson P, Maynard J, et al. Biallelic germline mutations in MYH predispose to multiple colorectal adenoma and somatic G: C–>T: a mutations. Hum Mol Genet 2002;11:2961–7.

104. Croitoru ME, Cleary SP, Di Nicola N, et al. Association between biallelic and monoallelic germline MYH gene mutations and colorectal cancer risk. J Natl Cancer Inst 2004;96:1631–4.

105. Jenkins MA, Croitoru ME, Monga N, et al. Risk of colorectal cancer in monoallelic and biallelic carriers of MYH mutations: a population-based case-family study. Cancer Epidemiol Biomarkers Prev 2006;15:312–4.

106. Eliason K, Hendrickson BC, Judkins T, et al. The potential for increased clinical sensitivity in genetic testing for polyposis colorectal cancer through the analysis of MYH mutations in North American patients. J Med Genet 2005;42:95–6.

107. Wang L, Baudhuin LM, Boardman LA, et al. MYH mutations in patients with attenuated and classic polyposis and with young-onset colorectal cancer without polyps. Gastroenterology 2004;127:9–16.

108. Marra G, Jiricny J. Multiple colorectal adenomas—is their number up? N Engl J Med 2003;348:845–7.

109. Farrington SM, Tenesa A, Barnetson R, et al. Germline susceptibility to colorectal cancer due to base-excision repair gene defects. Am J Hum Genet 2005;77:112–9.

110. Leite JS, Isidro G, Martins M, et al. Is prophylactic colectomy indicated in patients with MYH-associated polyposis? Colorectal Dis 2005;7:327–31.

111. Boardman LA. Heritable colorectal cancer syndromes: recognition and preventive management. Gastroenterol Clin North Am 2002;31:1107–31.

112. Giardiello FM, Trimbath JD. Peutz–Jeghers syndrome and management recommendations. Clin Gastroenterol Hepatol 2006;4:408–15.

113. Giardiello FM, Brensinger JD, Tersmette AC, et al. Very high risk of cancer in familial Peutz–Jeghers syndrome. Gastroenterology 2000;119:1447–53.

114. Hearle N, Schumacher V, Menko FH, et al. Frequency and spectrum of cancers in the Peutz–Jeghers syndrome. Clin Cancer Res 2006;12:3209–15.

115. Hemminki A. The molecular basis and clinical aspects of Peutz–Jeghers syndrome. Cell Mol Life Sci 1999;55:735–50.

116. Abdel-Rahman WM, Peltomaki P. Molecular basis and diagnostics of hereditary colorectal cancers. Ann Med 2004;36:379–88.

117. Boardman LA, Couch FJ, Burgart LJ, et al. Genetic heterogeneity in Peutz–Jeghers syndrome. Hum Mutat 2000;16:23–30.

118. Mehenni H, Blouin JL, Radhakrishna U, et al. Peutz–Jeghers syndrome: confirmation of linkage to chromosome 19p13.3 and identification of a potential second locus, on 19q13.4. Am J Hum Genet 1997;61:1327–34.

119. Sweet K, Willis J, Zhou XP, et al. Molecular classification of patients with unexplained hamartomatous and hyperplastic polyposis. JAMA 2005;294:2465–73.

120. McGrath DR, Spigelman AD. Preventive measures in Peutz–Jeghers syndrome. Fam Cancer 2001;1:121–5.
121. Saurin JC, Delvaux M, Gaudin JL, et al. Diagnostic value of endoscopic capsule in patients with obscure digestive bleeding: blinded comparison with video push-enteroscopy. Endoscopy 2003;35:576–84.
122. Rustgi AK. The genetics of hereditary colon cancer. Genes Dev 2007;21: 2525–38.
123. Hobert JA, Eng C. PTEN hamartoma tumor syndrome: an overview. Genet Med 2009;11:687–94.
124. Parsons DW, Wang TL, Samuels Y, et al. Colorectal cancer: mutations in a signalling pathway. Nature 2005;436:792.
125. Imai K, Yamamoto H. Carcinogenesis and microsatellite instability: the interrelationship between genetics and epigenetics. Carcinogenesis 2008;29: 673–80.
126. Lipkin SM, Afrasiabi K. Familial colorectal cancer syndrome X. Semin Oncol 2007;34:425–7.
127. Renkonen E, Zhang Y, Lohi H, et al. Altered expression of MLH1, MSH2, and MSH6 in predisposition to hereditary nonpolyposis colorectal cancer. J Clin Oncol 2003;21:3629–37.
128. Abdel-Rahman WM, Ollikainen M, Kariola R, et al. Comprehensive characterization of HNPCC-related colorectal cancers reveals striking molecular features in families with no germline mismatch repair gene mutations. Oncogene 2005;24: 1542–51.
129. Young J, Barker MA, Simms LA, et al. Evidence for BRAF mutation and variable levels of microsatellite instability in a syndrome of familial colorectal cancer. Clin Gastroenterol Hepatol 2005;3:254–63.
130. Lindor NM, Rabe K, Petersen GM, et al. Lower cancer incidence in Amsterdam-I criteria families without mismatch repair deficiency: familial colorectal cancer type X. JAMA 2005;293:1979–85.
131. Llor X, Pons E, Xicola RM, et al. Differential features of colorectal cancers fulfilling Amsterdam criteria without involvement of the mutator pathway. Clin Cancer Res 2005;11:7304–10.
132. Fearnhead NS, Winney B, Bodmer WF. Rare variant hypothesis for multifactorial inheritance: susceptibility to colorectal adenomas as a model. Cell Cycle 2005; 4:521–5.
133. Rennert G, Almog R, Tomsho LP, et al. Colorectal polyps in carriers of the APC I1307K polymorphism. Dis Colon Rectum 2005;48:2317–21.
134. Tenesa A, Dunlop MG. New insights into the aetiology of colorectal cancer from genome-wide association studies. Nat Rev Genet 2009;10:353–8.

Genitourinary Cancer Predisposition Syndromes

David J. Gallagher, MB, BCh, BAO[a,b,]*, Andrew Feifer, MD[c],
Jonathan A. Coleman, MD[c]

KEYWORDS

• Genitourinary • Cancer • Predisposition • Genetic

Genitourinary malignancies comprise a heterogenous group of cancers of the prostate, bladder, kidney, and testis that either, only (prostate and testis), or, more commonly (bladder male/female ratio 3:1; kidney male/female ratio 2:1),[1] occur in men. Early epidemiologic studies recognized a hereditary component to all 4 cancers, and subsequent linkage studies identified several rare syndromes whose phenotypes include a genitourinary malignancy (**Table 1**). Among these 4 cancers, testicular cancer seems to have the highest familial clustering, followed by prostate, kidney, and then bladder cancer.[2]

Prostate cancer is the most frequent nondermatologic malignancy in the United States and the second commonest cause of cancer death in men, after lung cancer.[1] Despite evidence from segregation analyses supporting the existence of prostate cancer susceptibility genes, few have been identified. BRCA is a rare exception that has been consistently replicated and seems to explain 2% to 5% of familial prostate cancer (**Table 2**). The discovery of germline determinants of bladder cancer has been similarly elusive. Familial bladder cancer is well recognized but its genetic cause has not yet been explained, and associations with rare predisposition syndromes such as Lynch syndrome (LS) or hereditary retinoblastoma (RB) explain only a minority of its inheritance. The incidence of renal cell cancer is increasing annually, largely because of the incidental discovery of small kidney tumors on imaging whose cause remains poorly understood. Birt-Hogg-Dubé (BHD) syndrome, hereditary leiomyomatosis

Supported by The Sidney Kimmel Center for Prostate and Urologic Cancers and funds provided by David H. Koch through the Prostate Cancer Foundation.

[a] Clinical Genetics Service, Department of Medicine, Memorial Sloan-Kettering Cancer Center, 1275 York Avenue, New York, NY 10021, USA

[b] Genitourinary Oncology Service, Division of Solid Tumor Oncology, Department of Medicine, Memorial Sloan-Kettering Cancer Center, 1275 York Avenue, New York, NY 10021, USA

[c] Urology Service, Department of Surgery, Memorial Sloan-Kettering Cancer Center, 1275 York Avenue, New York, NY 10021, USA

* Corresponding author. Clinical Genetics Service, Department of Medicine, Memorial Sloan-Kettering Cancer Center, 1275 York Avenue, New York, NY 10021.
E-mail address: gallaghd@mskcc.org

Hematol Oncol Clin N Am 24 (2010) 861–883
doi:10.1016/j.hoc.2010.06.002
0889-8588/10/$ – see front matter © 2010 Elsevier Inc. All rights reserved.

Table 1
Predisposition syndromes whose phenotype contains a genitourinary malignancy

Cancer	Predisposition Syndrome
Prostate	HBOC
Urothelial	Lynch
	Hereditary RB
	Costello
	Apert
Testicular	Peutz–Jeghers
	Carney complex
Kidney	Birt–Hogg–Dubé
	HLRCC
	Von Hippel–Lindau
	HPRCC
	WAGR
	Tuberous sclerosis

Abbreviations: HBOC, hereditary breast-ovarian cancer; HLRCC, hereditary leiomyomatosis and renal cell cancer; HPRCC, hereditary papillary renal carcinoma; RB, retinoblastoma; WAGR, Wilms tumor-aniridia-genitourinary anomalies-mental retardation.

and renal cell cancer syndrome (HLRCC), von Hippel-Lindau (VHL) syndrome and Wilms tumor-aniridia-genitourinary anomalies-mental retardation (WAGR) explain some, but, again, a minority of hereditary kidney cancer. Testicular cancer is most common in white men with a 75% lower incidence reported in African American men, and, like kidney cancer, its incidence is increasing annually. The cause of this increased incidence is unknown, but sons and brothers of affected men have a six- to tenfold increased risk of developing testicular cancer, and family history is the strongest risk factor for the disease, suggesting a strong genetic component.

PROSTATE CANCER
The Evidence for Hereditary Prostate Cancer

Prostate cancer is an umbrella term for a clinically heterogenous group of diseases with distinct natural histories.[3] Despite strong evidence for the existence of prostate cancer susceptibility genes,[4–8] family-based linkage studies have been unable to identify compelling candidates.[8–25] This raises the possibility that the clinical heterogeneity may be further complicated by an underlying genetic heterogeneity that the studies performed to date have been underpowered to detect.

Age, ethnicity, and family history are the principal risk factors for prostate cancer. Family history has been confirmed as a risk factor for prostate cancer irrespective of age, race, or ethnicity, with a reported odds ratio of 2.5 (95% confidence interval [CI], 1.9–3.3) after adjusting for age and ethnicity. In Sweden, a population-based study suggested that approximately 11.6% of all prostate cancer can be accounted for by familial factors alone.[26] A meta-analysis of 33 studies investigating familial clustering suggested that risk was greater for men with affected brothers (risk ratio [RR], 3.4; 95% CI, 1.8–5.7) than for men with affected fathers (RR, 2.2; 95% CI, 1.9–2.5), and risk increased with the number of close relatives affected. Second-degree relatives (RR, 1.7; 95% CI, 1.1–2.6) conferred a lower risk than first-degree relatives, and 2 or more first-degree relatives (RR, 5.1; 95% CI, 2.6–4.2) conferred increased risk compared with 1 (RR, 3.3; 95% CI, 2.6–4.2).[27] Twin studies have further investigated this familial clustering and confirmed a strong genetic component, with a concordance among monozygotic twins of 27% compared with 7.1% between

Table 2	
Candidate genes for prostate, bladder, testicular, and bladder cancer predisposition	
Cancer	**Candidate Genes**
Prostate	BRCA1 and 2
	HPC1
	PCAP
	HPCX
	CAPB
	ELAC2/HPC2
	HPC20
	KLF6
	AMACR
	MSR1
	NBS1
	CHEK2
Urothelial	MMR
	RB
	FGFR2
	HRAS
	NAT2
	GSTM1
Testicular	KITLG
	SPRY4
	PRKAR1A
	STK11(LKB1)
Kidney	FLCN
	FH
	MET
	VHL
	WT1
	TSC

dizygotic twins, suggesting that 42% (CI, 29%–50%) of prostate cancer risk is caused by hereditary factors.[4]

The incidence of prostate cancer is 24 to 60 times higher in Western compared with Asian countries, and in the United States, incidence rates are 60% higher for African American men than for whites.[28] Although the availability of screening may bias ethnic variations in disease incidence, the magnitude of the difference supports the credibility of this association. Dissecting the interplay of genetic, environmental, and social factors that contribute to these differences is challenging, but would undoubtedly be helped by an improved understanding of the genetic factors involved.

The later median age of onset of prostate cancer may support a polygenic inheritance pattern. With increasing age, somatic mutations accumulate in cells. Many predisposition syndromes, for example hereditary breast-ovarian cancer syndrome caused by germline *BRCA* mutations, manifest clinically when a second mutation occurs in a specific gene (the Knudson 2-hit hypothesis). Affected individuals inherit 1 abnormal copy of the gene, but the second normal copy of the gene must be knocked out, so that gene function is lost and the disease phenotype develops. If prostate cancer inheritance followed a similar pattern, and several different genes had to be lost before disease occurred, this may explain why early-onset prostate cancer is unusual and why individuals with inherited predisposition still develop late-onset disease.

Many segregation studies have been performed in an effort to explain the pattern of prostate cancer inheritance.[29–32] Data supporting autosomal recessive, X-linked, and multifactorial inheritance have been reported but the strongest evidence is for a rare autosomal dominantly inherited gene with an allele frequency of 0.3% to 1.7%. However, such a gene would only explain a minority of prostate cancer inheritance and it remains likely that many prostate cancer susceptibility genes exist.

Prostate Cancer Candidate Genes

BRCA-associated prostate cancer

Linkage studies of familial prostate cancer have identified many prostate cancer susceptibility loci, but few candidates have been replicated.[33,34] Linkage studies have compared genomic markers between cases and controls with the hope of detecting links between regions of the genome and disease, and many factors contribute to the disappointing results thus far. The phenotypic variation of prostate cancer makes linkage analysis difficult. Even within families, clinical presentation varies and natural history differs, suggesting that relatives may develop genetically heterogenous disease. Because of the prevalence of the disease, some individuals (phenocopies) may develop sporadic prostate cancer that is different from the hereditary disease in the family. Prostate cancer screening may also detect individuals who may not otherwise be diagnosed, further complicating the study of inheritance within families. More recent efforts have attempted to study a clinically homogenous population to increase the likelihood of identifying underlying genes; however, the predictive power of clinical variables in prostate cancer is limited, and accurate clinical definition of prostate cancer continues to hamper linkage analysis.[35] Molecular characterization of prostate cancer may facilitate more reliable disease classification and consequently aid the investigation of predisposition.

Although early studies of smaller subsets of patients were inconclusive,[36–40] recent studies have associated BRCA1 and BRCA2 mutations with a hereditary predisposition to prostate cancer, noting up to a 33% cumulative risk by age 80 years.[41–43] The evidence for BRCA2 is particularly compelling with a recent study in the United Kingdom attributing a 23-fold increase in risk of early-onset prostate cancer to BRCA2 mutations.[44] The role of BRCA1 in hereditary prostate cancer is less clear. Linkage studies have identified the BRCA1-containing region of chromosome 17q as a prostate cancer susceptibility region, but deleterious BRCA1 mutations have been inconsistently detected.[45] Furthermore, a study investigating loss of heterozygosity in prostate cancer specimens from BRCA1 and BRCA2 carriers confirmed loss of heterozygosity in 10 of the 14 BRCA2 carriers but in none of the BRCA1 carriers, suggesting that germline BRCA1 mutations may not have played a role in prostate cancer pathogenesis in these individuals.[46] It is possible that a prostate cancer susceptibility locus lies near (ie, is in linkage disequilibrium with) BRCA1, explaining the positive linkage studies but failed confirmatory BRCA1 mutation testing.

The association between BRCA and prostate cancer exists in both multiethnic cohorts, such as the Breast Cancer Linkage Consortium study of hereditary breast-ovarian cancer kindreds,[47,48] and in ethnic minorities such as men of Ashkenazi Jewish ancestry where founder mutation studies mirror the increased risk in broader population cohorts.[36,41,42] A study of 5000 Ashkenazi Jewish participants in the United States reported that BRCA carriers had a cumulative risk for prostate cancer of 16% compared with 3.8% for noncarriers.[42] This increased risk for male carriers was the same as the 16% absolute ovarian cancer risk for female BRCA carriers in the study. However, in men unselected for family history or ancestry, BRCA seems to contribute to a very small minority of prostate cancer risk, with a study of 290 men in the United

States with early-onset prostate cancer reporting a BRCA2 prevalence rate of only 0.78% (2 mutation carriers).[44] However, given the estimated 0.0069 BRCA2 mutation frequency in the population and the approximately threefold relative risk for prostate cancer, this translates to ˜1.5% of the 180,000 prostate cancer cases in the United States that are attributable to BRCA2 mutations, or 2790 cases each year that could benefit from treatments tailored to BRCA2 status.

Recent data suggest that BRCA-associated prostate cancer may represent an aggressive disease phenotype, and that carriers may require a unique management approach with earlier screening and more aggressive treatment.[49,50] BRCA carriers seem to progress earlier and die more commonly of prostate cancer than noncarriers, supporting the need for more aggressive therapy. A recent phase I study demonstrated that prostate cancer responds to poly-ADP ribose polymerase inhibition offering a relatively nontoxic therapeutic option for a genetically defined subset of prostate cancer,[51,52] and illustrating how germline variation may meaningfully contribute to prostate cancer management.

Other prostate cancer susceptibility loci

Few prostate cancer susceptibility loci have been as well studied as BRCA1 and BRCA2, but many others have been identified. Initial studies in Polish patients associated germline mutations in another breast cancer susceptibility locus, CHEK2, with prostate cancer, and reported that founder mutations explained up to 7% of prostate cancer in Poland.[52-55] A subsequent study in Ashkenazi Jewish men with prostate cancer failed to replicate these findings, and this pattern has been repeated with many other candidate genes.[56] A susceptibility locus at 1q24, termed HPC1, was initially linked with prostate cancer in high-risk families, and deleterious mutations in a nearby gene RNASEL at 1q25 were believed to be responsible for this association.[8,57,58] Numerous studies have attempted to verify this finding, with some confirming the initial reports and others refuting them,[11-14,22,59,60] suggesting that, if the association is real, it likely explains a very small percentage of familial prostate cancer, and again highlighting the pattern in linkage studies to date.

Recent advances, such as the HapMap project and the emergence of high-throughput genotyping, have facilitated more detailed scrutiny of the genome, and 8 independent prostate cancer genome-wide association studies (GWAS) have identified further susceptibility loci.[61-72] 8q24 is a region that contains no known genes (a gene desert) but has been consistently associated with prostate cancer in these studies, suggesting that it somehow plays a role in prostate cancer carcinogenesis. Recent evidence supports a possible role in regulation of the MYC proto-oncogene, which is found nearby.[73-75] An association between prostate cancer and the 8q21 region was previously made through the Nijmegen Breakage syndrome, caused by NBS1 mutations.[76] This rare autosomal recessive condition characterized by short stature, progressive microcephaly with loss of cognitive skills, premature ovarian failure in women, recurrent sinopulmonary infections, and an increased risk lymphoma and leukemia. Adult heterozygotes have an increased risk of breast cancer, prostate cancer, and melanoma, contributing to a tiny proportion of overall cases because of the rarity of this syndrome, but supporting the association between this chromosomal region and malignancy.

Accumulating data from GWAS is providing evidence for a polygenic inheritance pattern in prostate cancer. Many independent loci have been replicated in different studies. A recent population-based, case-control study from Sweden concluded that the population attributable risk (PAR) of a susceptibility single nucleotide polymorphism (SNP) panel was 4% to 21%, depending on the number of SNPs detected, and, when family history was added into the model, the PAR was 46%.[77] Available technology detects approximately 80% of common variation in the genome. This detection rate will improve, enabling more detailed scanning and further susceptibility loci will be identified. Explanation of prostate cancer inheritance will likely require an improved understanding of the interaction between these distinct genomic regions. The contribution of DNA structural variants (eg, copy number variation, microRNAs, long-range promoters, and epigenetics) to gene expression is being investigated and may also improve understanding of hereditary and familial prostate cancer.

Summary of Prostate Cancer Predisposition

Phenotypic variation and genetic heterogeneity have complicated the search for prostate cancer susceptibility genes. Many candidates have been identified but few results have been consistently replicated. BRCA2 is one exception that has repeatedly been associated with prostate cancer, and, more recently, with an aggressive subset of the disease, but accounts for a small percentage (<1%) of overall prostate cancer susceptibility. Recent GWAS have identified common variants associated with prostate cancer and, as this technology advances and our understanding of the genome improves, the role these loci play in prostate cancer susceptibility may emerge. It remains possible that rare, single-gene disorders explain familial predisposition to cancer, but more accurate clinical and/or molecular characterization of disease within families will be required to utilize recent technological advances and to identify these genes.

BLADDER CANCER
The Evidence for Hereditary Bladder Cancer

Bladder cancer is the fifth commonest malignancy in the United States and, because of the cost of screening, is the most expensive to manage, making it an important public health issue. Transitional cell carcinoma represents more than 90% of bladder cancer. It most commonly occurs in the bladder but also arises in the renal pelvis or ureter (upper urinary tract), and, irrespective of its site of origin, is collectively termed urothelial cancer (UC). Many environmental causes of UC have been reported,[78–83] among them smoking and exposure to aromatic amines, but epidemiologic data suggest that poorly defined genetic factors also play a role.

A population-based study in Utah reported that first-degree relatives of individuals with bladder cancer have an increased risk (RR, 1.51; 95% CI, 0.98–2.2) of developing the disease, and this increased to 5.07 (95% CI, 0.97–12.5) when the proband was less than 60 years of age.[2] There are 16 multiple-case UC reports in the literature, detailing 32 families with 86 affected individuals.[84] The early age of onset and co-occurrence of other malignancies seems to suggest a genetic predisposition, but it is difficult to separate this from shared environmental exposure. A large Dutch case-control study of 1193 UC cases and 853 controls reported a smoking-adjusted relative risk of 1.8 (95% CI, 1.3–2.7) for a positive family history of UC, suggesting that smoking history and genetic susceptibility are independent risk factors for the disease.[85] Other case-control and cohort studies completed to date support a modest hereditary component to UC, with most risk ratios lying between 1.4 and 1.9.[85–94]

High-penetrance UC Genes

The most common hereditary cancer syndrome with UC as a characteristic is LS. This is an autosomal dominantly inherited condition resulting from germline mutation in mismatch repair (MMR) genes.[23,24] It is the most common form of hereditary colorectal cancer and extracolonic manifestations include many malignancies, including UC. The revised Bethesda Guidelines, which were developed to help identify individuals and families who may be at risk for LS, include UC of the upper tract but not bladder among the syndrome-defining malignancies.[95] Although several reports of bladder cancer in LS exist, the association remains unclear. A Dutch LS study reported an RR of 14 (95% CI, 6.7–29.5) for upper-tract UC, but the risk for developing UC of the bladder was not increased in this cohort.[96] A discussion of screening for UC is beyond the scope of this manuscript, but guidelines for individuals with UC presently recommend considering annual urinary cytology.[97]

UC has been reported as a manifestation of other rare, high-penetrance syndromes. An association with hereditary RB was initially believed to be related to treatment effects from primary therapy for the RB[98,99]; however, survivors who did not receive radiation or chemotherapy had a considerably higher bladder cancer–specific mortality (standardized mortality ratio, 26.3; 95% CI, 8.5–61.4) than is seen in the general population, suggesting that UC of the bladder is a manifestation of hereditary RB.[100] This is consistent with data demonstrating somatic mutations in RB or p53 in 50% of high-grade UC.[101] Somatic mutations in HRAS and FGFR3 are commonly found in superficial UC. Costello syndrome is a hereditary condition with a large number of characteristic features, including UC of the bladder for adolescents and adults.[102] HRAS is the only known mutation associated with this syndrome and, again, this germline association is consistent with somatic alterations identified in superficial UC. Germline FGFR3 mutations cause achondroplasia that is not associated with an increased risk of UC, but Apert syndrome, which results from mutations in FGFR2, has been associated with UC.[103]

These high-penetrance predisposition syndromes explain a small minority of familial UC. Linkage studies have failed to identify other genes, and, although they have been small and underpowered, they seem to suggest a polygenic inheritance for the familial UC.

Low-penetrance UC Genes

Two candidate genes involved in carcinogen metabolism have been associated with an increased risk of bladder cancer. N-acetyltransferase 2 (NAT2) is a phase II enzyme that detoxifies aromatic amines, 1 family of carcinogens found in tobacco smoke, and glutathione S-transferase (GSTM1) is a phase II enzyme that detoxifies carcinogenic polycyclic aromatic hydrocarbons, such as benzopyrene.[104–106] The NAT2 slow acetylator phenotype and the GSTM1 null genotype increase bladder cancer risk by 1.4- and 1.5-fold respectively, but, because of their high prevalence in the white population (40%–60% and 40%–50% of whites respectively), have been estimated to account for 31% of bladder cancer in whites.[107]

Further support for the role of common genomic variation in bladder cancer predisposition was provided by recent GWAS. In a study of 4000 cases and 38,000 controls, Kiemeney and colleagues[108] identified 3 new susceptibility loci at 8q24, 3q28, and 5p15 that increase the risk of bladder cancer by 22%, 19%, and 16%, respectively. The same 8q24 locus has been associated with prostate cancer as discussed earlier,[109] as well as colorectal and breast cancer, suggesting that this poorly understood region may contain a common carcinogenic pathway. A second GWAS in 969 bladder cancer cases and 957 controls identified a second, independent SNP on 8q24 located in the promoter region of PSCA.[110]

Summary of Bladder Cancer Predisposition

Individuals with LS are screened for UC, but most familial UC remains unexplained. Candidate genes involved in carcinogen metabolism have been associated with increased risk of the disease, and recent GWAS have identified further common variants that confer increased risk of UC. Like prostate cancer, UC seems to be a polygenic disorder, although rare familial single-gene disorders may exist. More is known about environmental causes of bladder cancer than the other genitourinary malignancies discussed, and future studies investigating genetic susceptibility should consider gene-environment interaction in the analysis.

KIDNEY CANCER
Hereditary Kidney Cancer Syndromes

Conservative estimates suggest that 3% to 5% of kidney tumors are inherited.[111] Explanation of the genetic causes of hereditary renal cancer (HRC) identified important molecular pathways in renal cell cancer pathogenesis.[112] This understanding has proved instrumental in the development of clinical trials with targeted molecular therapies, which have become the new standards for medical therapies.[113] Several HRC syndromes have been characterized. These include VHL disease, BHD syndrome, hereditary papillary (type I) renal cancer (HPRC), HLRCC, and tuberous sclerosis (TS) (**Table 3**). Others, including familial renal oncocytoma and the association between lymphoma and kidney cancer, have been reported, although genetic evidence is lacking.

VHL disease
The VHL syndrome first reported in 1895 by a German ophthalmologist, Dr Eugene von Hippel,[114] and fully described by Davison and colleagues[115] in 1936, includes brain

Table 3
Biologic basis of hereditary renal tumor syndromes

Syndrome	Gene/Protein	Function	Pathway[a]	Phenotype
VHL	3p25/pVHL	TS	HIF	CNS/ocular hemangioblastoma ELST Pheochromocytoma Pancreatic NET Clear cell RCC
HPRC	7q31/c-Met Tyrosine kinase domain	OG	HGF/c-Met	Papillary type 1 RCC
BHD	17p12/folliculin	TS	mTOR	Fibrofolliculomas Pulmonary blebs Chromo/onco/clear RCC
HLRCC	1q42.3/fumarase	TS	HIF	Skin leiomyoma Uterine Leiomyoma/ sarcoma HLRCC renal cancer
TSC	TSC1 9q34 TSC2 16p13.3 tubulin/hamartin	TS	mTOR	Angiomyolipoma Clear cell RCC

Abbreviations: BHD, Birt-Hogg-Dubé; Chromo, chromophobe; CNS, central nervous system; ELST, endolymphatic sac tumors; HGF, hepatocyte growth factor; HIF, hypoxia inducible factor; HLRCC, hereditary leiomyomatosis renal cell carcinoma; HPRC, hereditary papillary renal cancer; mTOR, mammalian target of rapamycin; NET, neuroendocrine tumors; OG, oncogene; Onco, oncocytoma; RCC, renal cell carcinoma; TS, tumor suppressor; TSC, tuberous sclerosis complex; VHL, von Hippel-Lindau.
[a] Putative primary pathway for mechanism of action.

and retinal hemangioblastomas, endolymphatic sac tumors of the ear, clear cell renal cancer and renal cysts, pheochromocytoma, pancreatic neuroendocrine tumors and cysts, as well as cysts in the epididymis of the testis in men and of the broad ligament in women.

The VHL gene has been localized on the short arm of chromosome 3 (3p26–25) and functions as a classic tumor suppressor gene.[116] VHL syndrome is present in an estimated 1 in 36,000 individuals, and germline mutations are inherited in an autosomal dominant fashion. The VHL gene functions as part of a complex with other proteins that regulate hypoxia inducible factor (HIF)-1α and HIF-2α. Mutations which result in the inactivation of VHL, either directly or through epigenetic events such as methylation, allow for unregulated action of HIF even in conditions of normoxia.[111] Aberrant activation of HIF-dependent pathways creates a condition of pseudohypoxia believed to provide the environment for neovascularization and cellular proliferation associated with renal cell carcinoma.[117]

Four distinct VHL phenotypes have been described (**Table 4**). Type 1 families do not have pheochromocytomas. Those with type 2 may have pheochromocytoma found among family members and are further subdivided into 2a (low risk for renal cancer), 2b (high risk for renal cancer), and 2c (pheochromocytoma only).[118] Earliest manifestations of the disease are detectable among most affected individuals within the first 25 years of life.[119] Central nervous system (CNS) and ocular hemangiomas may be detected in children and infants.[120] The most common current cause of morbidity is from CNS hemangiomas, although, historically, complications of medical renal disease and kidney cancer have also been a major health risk. The renal manifestations of VHL are found in approximately 40% to 50% of patients, and vary from cystic to solid lesions, typically multifocal and bilateral. Organ-preserving approaches for control of VHL neoplasms are considered standard treatment and should be used when possible.

HPRC

HPRC is associated with mutation of the c-met oncogene.[121] C-met has been mapped to the long arm of chromosome 7 (7q31) and codes for a membrane-bound tyrosine kinase receptor whose ligand is hepatocyte growth factor (HGF).[121–123] In HPRC, kidney tumors are formed as a result of activating mutations, typically involving the intracellular domain of the c-met receptor, causing constitutive activation of the HGF/c-met pathway through its function as a tyrosine kinase.[124,125] Germline allelic imbalance through gains in chromosomes 7 and 17 has also been reported.[126,127] Analysis of families with identifiable germline mutations has revealed an autosomal dominant inheritance pattern with variable penetrance.

The clinical manifestations of HPRC, unlike the multiorgan involvement seen in VHL, seem isolated to papillary renal tumors only. Screening studies in affected families

Table 4
Clustered phenotypes of VHL (based on the presence of pheochromocytomas and renal tumors)

VHL Group	Phenotype
Type 1	Low risk of pheochromocytoma
Type 2	High risk of pheochromocytoma
2a	Hemangiomas, low-risk RCC
2b	Hemangiomas, high-risk RCC
2c	Pheochromocytoma predominant

have helped to describe details of the disease' natural history.[128,129] The median age for clinical presentation with tumors is in the fourth to fifth decade of life; older than that seen for VHL. Screening among families can be successful in detecting subclinical tumors earlier and can indicate a high degree of penetrance, with several hundred micropapillary tumors often present in resected kidneys.[128,130]

Management of patients with HPRC must strike a balance between the risks of intervention and those of distant disease progression. Nephron-sparing surgery is the preferred approach, but, because of the number of gross and macroscopic tumors encountered, repeated interventions are often necessary. Clinical trials investigating inhibitors of c-met are underway.[131]

BHD syndrome

BHD syndrome is characterized by skin fibrofolliculomas, pulmonary cysts, and renal tumors.[132,133] Several series evaluating familial disease clusters have identified variable penetrance patterns and phenotypes.[134,135] The largest series reported a 14% prevalence of renal tumors in mutation carriers.[134] Spontaneous pneumothoraces occurred in 23% of affected individuals and were most common in younger family members (<40 years old). Lung cysts were common and seen in 83% of screened patients as detected on high-resolution chest computed tomography (CT). A more recent study that screened 50 newly diagnosed families identified skin lesions in 90% of affected individuals and renal tumors in 34%.[136]

Variable renal manifestations have been described,[137] including chromophobe,[138] oncocytoma,[139] clear cell,[140] and hybrid oncocytic tumors composed of elements of oncocytoma and chromophobe,[140–142] and the average age of presentation is between 40 and 50 years. In the largest pathologic series to date, consisting of 130 tumors from 30 surgically managed patients, the distribution of renal tumor histopathology was as follows: hybrid onco/chromophobe 50%, chromophobe 34%, conventional clear cell 9%, oncocytoma 5%, and papillary 2%.[143] Other possibly related manifestations include multinodular goiter, medullary thyroid carcinoma, parotid oncocytoma, and colonic polyposis.[144]

BHD is an autosomal dominant condition caused by mutations in the folliculin, and has been mapped to chromosome 17 (17p12q11).[145,146] Folliculin has no known function but has been isolated in brain, parotid gland, lung, pancreas, breast, prostate, kidney, and skin.[147–150] It may play a role in the mTOR pathway, mediated though binding of the folliculin-interacting protein and the 5'-activated protein kinase.[151]

HLRCC

HLRCC is associated with a more malignant type II variant of papillary renal cancer.[152] HLRCC is an autosomal dominant condition caused by germline mutations of fumarate hydratase (FH), a Krebs cycle enzyme.[153] Detailed histologic descriptions facilitate identification of HLRCC renal tumors.[154] Symptomatic uterine fibroids are the commonest clinical presentation, often requiring early hysterectomy because of difficulties from menometrorrhagia.[155] In a recently described series in the United States, as many as 89% of affected women underwent hysterectomy, 44% before the age of 30 years.[156] Isolated cases of uterine leiomyosarcomas have been reported, and biallelic mutations in nonsyndromic leiomyomas have been described.[157] Cutaneous leiomyomas are common among affected individuals.

FH is located on chromosome 1 (1q42.3–43)[158,159] and loss of heterozygosity studies support its role as a tumor suppressor gene.[160] A genetic founder effect has been described for seemingly unrelated patients with similar clinicopathologic features.[161] Initial descriptions of the syndrome focused entirely on the uterine abnormalities and dermatologic manifestations, referring to the syndrome as multiple cutaneous and uterine leiomyomatosis or multiple leiomyomatosis.[158] Renal cortical tumors are typically found in 2% to 21% of affected individuals. The discrepancy between expressions of these 2 phenotypic findings has prompted some investigators to subclassify the disease based on phenotype.[159,162,163] Biallelic loss of FH in several published models indicates that aberrant signaling may be mediated through HIF-dependent pathways, suggesting that mechanisms of pseudohypoxia or apoptosis may play roles in tumorigenesis similar to VHL.[164,165] Reports of clear cell histology with FH mutation in a patient with HLRCC may support a common mechanism of tumorigenesis through HIF activation.[153,166,167]

Management Summary for HRCs

A therapeutic and preventive strategy in patients with HRC requires coordinated multi-modality care, which serves to minimize treatment related morbidity and preserve renal function. The general approach to HRC includes screening tests and physical examinations, as well as a regimented schedule of follow-up appointments.[119] Recent advances in nephron-sparing techniques that prioritize functional kidney preservation and expectant management of lesions have diminished kidney-related mortality and chronic renal dysfunction.[168,169] Retrospective studies have demonstrated the safety of observation of solid renal masses to a diameter of 3 cm.[168,170–172] Minimally invasive surgical procedures for multiple partial nephrectomies have also been used satisfactorily at experienced centers, including tumor ablation performed in prospective clinical trials.[171,173–176] Long-term outcomes with regard to efficacy and renal function have not been reported.[177]

Syndrome-specific management strategies have also been developed. VHL mutation carriers require neurologic, otologic, ophthalmologic, and endocrine follow-up involving magnetic resonance imaging (MRI)/CT scanning.[178–180] The development of pheochromocytomas can complicate patient management, increasing the risk of intracranial bleeding in patients at risk for CNS or ocular hemangiomas. Annual functional adrenal studies, and secondary meta-iodobenzylguanidine immunoscintigraphy are often indicated. Medical management before surgical resection is the most frequent management strategy. Partial adrenalectomy for a solitary adrenal gland or bilateral lesions can be safely performed to avoid steroid replacement therapy.[181,182]

HLRCC management differs from other HRC syndromes because of the aggressive nature of renal tumors. Among affected individuals, rapid distant disease progression, even when the primary tumors are small, is usually the case.[183–185] This is also evident in pediatric patients.[186] As a result, thorough and early imaging assessment, close follow-up, and rapid intervention is the management paradigm for these patients. Nephron-sparing surgery is less well established in this setting, and complete wide excision, including lymph node dissection, should be attempted.[187,188] Preoperative positron emission tomography scans may prove beneficial in cases where lymph node or nonlocalized disease is suspected.

TESTICULAR CANCER
Hereditary Germ Cell Tumors

Germ cell tumors (GCT) make up 95% of all testicular cancer and more than 90% of GCT occur in the testis, with a minority developing outside of the testes in the midline of the body along the embryologic development tract of the gonads. The incidence of GCT has increased 3% to 6% annually for the last 40 years.[189] This increase has occurred predominantly in white men, and GCT remains rare in African and Asian populations even after migration. There has been a simultaneous increase in cryptorchidism, hypospadias, and infertility, particularly among European men, and the term testicular dysgenesis syndrome has been proposed to describe this constellation of features,[190] although no unifying genetic or environmental causative factor has been identified. Initial efforts to link the epidemiologic observation that male infertility and GCTs commonly co-occur were unsuccessful until Nathanson and colleagues[191] identified an association between a Y-chromosome 1.6-Mb deletion, designated gr/gr, and familial testicular cancer. Presence of the gr/gr deletion was associated with a twofold increased risk of GCT and a threefold increased risk of testicular GCT among patients with a positive family history, confirming this locus as a low-penetrance susceptibility region. Candidate genes have not been identified despite associations of GCT with several syndromes that include abnormal testicular development, such as Klinefelter syndrome, XY dysgenesis, and Down syndrome (trisomy 21).

Perhaps the strongest evidence for a genetic predisposition to testicular cancer comes from epidemiologic studies of familial GCT that report a fourfold increased risk in sons of men with GCT, and eight- to tenfold increased risk in brothers of affected probands.[2,192–194] The higher familial risk for testicular cancer among brothers than father-son pairs may suggest the involvement of a recessive mode of inheritance or an X-linked susceptibility locus. Ovarian GCTs can also occur as part of this familial germ cell syndrome,[195] albeit with a much lower incidence. It is difficult to separate shared childhood environment and genetic causes, and linkage studies have been hampered by the rarity of familial testicular cancer.[196] Identification of predisposing genes is further complicated by the histologic variation in GCT presentation. GCTs are broadly categorized as seminomas (termed dysgerminomas in women) and nonseminomatous GCT (NSGCTs), which are further subclassified as yolk-sac tumors, choriocarcinomas, teratomas, and embryonal carcinoma. If each histologic presentation had a unique genetic cause, linkage would be extremely challenging given the rarity of this malignancy; however, GCTs seem to originate from a common precursor lesion termed intratubular germ cell neoplasia unclassified (ITGCNU),[197] suggesting a common genetic cause, and this is supported by the occurrence of varying histologies within families.

Further support is provided by 2 recent GWAS that identified the 12q22 locus as a GCT susceptibility locus in both seminomas and NSGCTs.[198,199] This association makes biologic sense because the 12q22 locus contains *KITLG*, which encodes the ligand for the receptor tyrosine kinase, c-KIT. ITGCNU cells, seminoma cells, and primordial germ cells all stain positively for KIT.[200] Primordial germ cell migration to the genital ridge is under the control of the KIT stem cell signaling pathway, and an activating mutation in the phosphotransferase region of KIT has been associated with bilateral GCTs.[201] A second association was identified at 5q31 just downstream of SPRY4. SPRY4 is a negative regulator of the RAS-ERK-MAPK pathway,[202] and tumor studies of imatinib-treated gastrointestinal stromal tumors that demonstrate downregulation of SPRY4 expression after KIT inhibition by imatinib, suggest a functional connection between KIT and SPRY4.[203]

Hereditary Sex Cord Stromal Tumors

Sex cord stromal tumors arise from the supporting tissues of the testis and comprise approximately 5% of all testicular tumors. They are subclassified as Leydig, Sertoli, and granulosa cell tumors, malignant mesothelioma of the tunica vaginalis, adenocarcinoma of the rete testis, and paratesticular rhabdomyosarcoma. Little is known about the genetic cause of these tumors except that Sertoli cell testicular tumors have been associated with Peutz-Jeghers syndrome and Carney complex,[204,205] and juvenile granulosa cell tumors, which are uniformly benign, have been associated with sex chromosome abnormalities, ambiguous genitalia, and ipsilateral cryptorchidism.[206]

Peutz-Jeghers syndrome is the commonest form of hamartomatous polyposis, with a reported prevalence of between 1 in 29,000 and 1 in 200,000. It is characterized by autosomal dominant inheritance, gastrointestinal hamartomas, and mucocutaneous freckling,[207] and an association with Sertoli cell tumors of the testis has been reported.[208] Carney complex is an autosomal dominantly inherited condition caused by mutations in *PRKAR1A* and an unknown gene at chromosomal locus 2p16. It is characterized by skin pigmentary abnormalities, myxomas, endocrine tumors or over-activity, and schwannomas, and one-third of men develop large cell calcifying Sertoli tumors within the first decade, and virtually all carriers by adulthood. These tumors are generally benign and commonly cured with orchiectomy. Rare metastases are often chemoresistant and difficult to treat. Clinical testing is available for *PRKAR1A*, and sequencing detects approximately 55% of mutations. More than two-thirds of patients with Carney complex inherit the mutation from a parent, but approximately 30% of mutations occur de novo.[209]

Summary of Testicular Cancer Predisposition

There is strong evidence supporting a hereditary component to testicular cancer; however, predisposing genes have only been identified for the rare pathologic subtype, Sertoli cell tumor. Large collaborative efforts may be required to overcome the challenge posed by the rarity of this tumor, and recent GWAS have used this approach to identify some novel candidate genes.

SUMMARY

Despite epidemiologic data supporting a significant genetic contribution to the cause of genitourinary malignancies, their diagnosis rarely results in clinical genetics referral and the heritability of prostate, bladder, kidney, and testicular cancer remains poorly understood. Little of this inheritance has been explained by rare, high-penetrance predisposition syndromes and, although rare genetic variation may explain some of the remaining familial predisposition, recent GWAS support an important causal role for more common genomic variation and other structural variants. Susceptibility loci associated with risk of prostate, bladder, and testicular cancer have been identified that may improve our understanding of the cause and natural history of these malignancies. It remains to be seen whether this emerging knowledge of genetic predisposition can meaningfully contribute to the clinical management of genitourinary malignancies.

REFERENCES

1. Jemal A, Siegel R, Ward E, et al. Cancer statistics, 2009. CA Cancer J Clin 2009; 59:225–49.
2. Goldgar DE, Easton DF, Cannon-Albright LA, et al. Systematic population-based assessment of cancer risk in first-degree relatives of cancer probands. J Natl Cancer Inst 1994;86:1600–8.
3. Mackinnon AC, Yan BC, Joseph LJ, et al. Molecular biology underlying the clinical heterogeneity of prostate cancer: an update. Arch Pathol Lab Med 2009; 133:1033–40.
4. Lichtenstein P, Holm NV, Verkasalo PK, et al. Environmental and heritable factors in the causation of cancer-analyses of cohorts of twins from Sweden, Denmark, and Finland. N Engl J Med 2000;343:78–85.

5. Schaid DJ. The complex genetic epidemiology of prostate cancer. Hum Mol Genet 2004;13(1):R103–21.
6. Gronberg H, Damber L, Damber JE. Studies of genetic factors in prostate cancer in a twin population. J Urol 1994;152:1484–7 [discussion: 1487–9].
7. Page WF, Braun MM, Partin AW, et al. Heredity and prostate cancer: a study of World War II veteran twins. Prostate 1997;33:240–5.
8. Smith JR, Freije D, Carpten JD, et al. Major susceptibility locus for prostate cancer on chromosome 1 suggested by a genome-wide search. Science 1996;274:1371–4.
9. Gronberg H, Xu J, Smith JR, et al. Early age at diagnosis in families providing evidence of linkage to the hereditary prostate cancer locus (HPC1) on chromosome 1. Cancer Res 1997;57:4707–9.
10. Carpten J, Nupponen N, Isaacs S, et al. Germline mutations in the ribonuclease L gene in families showing linkage with HPC1. Nat Genet 2002;30:181–4.
11. Cooney KA, McCarthy JD, Lange E, et al. Prostate cancer susceptibility locus on chromosome 1q: a confirmatory study. J Natl Cancer Inst 1997;89:955–9.
12. Hsieh CL, Oakley-Girvan I, Gallagher RP, et al. Re: prostate cancer susceptibility locus on chromosome 1q: a confirmatory study. J Natl Cancer Inst 1997;89:1893–4.
13. McIndoe RA, Stanford JL, Gibbs M, et al. Linkage analysis of 49 high-risk families does not support a common familial prostate cancer-susceptibility gene at 1q24–25. Am J Hum Genet 1997;61:347–53.
14. Eeles RA, Durocher F, Edwards S, et al. Linkage analysis of chromosome 1q markers in 136 prostate cancer families. The Cancer Research Campaign/ British Prostate Group U.K. Familial Prostate Cancer Study Collaborators. Am J Hum Genet 1998;62:653–8.
15. Bergthorsson JT, Johannesdottir G, Arason A, et al. Analysis of HPC1, HPCX, and PCaP in Icelandic hereditary prostate cancer. Hum Genet 2000;107:372–5.
16. Cancel-Tassin G, Latil A, Valeri A, et al. PCAP is the major known prostate cancer predisposing locus in families from south and west Europe. Eur J Hum Genet 2001;9:135–42.
17. Suarez BK, Lin J, Witte JS, et al. Replication linkage study for prostate cancer susceptibility genes. Prostate 2000;45:106–14.
18. Berry R, Schaid DJ, Smith JR, et al. Linkage analyses at the chromosome 1 loci 1q24–25 (HPC1), 1q42.2–43 (PCAP), and 1p36 (CAPB) in families with hereditary prostate cancer. Am J Hum Genet 2000;66:539–46.
19. Farnham JM, Camp NJ, Swensen J, et al. Confirmation of the HPCX prostate cancer predisposition locus in large Utah prostate cancer pedigrees. Hum Genet 2005;116:179–85.
20. Xu J, Meyers D, Freije D, et al. Evidence for a prostate cancer susceptibility locus on the X chromosome. Nat Genet 1998;20:175–9.
21. Xu J. Combined analysis of hereditary prostate cancer linkage to 1q24–25: results from 772 hereditary prostate cancer families from the International Consortium for Prostate Cancer Genetics. Am J Hum Genet 2000;66:945–57.
22. Berthon P, Valeri A, Cohen-Akenine A, et al. Predisposing gene for early-onset prostate cancer, localized on chromosome 1q42.2–43. Am J Hum Genet 1998;62:1416–24.
23. Gibbs M, Chakrabarti L, Stanford JL, et al. Analysis of chromosome 1q42.2–43 in 152 families with high risk of prostate cancer. Am J Hum Genet 1999;64: 1087–95.
24. Gibbs M, Stanford JL, McIndoe RA, et al. Evidence for a rare prostate cancer-susceptibility locus at chromosome 1p36. Am J Hum Genet 1999;64:776–87.

25. Whittemore AS, Lin IG, Oakley-Girvan I, et al. No evidence of linkage for chromosome 1q42.2–43 in prostate cancer. Am J Hum Genet 1999;65:254–6.
26. Gronberg H, Wiklund F, Damber JE. Age specific risks of familial prostate carcinoma: a basis for screening recommendations in high risk populations. Cancer 1999;86:477–83.
27. Zeegers MP, Jellema A, Ostrer H. Empiric risk of prostate carcinoma for relatives of patients with prostate carcinoma: a meta-analysis. Cancer 2003;97:1894–903.
28. Haas GP, Sakr WA. Epidemiology of prostate cancer. CA Cancer J Clin 1997;47: 273–87.
29. Valeri A, Briollais L, Azzouzi R, et al. Segregation analysis of prostate cancer in France: evidence for autosomal dominant inheritance and residual brother–brother dependence. Ann Hum Genet 2003;67:125–37.
30. Schaid DJ, McDonnell SK, Blute ML, et al. Evidence for autosomal dominant inheritance of prostate cancer. Am J Hum Genet 1998;62:1425–38.
31. Verhage BA, Baffoe-Bonnie AB, Baglietto L, et al. Autosomal dominant inheritance of prostate cancer: a confirmatory study. Urology 2001;57:97–101.
32. Carter BS, Beaty TH, Steinberg GD, et al. Mendelian inheritance of familial prostate cancer. Proc Natl Acad Sci U S A 1992;89:3367–71.
33. Ostrander EA, Markianos K, Stanford JL. Finding prostate cancer susceptibility genes. Annu Rev Genomics Hum Genet 2004;5:151–75.
34. Langeberg WJ, Isaacs WB, Stanford JL. Genetic etiology of hereditary prostate cancer. Front Biosci 2007;12:4101–10.
35. Walz J, Gallina A, Perrotte P, et al. Clinicians are poor raters of life-expectancy before radical prostatectomy or definitive radiotherapy for localized prostate cancer. BJU Int 2007;100:1254–8.
36. Kirchhoff T, Kauff ND, Mitra N, et al. BRCA mutations and risk of prostate cancer in Ashkenazi Jews. Clin Cancer Res 2004;10:2918–21.
37. Hubert A, Peretz T, Manor O, et al. The Jewish Ashkenazi founder mutations in the BRCA1/BRCA2 genes are not found at an increased frequency in Ashkenazi patients with prostate cancer. Am J Hum Genet 1999;65:921–4.
38. Lehrer S, Fodor F, Stock RG, et al. Absence of 185delAG mutation of the BRCA1 gene and 6174delT mutation of the BRCA2 gene in Ashkenazi Jewish men with prostate cancer. Br J Cancer 1998;78:771–3.
39. Nastiuk KL, Mansukhani M, Terry MB, et al. Common mutations in BRCA1 and BRCA2 do not contribute to early prostate cancer in Jewish men. Prostate 1999;40:172–7.
40. Vazina A, Baniel J, Yaacobi Y, et al. The rate of the founder Jewish mutations in BRCA1 and BRCA2 in prostate cancer patients in Israel. Br J Cancer 2000;83: 463–6.
41. Giusti RM, Rutter JL, Duray PH, et al. A twofold increase in BRCA mutation related prostate cancer among Ashkenazi Israelis is not associated with distinctive histopathology. J Med Genet 2003;40:787–92.
42. Struewing JP, Hartge P, Wacholder S, et al. The risk of cancer associated with specific mutations of BRCA1 and BRCA2 among Ashkenazi Jews. N Engl J Med 1997;336:1401–8.
43. Warner E, Foulkes W, Goodwin P, et al. Prevalence and penetrance of BRCA1 and BRCA2 gene mutations in unselected Ashkenazi Jewish women with breast cancer. J Natl Cancer Inst 1999;91:1241–7.
44. Agalliu I, Karlins E, Kwon EM, et al. Rare germline mutations in the BRCA2 gene are associated with early-onset prostate cancer. Br J Cancer 2007; 97:826–31.

45. Douglas JA, Levin AM, Zuhlke KA, et al. Common variation in the BRCA1 gene and prostate cancer risk. Cancer Epidemiol Biomarkers Prev 2007;16: 1510–6.

46. Willems AJ, Dawson SJ, Samaratunga H, et al. Loss of heterozygosity at the BRCA2 locus detected by multiplex ligation-dependent probe amplification is common in prostate cancers from men with a germline BRCA2 mutation. Clin Cancer Res 2008;14:2953–61.

47. Thompson D, Easton DF. Cancer incidence in BRCA1 mutation carriers. J Natl Cancer Inst 2002;94:1358–65.

48. Cancer risks in BRCA2 mutation carriers. The Breast Cancer Linkage Consortium. J Natl Cancer Inst 1999;91:1310–6.

49. Tryggvadóttir L, Vidarsdóttir L, Thorgeirsson T, et al. Prostate cancer progression and survival in BRCA2 mutation carriers. J Natl Cancer Inst 2007;99:929–35.

50. Gallagher DJ, Gaudet MM, Pal P, et al. Germline BRCA mutations denote a clinicopathologic subset of prostate cancer. Clin Cancer Res 2010;16(7):2115–21.

51. Fong PC, Boss DS, Yap TA, et al. Inhibition of poly(ADP-ribose) polymerase in tumors from BRCA mutation carriers. N Engl J Med 2009;361:123–34.

52. Dong X, Wang L, Taniguchi K, et al. Mutations in CHEK2 associated with prostate cancer risk. Am J Hum Genet 2003;72:270–80.

53. Wu X, Dong X, Liu W, et al. Characterization of CHEK2 mutations in prostate cancer. Hum Mutat 2006;27:742–7.

54. Cybulski C, Wokolorczyk D, Huzarski T, et al. A large germline deletion in the Chek2 kinase gene is associated with an increased risk of prostate cancer. J Med Genet 2006;43:863–6.

55. Cybulski C, Huzarski T, Gorski B, et al. A novel founder CHEK2 mutation is associated with increased prostate cancer risk. Cancer Res 2004;64:2677–9.

56. Tischkowitz MD, Yilmaz A, Chen LQ, et al. Identification and characterization of novel SNPs in CHEK2 in Ashkenazi Jewish men with prostate cancer. Cancer Lett 2008;270:173–80.

57. Rokman A, Ikonen T, Seppala EH, et al. Germline alterations of the RNASEL gene, a candidate HPC1 gene at 1q25, in patients and families with prostate cancer. Am J Hum Genet 2002;70:1299–304.

58. Rennert H, Bercovich D, Hubert A, et al. A novel founder mutation in the RNASEL gene, 471delAAAG, is associated with prostate cancer in Ashkenazi Jews. Am J Hum Genet 2002;71:981–4.

59. Gronberg H, Isaacs SD, Smith JR, et al. Characteristics of prostate cancer in families potentially linked to the hereditary prostate cancer 1 (HPC1) locus. JAMA 1997;278:1251–5.

60. Goode EL, Stanford JL, Chakrabarti L, et al. Linkage analysis of 150 high-risk prostate cancer families at 1q24-25. Genet Epidemiol 2000;18:251–75.

61. Eeles RA, Kote-Jarai Z, Giles GG, et al. Multiple newly identified loci associated with prostate cancer susceptibility. Nat Genet 2008;40:316–21.

62. Thomas G, Jacobs KB, Yeager M, et al. Multiple loci identified in a genome-wide association study of prostate cancer. Nat Genet 2008;40:310–5.

63. Yeager M, Orr N, Hayes RB, et al. Genome-wide association study of prostate cancer identifies a second risk locus at 8q24. Nat Genet 2007;39:645–9.

64. Yeager M, Chatterjee N, Ciampa J, et al. Identification of a new prostate cancer susceptibility locus on chromosome 8q24. Nat Genet 2009;41:1055–7.

65. Eeles RA, Kote-Jarai Z, Al Olama AA, et al. Identification of seven new prostate cancer susceptibility loci through a genome-wide association study. Nat Genet 2009;41:1116–21.

66. Gudmundsson J, Sulem P, Manolescu A, et al. Genome-wide association study identifies a second prostate cancer susceptibility variant at 8q24. Nat Genet 2007;39:631–7.
67. Gudmundsson J, Sulem P, Rafnar T, et al. Common sequence variants on 2p15 and Xp11.22 confer susceptibility to prostate cancer. Nat Genet 2008;40:281–3.
68. Gudmundsson J, Sulem P, Gudbjartsson DF, et al. Genome-wide association and replication studies identify four variants associated with prostate cancer susceptibility. Nat Genet 2009;41:1122–6.
69. Amundadottir LT, Sulem P, Gudmundsson J, et al. A common variant associated with prostate cancer in European and African populations. Nat Genet 2006;38:652–8.
70. Freedman ML, Haiman CA, Patterson N, et al. Admixture mapping identifies 8q24 as a prostate cancer risk locus in African-American men. Proc Natl Acad Sci U S A 2006;103:14068–73.
71. Al Olama AA, Kote-Jarai Z, Giles GG, et al. Multiple loci on 8q24 associated with prostate cancer susceptibility. Nat Genet 2009;41:1058–60.
72. Sun J, Zheng SL, Wiklund F, et al. Evidence for two independent prostate cancer risk-associated loci in the HNF1B gene at 17q12. Nat Genet 2008;40:1153–5.
73. Sole X, Hernandez P, de Heredia ML, et al. Genetic and genomic analysis modeling of germline c-MYC overexpression and cancer susceptibility. BMC Genomics 2008;9:12.
74. Pomerantz MM, Ahmadiyeh N, Jia L, et al. The 8q24 cancer risk variant rs6983267 shows long-range interaction with MYC in colorectal cancer. Nat Genet 2009;41:882–4.
75. Tuupanen S, Turunen M, Lehtonen R, et al. The common colorectal cancer predisposition SNP rs6983267 at chromosome 8q24 confers potential to enhanced Wnt signaling. Nat Genet 2009;41:885–90.
76. Cybulski C, Gorski B, Debniak T, et al. NBS1 is a prostate cancer susceptibility gene. Cancer Res 2004;64:1215–9.
77. Beebe-Dimmer JL, Levin AM, Ray AM, et al. Chromosome 8q24 markers: risk of early-onset and familial prostate cancer. Int J Cancer 2008;122:2876–9.
78. Jung I, Messing E. Molecular mechanisms and pathways in bladder cancer development and progression. Cancer Control 2000;7:325–34.
79. Kogevinas M, Fernandez F, Garcia-Closas M, et al. Hair dye use is not associated with risk for bladder cancer: evidence from a case-control study in Spain. Eur J Cancer 2006;42:1448–54.
80. Morris RD, Audet AM, Angelillo IF, et al. Chlorination, chlorination by-products, and cancer: a meta-analysis. Am J Public Health 1992;82:955–63.
81. Marshall G, Ferreccio C, Yuan Y, et al. Fifty-year study of lung and bladder cancer mortality in Chile related to arsenic in drinking water. J Natl Cancer Inst 2007;99:920–8.
82. Cantor KP, Lynch CF, Hildesheim ME, et al. Drinking water source and chlorination byproducts. I. Risk of bladder cancer. Epidemiology 1998;9:21–8.
83. Lillienfeld A, Levin M. The association of smoking with cancer of the urinary bladder in humans. Arch Intern Med 1956;98:129–35.
84. Mueller CM, Caporaso N, Greene MH. Familial and genetic risk of transitional cell carcinoma of the urinary tract. Urol Oncol 2008;26:451–64.
85. Aben KK, Witjes JA, Schoenberg MP, et al. Familial aggregation of urothelial cell carcinoma. Int J Cancer 2002;98:274–8.
86. Randi G, Pelucchi C, Negri E, et al. Family history of urogenital cancers in patients with bladder, renal cell and prostate cancers. Int J Cancer 2007;121:2748–52.
87. Cartwright RA. Genetic association with bladder cancer. Br Med J 1979;2:798.

88. Kantor AF, Hartge P, Hoover RN, et al. Familial and environmental interactions in bladder cancer risk. Int J Cancer 1985;35:703–6.
89. Kiemeney LA, Moret NC, Witjes JA, et al. Familial transitional cell carcinoma among the population of Iceland. J Urol 1997;157:1649–51.
90. Kramer AA, Graham S, Burnett WS, et al. Familial aggregation of bladder cancer stratified by smoking status. Epidemiology 1991;2:145–8.
91. Kunze E, Chang-Claude J, Frentzel-Beyme R. Life style and occupational risk factors for bladder cancer in Germany. A case-control study. Cancer 1992;69:1776–90.
92. Lin J, Spitz MR, Dinney CP, et al. Bladder cancer risk as modified by family history and smoking. Cancer 2006;107:705–11.
93. Lynch HT, Kimberling WJ, Lynch JF, et al. Familial bladder cancer in an oncology clinic. Cancer Genet Cytogenet 1987;27:161–5.
94. Piper JM, Matanoski GM, Tonascia J. Bladder cancer in young women. Am J Epidemiol 1986;123:1033–42.
95. Umar A, Boland CR, Terdiman JP, et al. Revised Bethesda Guidelines for hereditary nonpolyposis colorectal cancer (Lynch syndrome) and microsatellite instability. J Natl Cancer Inst 2004;96:261–8.
96. Sijmons RH, Kiemeney LA, Witjes JA, et al. Urinary tract cancer and hereditary nonpolyposis colorectal cancer: risks and screening options. J Urol 1998;160:466–70.
97. Burt RW, Barthel JS, Dunn KB, et al. NCCN clinical practice guidelines in oncology. Colorectal cancer screening. J Natl Compr Canc Netw 2010;8:8–61.
98. Draper GJ, Sanders BM, Kingston JE. Second primary neoplasms in patients with retinoblastoma. Br J Cancer 1986;53:661–71.
99. Schlienger P, Campana F, Vilcoq JR, et al. Nonocular second primary tumors after retinoblastoma: retrospective study of 111 patients treated by electron beam radiotherapy with or without TEM. Am J Clin Oncol 2004;27:411–9.
100. Fletcher O, Easton D, Anderson K, et al. Lifetime risks of common cancers among retinoblastoma survivors. J Natl Cancer Inst 2004;96:357–63.
101. Wu XR. Urothelial tumorigenesis: a tale of divergent pathways. Nat Rev Cancer 2005;5:713–25.
102. Hennekam RC. Costello syndrome: an overview. Am J Med Genet C Semin Med Genet 2003;117C:42–8.
103. Aoki Y, Niihori T, Kawame H, et al. Germline mutations in HRAS proto-oncogene cause Costello syndrome. Nat Genet 2005;37:1038–40.
104. Silverman DT, Devesa SS, Moore LE, et al. Bladder cancer. 3rd edition. New York: Oxford University Press; 2006.
105. Garte S, Gaspari L, Alexandrie AK, et al. Metabolic gene polymorphism frequencies in control populations. Cancer Epidemiol Biomarkers Prev 2001;10:1239–48.
106. Hein DW, Doll MA, Fretland AJ, et al. Molecular genetics and epidemiology of the NAT1 and NAT2 acetylation polymorphisms. Cancer Epidemiol Biomarkers Prev 2000;9:29–42.
107. Garcia-Closas M, Malats N, Silverman D, et al. NAT2 slow acetylation, GSTM1 null genotype, and risk of bladder cancer: results from the Spanish Bladder Cancer Study and meta-analyses. Lancet 2005;366:649–59.
108. Kiemeney LA, Thorlacius S, Sulem P, et al. Sequence variant on 8q24 confers susceptibility to urinary bladder cancer. Nat Genet 2008;40:1307–12.
109. Witte JS. Prostate cancer genomics: towards a new understanding. Nat Rev Genet 2009;10:77–82.
110. Wu X, Ye Y, Kiemeney LA, et al. Genetic variation in the prostate stem cell antigen gene PSCA confers susceptibility to urinary bladder cancer. Nat Genet 2009;41:991–5.

111. Zbar B, Glenn G, Merino M, et al. Familial renal carcinoma: clinical evaluation, clinical subtypes and risk of renal carcinoma development. J Urol 2007;177: 461–5 [discussion: 465].

112. Duan DR, Humphrey JS, Chen DY, et al. Characterization of the VHL tumor suppressor gene product: localization, complex formation, and the effect of natural inactivating mutations. Proc Natl Acad Sci U S A 1995;92:6459–63.

113. Motzer RJ, Hutson TE, Tomczak P, et al. Sunitinib versus interferon alfa in metastatic renal-cell carcinoma. N Engl J Med 2007;356:115–24.

114. Molino D, Sepe J, Anastasio P, et al. The history of von Hippel–Lindau disease. J Nephrol 2006;19(Suppl 10):S119–23.

115. Davison C, Brock S, Dyke CG. Retinal and central nervous hemangioblastomatosis with visceral changes (von Hippel-Lindau's disease). Bull Neurol Instit NY 1936;5:72–93.

116. Seizinger BR, Rouleau GA, Ozelius LJ, et al. Von Hippel–Lindau disease maps to the region of chromosome 3 associated with renal cell carcinoma. Nature 1988;332:268–9.

117. Pfaffenroth EC, Linehan WM. Genetic basis for kidney cancer: opportunity for disease-specific approaches to therapy. Expert Opin Biol Ther 2008;8:779–90.

118. Zbar B, Kishida T, Chen F, et al. Germline mutations in the Von Hippel–Lindau disease (VHL) gene in families from North America, Europe, and Japan. Hum Mutat 1996;8:348–57.

119. Lonser RR, Glenn GM, Walther M, et al. von Hippel–Lindau disease. Lancet 2003;361:2059–67.

120. Wong WT, Agron E, Coleman HR, et al. Genotype–phenotype correlation in von Hippel–Lindau disease with retinal angiomatosis. Arch Ophthalmol 2007;125:239–45.

121. Schmidt L, Duh FM, Chen F, et al. Germline and somatic mutations in the tyrosine kinase domain of the MET proto-oncogene in papillary renal carcinomas. Nat Genet 1997;16:68–73.

122. Lindor NM, Dechet CB, Greene MH, et al. Papillary renal cell carcinoma: analysis of germline mutations in the MET proto-oncogene in a clinic-based population. Genet Test 2001;5:101–6.

123. Schmidt LS, Nickerson ML, Angeloni D, et al. Early onset hereditary papillary renal carcinoma: germline missense mutations in the tyrosine kinase domain of the met proto-oncogene. J Urol 2004;172:1256–61.

124. Miyata Y, Kanetake H, Kanda S. Presence of phosphorylated hepatocyte growth factor receptor/c-Met is associated with tumor progression and survival in patients with conventional renal cell carcinoma. Clin Cancer Res 2006;12:4876–81.

125. Dharmawardana PG, Giubellino A, Bottaro DP. Hereditary papillary renal carcinoma type I. Curr Mol Med 2004;4:855–68.

126. Fischer J, Palmedo G, von Knobloch R, et al. Duplication and overexpression of the mutant allele of the MET proto-oncogene in multiple hereditary papillary renal cell tumours. Oncogene 1998;17:733–9.

127. Palmedo G, Fischer J, Kovacs G. Duplications of DNA sequences between loci D20S478 and D20S206 at 20q11.2 and between loci D20S902 and D20S480 at 20q13.2 mark new tumor genes in papillary renal cell carcinoma. Lab Invest 1999;79:311–6.

128. Zbar B, Glenn G, Lubensky I, et al. Hereditary papillary renal cell carcinoma: clinical studies in 10 families. J Urol 1995;153:907–12.

129. Schmidt L, Junker K, Weirich G, et al. Two North American families with hereditary papillary renal carcinoma and identical novel mutations in the MET proto-oncogene. Cancer Res 1998;58:1719–22.

130. Ornstein DK, Lubensky IA, Venzon D, et al. Prevalence of microscopic tumors in normal appearing renal parenchyma of patients with hereditary papillary renal cancer. J Urol 2000;163:431–3.
131. Bellon SF, Kaplan-Lefko P, Yang Y, et al. c-Met inhibitors with novel binding mode show activity against several hereditary papillary renal cell carcinoma-related mutations. J Biol Chem 2008;283:2675–83.
132. Menko FH, van Steensel MA, Giraud S, et al. Birt–Hogg–Dube syndrome: diagnosis and management. Lancet Oncol 2009;10:1199–206.
133. Linehan WM, Pinto PA, Bratslavsky G, et al. Hereditary kidney cancer: unique opportunity for disease-based therapy. Cancer 2009;115:2252–61.
134. Zbar B, Alvord WG, Glenn G, et al. Risk of renal and colonic neoplasms and spontaneous pneumothorax in the Birt–Hogg–Dube syndrome. Cancer Epidemiol Biomarkers Prev 2002;11:393–400.
135. Wei MH, Toure O, Glenn GM, et al. Novel mutations in FH and expansion of the spectrum of phenotypes expressed in families with hereditary leiomyomatosis and renal cell cancer. J Med Genet 2006;43:18–27.
136. Toro JR, Wei MH, Glenn GM, et al. BHD mutations, clinical and molecular genetic investigations of Birt–Hogg–Dube syndrome: a new series of 50 families and a review of published reports. J Med Genet 2008;45:321–31.
137. Murakami T, Sano F, Huang Y, et al. Identification and characterization of Birt–Hogg–Dube associated renal carcinoma. J Pathol 2007;211:524–31.
138. Durrani OH, Ng L, Bihrle W 3rd. Chromophobe renal cell carcinoma in a patient with the Birt–Hogg–Dube syndrome. J Urol 2002;168:1484–5.
139. Nagashima Y, Mitsuya T, Shioi KI, et al. Renal oncocytosis. Pathol Int 2005;55:210–5.
140. Imada K, Dainichi T, Yokomizo A, et al. Birt–Hogg–Dube syndrome with clear-cell and oncocytic renal tumour and trichoblastoma associated with a novel FLCN mutation. Br J Dermatol 2009;160:1350–3.
141. Mai KT, Dhamanaskar P, Belanger E, et al. Hybrid chromophobe renal cell neoplasm. Pathol Res Pract 2005;201:385–9.
142. Adley BP, Schafernak KT, Yeldandi AV, et al. Cytologic and histologic findings in multiple renal hybrid oncocytic tumors in a patient with Birt–Hogg–Dube syndrome: a case report. Acta Cytol 2006;50:584–8.
143. Pavlovich CP, Walther MM, Eyler RA, et al. Renal tumors in the Birt–Hogg–Dube syndrome. Am J Surg Pathol 2002;26:1542–52.
144. Adley BP, Smith ND, Nayar R, et al. Birt–Hogg–Dube syndrome: clinicopathologic findings and genetic alterations. Arch Pathol Lab Med 2006;130:1865–70.
145. Khoo SK, Bradley M, Wong FK, et al. Birt–Hogg–Dube syndrome: mapping of a novel hereditary neoplasia gene to chromosome 17p12–q11.2. Oncogene 2001;20:5239–42.
146. Hudon V, Sabourin S, Dydensborg AB, et al. Renal tumor suppressor function of the Birt–Hogg–Dube syndrome gene product folliculin. J Med Genet 2009;47(3):182–9.
147. Schmidt LS, Warren MB, Nickerson ML, et al. Birt–Hogg–Dube syndrome, a genodermatosis associated with spontaneous pneumothorax and kidney neoplasia, maps to chromosome 17p11.2. Am J Hum Genet 2001;69:876–82.
148. Warren MB, Torres-Cabala CA, Turner ML, et al. Expression of Birt–Hogg–Dube gene mRNA in normal and neoplastic human tissues. Mod Pathol 2004;17:998–1011.
149. Nickerson ML, Warren MB, Toro JR, et al. Mutations in a novel gene lead to kidney tumors, lung wall defects, and benign tumors of the hair follicle in patients with the Birt–Hogg–Dube syndrome. Cancer Cell 2002;2:157–64.

150. Schmidt LS, Nickerson ML, Warren MB, et al. Germline BHD-mutation spectrum and phenotype analysis of a large cohort of families with Birt–Hogg–Dube syndrome. Am J Hum Genet 2005;76:1023–33.

151. Baba M, Hong SB, Sharma N, et al. Folliculin encoded by the BHD gene interacts with a binding protein, FNIP1, and AMPK, and is involved in AMPK and mTOR signaling. Proc Natl Acad Sci U S A 2006;103:15552–7.

152. Kiuru M, Launonen V. Hereditary leiomyomatosis and renal cell cancer (HLRCC). Curr Mol Med 2004;4:869–75.

153. Sudarshan S, Linehan WM, Neckers L. HIF and fumarate hydratase in renal cancer. Br J Cancer 2007;96:403–7.

154. Merino MJ, Torres-Cabala C, Pinto P, et al. The morphologic spectrum of kidney tumors in hereditary leiomyomatosis and renal cell carcinoma (HLRCC) syndrome. Am J Surg Pathol 2007;31:1578–85.

155. Stewart L, Glenn GM, Stratton P, et al. Association of germline mutations in the fumarate hydratase gene and uterine fibroids in women with hereditary leiomyomatosis and renal cell cancer. Arch Dermatol 2008;144:1584–92.

156. Toro JR, Nickerson ML, Wei MH, et al. Mutations in the fumarate hydratase gene cause hereditary leiomyomatosis and renal cell cancer in families in North America. Am J Hum Genet 2003;73:95–106.

157. Lehtonen R, Kiuru M, Vanharanta S, et al. Biallelic inactivation of fumarate hydratase (FH) occurs in nonsyndromic uterine leiomyomas but is rare in other tumors. Am J Pathol 2004;164:17–22.

158. Alam NA, Bevan S, Churchman M, et al. Localization of a gene (MCUL1) for multiple cutaneous leiomyomata and uterine fibroids to chromosome 1q42.3–q43. Am J Hum Genet 2001;68:1264–9.

159. Alam NA, Olpin S, Rowan A, et al. Missense mutations in fumarate hydratase in multiple cutaneous and uterine leiomyomatosis and renal cell cancer. J Mol Diagn 2005;7:437–43.

160. Pollard PJ, Briere JJ, Alam NA, et al. Accumulation of Krebs cycle intermediates and over-expression of HIF1alpha in tumours which result from germline FH and SDH mutations. Hum Mol Genet 2005;14:2231–9.

161. Heinritz W, Paasch U, Sticherling M, et al. Evidence for a founder effect of the germline fumarate hydratase gene mutation R58P causing hereditary leiomyomatosis and renal cell cancer (HLRCC). Ann Hum Genet 2008;72:35–40.

162. Tomlinson IP, Alam NA, Rowan AJ, et al. Germline mutations in FH predispose to dominantly inherited uterine fibroids, skin leiomyomata and papillary renal cell cancer. Nat Genet 2002;30:406–10.

163. Alam NA, Rowan AJ, Wortham NC, et al. Genetic and functional analyses of FH mutations in multiple cutaneous and uterine leiomyomatosis, hereditary leiomyomatosis and renal cancer, and fumarate hydratase deficiency. Hum Mol Genet 2003;12:1241–52.

164. Wortham NC, Alam NA, Barclay E, et al. Aberrant expression of apoptosis proteins and ultrastructural aberrations in uterine leiomyomas from patients with hereditary leiomyomatosis and renal cell carcinoma. Fertil Steril 2006;86:961–71.

165. Pollard P, Wortham N, Barclay E, et al. Evidence of increased microvessel density and activation of the hypoxia pathway in tumours from the hereditary leiomyomatosis and renal cell cancer syndrome. J Pathol 2005;205:41–9.

166. Lehtonen HJ, Blanco I, Piulats JM, et al. Conventional renal cancer in a patient with fumarate hydratase mutation. Hum Pathol 2007;38:793–6.

167. Sudarshan S, Linehan WM. Genetic basis of cancer of the kidney. Semin Oncol 2006;33:544–51.

168. Hwang JJ, Walther MM, Pautler SE, et al. Radio frequency ablation of small renal tumors: intermediate results. J Urol 2004;171:1814–8.

169. Huang WC, Levey AS, Serio AM, et al. Chronic kidney disease after nephrectomy in patients with renal cortical tumours: a retrospective cohort study. Lancet Oncol 2006;7:735–40.

170. Coleman J, Singh A, Pinto P, et al. Radiofrequency-assisted laparoscopic partial nephrectomy: clinical and histologic results. J Endourol 2007;21:600–5.

171. Hwang JJ, Uchio EM, Pavlovich CP, et al. Surgical management of multi-organ visceral tumors in patients with von Hippel–Lindau disease: a single stage approach. J Urol 2003;169:895–8.

172. Grubb RL, Corbin NS, Choyke P, et al. Analysis of 3-cm tumor size threshold for intervention in patients with Birt–Hogg–Dubé and hereditary papillary renal cancer [abstract 980]. American Urological Association National Conference; 2005.

173. Bratslavsky G, Liu JJ, Johnson AD, et al. Salvage partial nephrectomy for hereditary renal cancer: feasibility and outcomes. J Urol 2008;179:67–70.

174. Herring JC, Enquist EG, Chernoff A, et al. Parenchymal sparing surgery in patients with hereditary renal cell carcinoma: 10-year experience. J Urol 2001; 165:777–81.

175. Pinto PA. Renal carcinoma: minimally invasive surgery of the small renal mass. Urol Oncol 2009;27:335–6.

176. Hsieh TC, Jarrett TW, Pinto PA. Current status of nephron-sparing robotic partial nephrectomy. Curr Opin Urol 2010;20:65–9.

177. Russo P. Partial nephrectomy achieves local tumor control and prevents chronic kidney disease. Expert Rev Anticancer Ther 2006;6:1745–51.

178. Webster AR, Maher ER, Moore AT. Clinical characteristics of ocular angiomatosis in von Hippel–Lindau disease and correlation with germline mutation. Arch Ophthalmol 1999;117:371–8.

179. Butman JA, Linehan WM, Lonser RR. Neurologic manifestations of von Hippel–Lindau disease. JAMA 2008;300:1334–42.

180. Ammerman JM, Lonser RR, Dambrosia J, et al. Long-term natural history of hemangioblastomas in patients with von Hippel–Lindau disease: implications for treatment. J Neurosurg 2006;105:248–55.

181. Baghai M, Thompson GB, Young WF Jr, et al. Pheochromocytomas and paragangliomas in von Hippel–Lindau disease: a role for laparoscopic and cortical-sparing surgery. Arch Surg 2002;137:682–8 [discussion: 688–9].

182. Diner EK, Franks ME, Behari A, et al. Partial adrenalectomy: the National Cancer Institute experience. Urology 2005;66:19–23.

183. Launonen V, Vierimaa O, Kiuru M, et al. Inherited susceptibility to uterine leiomyomas and renal cell cancer. Proc Natl Acad Sci U S A 2001;98:3387–92.

184. Refae MA, Wong N, Patenaude F, et al. Hereditary leiomyomatosis and renal cell cancer: an unusual and aggressive form of hereditary renal carcinoma. Nat Clin Pract Oncol 2007;4:256–61.

185. Grubb RL 3rd, Franks ME, Toro J, et al. Hereditary leiomyomatosis and renal cell cancer: a syndrome associated with an aggressive form of inherited renal cancer. J Urol 2007;177:2074–9 [discussion: 2079–80].

186. Alrashdi I, Levine S, Paterson J, et al. Hereditary leiomyomatosis and renal cell carcinoma: very early diagnosis of renal cancer in a paediatric patient. Fam Cancer 2009;9(2):239–43.

187. Sudarshan S, Pinto PA, Neckers L, et al. Mechanisms of disease: hereditary leiomyomatosis and renal cell cancer–a distinct form of hereditary kidney cancer. Nat Clin Pract Urol 2007;4:104–10.

188. Rosner I, Bratslavsky G, Pinto PA, et al. The clinical implications of the genetics of renal cell carcinoma. Urol Oncol 2009;27:131–6.
189. Houldsworth J, Korkola JE, Bosl GJ, et al. Biology and genetics of adult male germ cell tumors. J Clin Oncol 2006;24:5512–8.
190. Sharpe RM, Skakkebaek NE. Testicular dysgenesis syndrome: mechanistic insights and potential new downstream effects. Fertil Steril 2008;89:e33–8.
191. Nathanson KL, Kanetsky PA, Hawes R, et al. The Y deletion gr/gr and susceptibility to testicular germ cell tumor. Am J Hum Genet 2005;77:1034–43.
192. Heimdal K, Olsson H, Tretli S, et al. Familial testicular cancer in Norway and southern Sweden. Br J Cancer 1996;73:964–9.
193. Hemminki K, Li X. Familial risk in testicular cancer as a clue to a heritable and environmental aetiology. Br J Cancer 2004;90:1765–70.
194. Westergaard T, Olsen JH, Frisch M, et al. Cancer risk in fathers and brothers of testicular cancer patients in Denmark. A population-based study. Int J Cancer 1996;66:627–31.
195. Giambartolomei C, Mueller CM, Greene MH, et al. A mini-review of familial ovarian germ cell tumors: an additional manifestation of the familial testicular germ cell tumor syndrome. Cancer Epidemiol 2009;33:31–6.
196. Crockford GP, Linger R, Hockley S, et al. Genome-wide linkage screen for testicular germ cell tumour susceptibility loci. Hum Mol Genet 2006;15:443–51.
197. Skakkebaek NE. Possible carcinoma-in-situ of the testis. Lancet 1972;2:516–7.
198. Kanetsky PA, Mitra N, Vardhanabhuti S, et al. Common variation in KITLG and at 5q31.3 predisposes to testicular germ cell cancer. Nat Genet 2009;41:811–5.
199. Rapley EA, Turnbull C, Al Olama AA, et al. A genome-wide association study of testicular germ cell tumor. Nat Genet 2009;41:807–10.
200. Rajpert-De Meyts E, Skakkebaek NE. Expression of the c-kit protein product in carcinoma-in-situ and invasive testicular germ cell tumours. Int J Androl 1994; 17:85–92.
201. Dieckmann KP, Loy V. Prevalence of contralateral testicular intraepithelial neoplasia in patients with testicular germ cell neoplasms. J Clin Oncol 1996; 14:3126–32.
202. Sasaki A, Taketomi T, Kato R, et al. Mammalian Sprouty4 suppresses Ras-independent ERK activation by binding to Raf1. Nat Cell Biol 2003;5:427–32.
203. Frolov A, Chahwan S, Ochs M, et al. Response markers and the molecular mechanisms of action of Gleevec in gastrointestinal stromal tumors. Mol Cancer Ther 2003;2:699–709.
204. Washecka R, Dresner MI, Honda SA. Testicular tumors in Carney's complex. J Urol 2002;167:1299–302.
205. Proppe KH, Scully RE. Large-cell calcifying Sertoli cell tumor of the testis. Am J Clin Pathol 1980;74:607–19.
206. Gourlay WA, Johnson HW, Pantzar JT, et al. Gonadal tumors in disorders of sexual differentiation. Urology 1994;43:537–40.
207. Jeghers H, Mc KV, Katz KH. Generalized intestinal polyposis and melanin spots of the oral mucosa, lips and digits; a syndrome of diagnostic significance. N Engl J Med 1949;241:1031–6.
208. Ulbright TM, Amin MB, Young RH. Intratubular large cell hyalinizing Sertoli cell neoplasia of the testis: a report of 8 cases of a distinctive lesion of the Peutz–Jeghers syndrome. Am J Surg Pathol 2007;31:827–35.
209. Boikos SA, Stratakis CA. Carney complex: the first 20 years. Curr Opin Oncol 2007;19:24–9.

Hereditary Genodermatoses with Cancer Predisposition

Meg R. Gerstenblith, MD[a],*, Alisa M. Goldstein, PhD[b],
Margaret A. Tucker, MD[c]

KEYWORDS

- Genodermatoses • Nevoid basal cell carcinoma syndrome
- Neurofibromatosis type 1 • Neurofibromatosis type 2
- Tuberous sclerosis • Melanoma • Xeroderma pigmentosum
- Dyskeratosis congenita

NEVOID BASAL CELL CARCINOMA SYNDROME (GORLIN SYNDROME)
History and Overview

A relationship between multiple basal cell carcinomas and developmental defects was suggested by Binkley and Johnson[1] in 1951 and Howell and Caro[2] in 1959, but it was Gorlin and Goltz[3] who, in 1960, first described a distinct syndrome consisting of the presence of multiple nevoid basal cell epitheliomas, jaw cysts, and bifid ribs. Nevoid basal cell carcinoma syndrome (NBCCS), or Gorlin syndrome, is a rare condition, with an estimated prevalence of 1 per 40,000 to 57,000,[4] though the figure may be higher.[5] Two major features characterize the phenotype of NBCCS: developmental abnormalities and multiple neoplasms. Developmental abnormalities include palmar and plantar pits, coarse facies with frontal bossing, cleft palate, strabismus, corpus callosum dysgenesis, falx cerebri calcification, spina bifida occulta, bifid ribs, mesenteric cysts,

This study was supported by the Intramural Research Program of NIH, National Cancer Institute, Division of Cancer Epidemiology and Genetics.

[a] Genetic Epidemiology Branch, Division of Cancer Epidemiology and Genetics, National Cancer Institute, National Institutes of Health, Building EPS, Room 7003, 6120 Executive Boulevard, Rockville, MD 20892-7236, USA

[b] Genetic Epidemiology Branch, Division of Cancer Epidemiology and Genetics, National Cancer Institute, National Institutes of Health, Building EPS, Room 7004, 6120 Executive Boulevard, Rockville, MD 20892-7236, USA

[c] Genetic Epidemiology Branch, Division of Cancer Epidemiology and Genetics, National Cancer Institute, National Institutes of Health, Building EPS, Room 7122, 6120 Executive Boulevard, Rockville, MD 20892-7236, USA

* Corresponding author.
E-mail address: gerstenblithm@gmail.com

macrocephaly, and polydactyly. Neoplasms include basal cell carcinomas (BCCs), medulloblastomas, rhabdomyosarcomas, odontogenic keratocysts, fibrosarcomas, meningiomas, and ovarian fibromas, among other benign and malignant neoplasms. In a study of 105 individuals with NBCCS, mostly from multiple case families, palmar pits, jaw cysts, BCCs, and calcification of the falx cerebri were present in more than 50% of cases, and bifid ribs were present in 42% of cases.[6] Clinical studies have led to revisions of the diagnostic criteria over time. Diagnosis of NBCCS may be made by the presence of 2 major and 1 minor or 1 major and 3 minor criteria. Major criteria include: (1) lamellar calcification of the falx cerebri in persons younger than 20 years, (2) histologically confirmed odontogenic (jaw) keratocyst, (3) 2 or more palmar/plantar pits, (4) greater than 5 BCCs in a lifetime or a BCC before age 30 years, and (5) a first-degree relative with NBCCS. Minor criteria include: (1) childhood medulloblastoma, (2) lymphomesenteric or pleural cysts, (3) macrocephaly, (4) cleft lip/palate, (5) vertebral/rib anomalies including bifid vertebrae/ribs, extra ribs, and/or splayed ribs, (6) polydactyly, (7) ovarian/cardiac fibromas, and (8) ocular abnormalities including cataracts.[5,6] Of note, making the diagnosis may be difficult in African Americans because those affected with NBCCS have fewer BCCs than their Caucasian counterparts.[7]

Genetics

Chromosomal mapping and genetic studies elucidated the role of inactivating mutations in the human homologue of Drosophila Patched gene (PTCH1) on chromosome 9q22.3 as the cause of almost all cases of NBCCS. Approximately 70% of germline PTCH1 mutations are rearrangements leading to formation of a truncated protein, although deletions, insertions, splice site alterations, nonsense and missense mutations of PTCH1 are also reported.[8-11] About 6% of mutations are whole gene deletions.[5] Mutations in PTCH1 are inherited in an autosomal dominant manner, and although penetrance is nearly complete, phenotypic expression of the syndrome is widely variable.[12] This phenotypic variation does not appear to be related to the type of PTCH1 mutation present.[8,13] PTCH1 inactivation has been proposed to occur in 2 steps—the first "hit" occurs in the germline and the second, postnatally. Heterozygosity for PTCH1 due to the inherited germline mutation is likely to give rise to the developmental abnormalities seen in NBCCS. Subsequent postnatal loss of the normal Patched allele by mutation or silencing may lead to multiple BCCs and other neoplasms.[14] Thus, PTCH1 acts as a tumor suppressor. Reports of segmental cases of NBCCS, hypothesized to be caused by postzygotic mutations, are rare.[15] A few cases of NBCCS are caused by mutations in PTCH2 on chromosome 1p32, which is also a tumor suppressor, and suppressor of fused (SUFU) on chromosome 10q24-q25.[16,17]

PTCH1, PTCH2, and SUFU are components of the Hedgehog (Hh) signaling pathway, which was first elucidated in Drosophila.[4,18,19] Two transmembrane proteins—Patched and Smoothened—transduce the secreted Hh protein signal. In the absence of Hh, Patched catalytically inhibits Smoothened.[20] Secreted Hh binds to Patched, releasing inhibition of Smoothened and effecting downstream events including cell cycle regulation via the transcription factor Ci and a complex of cytoplasmic proteins including Fused (Fu), Suppressor of Fused (Su(fu)), and Costal-2 (Cos2).[21] In this model, Patched inactivation or the constitutive activity of Smoothened leads to overactivity of the Hh pathway resulting in neoplasm formation, though the mechanism connecting pathway overactivity and tumor formation is not yet defined. Not surprisingly, PTCH1, Smoothened (SMO), and SUFU mutations have been identified in sporadic BCCs, medulloblastomas, and odontogenic keratocysts, further implicating the role of the Hh signaling pathway in the development of these tumors.[19,22–26]

Genetic Testing and Treatment

Molecular genetic testing can confirm the diagnosis in individuals when the diagnosis is clinically considered. Prenatal diagnosis of NBCCS is possible, though knowledge of the disease-causing mutation in a given family is required.[5,27]

There are many current treatments for BCCs such as surgical excision and topical immunomodulation. However, the application of these traditional treatments to the BCCs that occur in NBCCS is problematic because of the multiplicity and recurrent nature of the tumors. Photodynamic therapy is emerging as a promising treatment for BCCs in patients with NBCCS.[28] A recent trial with oral nonsteroidal anti-inflammatory drugs in patients with NBCCS with less severe disease showed significantly reduced numbers of BCC in the treated as compared with the placebo group.[29] Because BCCs arise in NBCCS as a result of overactivation of the Hh pathway, novel therapies inhibiting this pathway might be expected to suppress tumor growth. Cyclopamine, a Hh pathway antagonist, inhibited growth of medulloblastomas in a mouse model of NBCCS.[30] In recent clinical trials, the effects of Hh inhibitors were studied in 1 patient with sporadic metastatic medulloblastoma and 33 patients with locally advanced or metastatic BCC, one of whom had NBCCS.[31,32] Rapid reductions of tumor size and associated symptoms were noted in the patient with metastatic medulloblastoma. Eighteen of 33 patients with locally advanced or metastatic BCC had a partial or complete response, and 11 had stable disease. These studies are promising; however, further research is needed to guide recommendations for use of these Hh inhibitors in individuals with NBCCS.

NEUROFIBROMATOSIS TYPE 1
History and Overview

Neurofibromatosis type 1 (NF1), first described by von Recklinghausen in 1882,[33] occurs in approximately 1 in 3500 individuals.[34] NF1 is characterized by a combination of cutaneous, neurologic, skeletal, and ocular findings, including benign and malignant tumors primarily of the nerve sheath. To date, the National Institutes of Health (NIH) diagnostic criteria for NF1 includes at least 2 of the following features: (1) 6 or more café-au-lait macules (with largest diameter >0.5 cm in prepubertal individuals or >1.5 cm in postpubertal individuals), (2) axillary or inguinal freckling (Crowe sign), (3) 2 or more neurofibromas of any type or at least 1 plexiform neurofibroma, (4) 2 or more iris hamartomas (Lisch nodules), (5) a distinctive bony lesion, such as sphenoid wing dysplasia or long bone cortical thinning with or without pseudoarthrosis, and (6) a first-degree relative with NF1.[35] The majority of individuals can be diagnosed by age 3 years.[36]

Café-au-lait macules are the most common feature of NF1, occurring in 95% of individuals and typically appearing by age 3 years.[36] Other cutaneous manifestations include axillary and/or inguinal freckling, present in most children; xanthogranulomas, observed in early childhood and possibly associated with chronic myeloid leukemia in children; and diffuse hyperpigmentation.[34,37] Neurofibromas, benign nerve sheath tumors arising from Schwann cells, are a hallmark finding of NF1, though their numbers vary across affected patients. Dermal, spinal, and plexiform neurofibromas may occur in NF1. The number of neurofibromas varies among patients with NF1. Spinal neurofibromas may cause nerve compression.[38] Dermal and plexiform neurofibromas can lead to significant cosmetic deformity; additionally, plexiform neurofibromas may develop into malignant peripheral nerve sheath tumors (MPNST), which may metastasize extensively and be fatal.[36,39] The lifetime risk for development of MPNST is 10%.[36] Additional neurologic findings include optic pathway gliomas, cognitive deficits including learning disabilities, and epilepsy. Optic pathway gliomas are low-grade pilocytic astrocytomas capable of involving the optic nerve, chiasm, tract, and/or hypothalamus, which may cause visual loss and/or endocrine dysregulation.[39] Vascular abnormalities cause significant mortality and include severe hypertension, usually secondary to renal artery stenosis; cerebrovascular disease, possibly leading to cerebral hemorrhage; and pulmonary arterial hypertension.[40] Skeletal abnormalities associated with significant morbidity include scoliosis, pseudoarthroses, sphenoid wing dysplasia, macrocephaly, and short stature. Additional malignancies that may occur in patients with NF1 include pheochromocytoma, pancreatic endocrine tumors, rhabdomyosarcomas, and duodenal somatostatinomas.[41,42] Glomus tumors were also recently associated with NF1.[43]

Genetics

NF1 is caused by an approximately equal number of spontaneous and autosomal dominantly inherited germline mutations in the *NF1* gene, located on chromosome 17q11.2, encoding neurofibromin, a tumor suppressor predominantly expressed in neural crest cells including neurons, Schwann cells, and early melanocytes.[44,45] Similar to BCCs in Gorlin syndrome, neurofibromas are thought to arise after a "second hit" to *NF1*, leading to loss of heterozygosity.[46] Neurofibromin regulates Ras guanosine triphosphatase activity by converting Ras into its inactive form and suppressing cell growth.[34,47,48] In NF1, the Ras/Raf/ERK signaling pathway is unchecked, leading to unregulated cell proliferation. One important protein activated by Ras is the mammalian target of rapamycin (mTOR) protein. Of interest is that another protein in this signaling pathway, SPRED1, inhibits the Raf protein, and mutations in *SPRED1* account for an NF1-like syndrome consisting of multiple café-au-lait macules, axillary freckling, and macrocephaly.[35,49]

In individuals with NF1, there is complete penetrance by age 20 years, although there is variable phenotypic expression.[34] Even among individuals from the same family sharing the same mutation, phenotypes can differ substantially. Partial and complete gene deletions, insertions, nonsense, frameshift, and splice mutations as well as amino acid substitutions and chromosomal rearrangements affecting the *NF1* gene may cause NF1.[34,50] Of note, NF1 can be manifested by somatic mosaicism due to mutations in the *NF1* gene that occur postzygotically during development.[51,52]

Genetic Testing and Treatment

A comprehensive genetic screening test identified mutations in more than 95% of subjects who fulfilled the NIH diagnostic criteria.[50] Genetic testing is indicated for prenatal testing, preimplantation genetic diagnosis, and for confirmation in individuals with suspected NF1 who do not meet the full diagnostic criteria.[34] One caveat of genetic testing, however, is that in most cases the disease phenotype cannot be predicted by the genotype. Exceptions are for patients with complete deletions of the *NF1* gene and a 3–base-pair inframe deletion in exon 17, which do result in predictable phenotypes. Complete deletions are associated with a severe NF1 phenotype including numerous neurofibromas, significant cognitive deficits, dysmorphic facies, and an elevated risk of MPNST development.[53,54] The 3–base-pair inframe deletion is associated with a mild phenotype, including even the absence of cutaneous neurofibromas.[55]

Affected individuals should be followed annually with physical examinations, including fundoscopy at least until age 7 years, with assessment and workup of symptoms that may indicate MPNST development; routine imaging in asymptomatic individuals is not recommended.[42] Thalidomide and a vascular endothelial growth factor receptor (VEGFR) inhibitor, both angiogenesis inhibitors, are being tested to treat MPNSTs and plexiform neurofibromas, because both tumors require intact vascular supplies.[35,56] Novel treatments for NF1 are emerging from advances in understanding the functional consequences of the genetic mutations, specifically altering the Ras/Raf/ERK signaling pathway. Ras inhibitors, for example, are postulated to inhibit the pathway, and in this manner substitute for neurofibromin. Tipifarnib, a farnesyltransferase inhibitor that targets Ras, is currently being investigated for treatment in NF1 patients with plexiform neurofibromas.[57] Rapamycin, though primarily used for its immunosuppressive properties, is now being considered for use in NF1 patients because it, like neurofibromin, inhibits mTOR signaling and may substitute for NF1 in this way.[58,59]

NEUROFIBROMATOSIS TYPE 2
History and Overview

Neurofibromatosis type 2 (NF2), like NF1, is a neurocutaneous disorder. Although NF2 shares some features with NF1, they are distinct syndromes with many differences firmly distinguished in 1987, with the discovery that the gene causing NF1 mapped to chromosome 17q whereas tumor DNA from individuals with NF2 showed loss of heterozygosity for markers on chromosome 22q.[60–62] First described in 1822, NF2 is rare, affecting 1 in 25,000 individuals.[63,64] Bilateral vestibular schwannomas are the most frequent clinical feature, present in up to 95% of cases. According to the most commonly used Manchester diagnostic criteria, NF2 can be diagnosed by this feature alone.[63,64] NF2, however, is a multiple neoplasia syndrome, and other tumors affecting the nervous system, skin, and eyes also occur. Diagnostic criteria, in addition to bilateral vestibular schwannomas, include: (1) a family history of NF2 and a unilateral vestibular schwannoma or 2 NF2-associated nervous system tumors or cataracts, (2) a unilateral vestibular schwannoma and 2 NF2-associated nervous system tumors or cataracts, or (3) multiple meningiomas and a unilateral vestibular schwannoma or 2 other NF2-associated nervous system tumors or cataracts.[64] Nervous system tumors include schwannomas developing in cranial nerves other than 8, spinal nerves, and peripheral nerves; meningiomas, ependymomas, pilocytic astrocytomas, and occasionally, neurofibromas as in NF1.[64,65] Bilateral hearing loss, secondary to vestibular schwannomas, is common. Peripheral neuropathy, though not one of the diagnostic criteria for NF2, can develop in affected individuals, both in association with and independent of nerve-compressing tumors.[64] The most common ocular finding is early cataracts, which may lead to loss of vision.[66] Other ocular manifestations include epiretinal membranes and retinal hamartomas.[67] Cutaneous findings include rough, slightly hyperpigmented plaques with overlying hypertrichosis as well as subcutaneous and intradermal tumors, typically schwannomas, although as previously mentioned, neurofibromas may occur.[68,69] Café-au-lait macules, typical of NF1, may be seen in NF2 as well, though in one series no patient had more than 6.[68–72]

Genetics

NF2 is caused by mutations in the tumor suppressor *NF2* gene on chromosome 22q12. The NF2 protein (named merlin or alternatively schwannomin) normally regulates mitogenic intracellular pathways including the phosphoinositide-3-kinase (PI3K) signaling pathway, which includes Akt and mTOR, and the mitogen-activated protein kinase (MAPK) signaling pathway, which includes Ras/Raf/MEK/ERK. Inherited in an autosomal dominant fashion, NF2 has nearly complete penetrance by age 60 years.[63,73] Age of onset is typically around 18 years.[74] Affected individuals in the same family usually share similar phenotypic features, but there is variable expressivity among families, which can largely be attributed to the type of NF2 mutations segregating in each family. Severe disease and a higher mortality are associated with constitutional nonsense or frameshift mutations, which result in a truncated protein, as well as splice-site mutations within exons 1 to 5.[75] Mild disease and a lower mortality are associated with missense mutations and inframe or large deletions as well as splice-site mutations within exons 11 to 15.[76–78] Fifty percent of NF2 patients have a de novo mutation,[74] and mosaic forms of NF2 occur with high frequency in these patients.[79] Most patients with mosaic forms of NF2 have mild disease or limited involvement; there is also a lower risk of transmission to offspring from individuals with mosaic forms of NF2 because it is likely that less than 50% of germ cells carry the mutation.[64]

Genetic Testing and Treatment

Genetic testing of individuals without symptoms from affected families is recommended and allows for early diagnosis, which can improve clinical care. For asymptomatic individuals with an affected parent, screening guidelines recommend: annual follow-up by an ophthalmologist, neurologist, and audiologist from infancy; head and spinal magnetic resonance imaging (MRI) starting at around age 10 years repeated every 2 to 3 years for spinal MRI; and presymptomatic genetic testing at around age 10 if not performed earlier by request of the parents. For asymptomatic individuals from families with severe disease, MRI and genetic testing are recommended at an earlier age, and MRI may be performed annually.[64,80]

Treatment for NF2 is directed at early and complete removal of bilateral vestibular schwannomas to preserve hearing. In patients with an intact cochlear nerve following vestibular schwannoma surgery, cochlear implants may improve hearing. Meningiomas are typically managed by neurosurgical intervention. These tumors may or may not be fully resectable, depending on their location in the nervous system; furthermore, resection of meningiomas in some locations, such as the skull base or optic nerve sheath, carries greater risks than other locations, such as the cerebral hemisphere or spinal canal.[81,82] With close ophthalmologic follow-up, cataracts may be found early and those associated with significant loss of visual acuity extracted.[66] Skin tumors, when symptomatic, may be excised. The use of mTOR inhibitors is currently being investigated for individuals with NF2.[83]

TUBEROUS SCLEROSIS COMPLEX
History and Overview

Similar to NF1 and NF2, tuberous sclerosis complex (TSC) is a neurocutaneous disorder affecting multiple systems. First reported by Bourneville in 1880, TSC was named after the cerebral cortical lesions resembling tubers and the periventricular calcification characteristic of the disorder.[84] Multiple hamartomas, or tumors, can develop in multiple organs, such as the brain, skin, kidney, eye, lung, and liver in TSC patients. The incidence is estimated to be 1 per 6000 live births.[85] Diagnostic criteria for TSC endorsed by the Tuberous Sclerosis Alliance organization include both major and minor categories. The diagnosis is made with 2 major features (excluding lymphangioleiomyomatosis and renal angiomyolipoma alone) or 1 major and 2 minor features. Major diagnostic criteria include: (1) facial angiofibromas ("adenoma sebaceum") or forehead plaque, (2) nontraumatic ungual or periungual fibroma ("Koenen tumor"), (3) 3 or more hypomelanotic macules ("ash leaf spots" or "Fitzpatrick patches"), (4) connective tissue nevus ("Shagreen patch"), (5) multiple retinal nodular hamartomas, (6) cortical tuber, (7) subependymal nodule, (8) subependymal giant cell astrocytoma, (9) single or multiple cardiac rhabdomyoma, (10) lymphangioleiomyomatosis, and (11) renal angiomyolipoma.[86] Minor criteria include: (1) multiple dental enamel pits, (2) hamartomatous rectal polyps, (3) bone cysts, (4) cerebral white matter radial migration lines, (5) gingival fibromas, (6) nonrenal hamartomas, (7) retinal achromic patch, (8) cutaneous symmetric hypopigmented macules ("confetti" macules), and (9) multiple renal cysts.[86]

Neurologic manifestations are present in approximately 85% of children and adolescents with TSC and include epilepsy, cognitive impairment, behavioral problems, and autism. These neurologic problems are the primary cause of morbidity and mortality in affected individuals, and are likely caused by the presence of brain lesions including cortical tubers, subependymal nodules, subependymal giant cell tumors, and white matter abnormalities.[87–90] In familial cases of TSC, nodules have a high likelihood of transforming into an ependymal giant cell tumor, with a prevalence of about 11% in affected individuals.[91] Epilepsy, caused by diminished γ-aminobutyric acid (GABA) neuronal inhibition, typically starts in the first few months of life and affects 90% to 96% of TSC patients.[92] Control of seizures is necessary to reduce the risk of cognitive impairment. Mental retardation (MR) is seen in up to 50% of affected individuals, almost all of whom have seizures; however, not all patients with seizures have MR.[93,94]

After neurologic complications, those from renal involvement are the major contributors to mortality in TSC.[95] Angiomyolipomas, the most common renal abnormality, affect about 80% of individuals with TSC, increase in incidence with age, and are usually treated with embolization or renal-sparing surgery if necessary.[95–98] Angiomyolipomas are typically bilateral and may be symptomatic, especially in women.[95,98] Renal cysts and renal cell carcinoma can also occur. Cardiac rhabdomyomas are often the first manifestation of TSC; they are benign, largely asymptomatic tumors that regress with age and rarely require surgery. MRI can diagnose cardiac rhabdomyomas in utero; most of these cases are affected with TSC.[99,100] Pulmonary involvement is rare in TSC; the most common lesion is lymphangioleiomyomatosis, typically affecting premenopausal adult women.[101,102] Ocular findings include retinal astrocytic hamartomas (also called "mulberry lesions"), which occur in 40% to 50% of TSC patients and increase with age.[103] Oral involvement includes pitting of dental enamel, occurring in about 50% to 100% of cases, and gingival fibromas, noted mostly on the anterior upper jaw.[86,101,104,105] Surgery may be needed for large gingival lesions.

TSC patients typically have a variety of dermatologic manifestations. Small, confetti-like hypopigmented macules and medium to large hypopigmented patches with an ash leaf, round, or polygonal shape may be observed. The "ash leaf spot" is typically present at birth, and so can help to confirm the diagnosis.[101,106] Facial angiofibromas, small pink papules, are typically found around the central face, particularly the nasolabial folds, and can be removed with carbon dioxide or other destructive lasers.[101] Fibrous plaques, resembling angiofibromas histologically, are large plaques typically found on the forehead or scalp. Whereas angiofibromas typically appear around age 5 years, fibrous plaques may be present in affected individuals younger than 2 years or even at birth.[86,92,107] Many consider angiofibromas and fibrous plaques the same in terms of diagnostic criteria for TSC. Ungual or periungual fibromas, pink papulonodules arising from the nail bed and also resembling angiofibromas histologically, become apparent at puberty and increase in number with age; they affect toenails more commonly than fingernails and may be symptomatic, requiring surgery. Connective tissue nevi, or Shagreen patches, can be found on the trunk, especially the lumbosacral region, and may also increase in size with age.[101] Café-au-lait macules may also occur in up to 30% of TSC patients, although their frequency in TSC patients compared with unaffected individuals is the same.[108,109] Molluscum fibrosum pendulum, pedunculated skin-colored papules, may also develop.[101]

Genetics

TSC is caused by autosomal dominantly inherited and sporadic mutations in 2 genes: *TSC1*, located on chromosome 9q34, encoding tuberin, and *TSC2*, located on chromosome 16p13.3, encoding hamartin. Tuberin and hamartin proteins bind tightly to form a heterodimer with tumor suppressor properties including regulation of cell growth by inhibiting mTOR via the Rheb (Ras homologue enriched in brain) protein.[110–113] Studies in *Drosophila* have exposed the role of the tuberin and hamartin genes downstream of the insulin receptor in regulation of cell size.[114–116]

TSC exhibits complete penetrance with wide phenotypic variability, even within families sharing the same mutation.[101,117] In TSC, germline mosaicism is possible. In large, multigeneration TSC families, *TSC1* and *TSC2* gene mutations occur in a 1:1 ratio; however, *TSC2* mutations account for the majority of sporadic cases, apparently because of an increased rate of second-hit events.[118–120] *TSC1* mutations are generally small deletions and insertions as well as nonsense mutations, whereas *TSC2* mutations can include these as well as large deletions and rearrangements. Phenotype severity generally cannot be predicted by the type and location of the mutation, although some missense mutations in *TSC2* are associated with a mild phenotype.[117,121–123] Of note, large deletions of *TSC2* can also result in deletions of the nearby gene responsible for polycystic kidney disease, *PDK1*, resulting in individuals with TSC and multiple renal cysts in infancy.[124,125] Disease phenotype has been found to differ among TSC patients with *TSC1* versus *TSC2* mutations; individuals with *TSC2* mutations have a similar but more severe phenotype, including more severe mental retardation and increased numbers of cortical tubers, retinal hamartomas, and facial angiofibromas, than those with *TSC1* mutations.[118–120,126]

Genetic Testing and Treatment

DNA testing can be performed to confirm a diagnosis as well as for prenatal diagnosis.[92] Identification of affected individuals before or at birth, or during infancy allows for prompt diagnostic evaluation with neuroimaging studies, cardiac evaluation, and renal ultrasonography as well as early intervention with seizure-controlling medications, reducing the potential for intellectual impairment.[127] When TSC-associated seizures are intractable despite standard antiepileptic medication, vigabatrin (γ-vinyl-γ-aminobutyric acid), a selective GABA-transaminase inhibitor, may be used to reduce infantile spasms; however, this medication is not available in the United States.[128,129] TSC patients should be managed by a team of physicians, including neurologists, dermatologists, urologists, pediatricians, and geneticists.

Because mTOR is unregulated in TSC as in NF1, rapamycin may play a role in the treatment of TSC-related tumors.[113] Studies in animal models demonstrate that rapamycin and other mTOR inhibitors are effective treatments for renal tumors, liver hemangiomas, epilepsy, and cutaneous tumors.[130–132] In human studies, rapamycin decreases the volume of renal angiomyolipomas and subependymal giant cell astrocytomas. Further studies are needed to evaluate this promising therapy for individuals affected with TSC.[133–135]

XERODERMA PIGMENTOSUM
History and Overview

Xeroderma pigmentosum (XP) is characterized by severe ultraviolet (UV) light photosensitivity and a greater than 1000-fold increase in frequency of squamous cell carcinoma, basal cell carcinoma, and melanoma. Sun sensitivity and freckling are typically seen by 2 years of age.[136] Skin cancers can develop in the first decade of life, with the majority occurring on the head, neck, or face.[137] In addition to cutaneous findings, patients often have ocular abnormalities including ectropion, corneal opacities, and neoplasms; these may cause blindness.[136] Neurologic abnormalities may also occur, depending on the underlying genetic abnormality. XP patients also have increased risks of other cancers, especially oral cancer, most commonly affecting the anterior tongue.[138]

Genetics

XP is an autosomal recessive disorder caused by mutations in nucleotide excision repair complementation groups, of which there are 7, A to G; there is also an XP-variant type caused by mutations in the DNA polymerase eta gene. XP variant type is characterized by photosensitivity, skin cancers, and absence of neurologic abnormalities. The complementation groups and DNA polymerase function in DNA repair, particularly after UV damage. Mutations in *XPA* and *XPC* account for approximately 50% of cases of XP.[138] The relationship between defects in these complementation groups and the clinical disease phenotype is complex; whereas mutations in several genes can cause the same phenotype, different mutations in the same gene can cause different phenotypes.[138,139] For example, some forms of XP are associated with neurologic problems including mental retardation, sensorineural deafness, spasticity, and hyporeflexia due to progressive neuronal degeneration.[139] Furthermore, Cockayne syndrome (CS) and trichothiodystrophy (TTD), other autosomal recessive disorders, are also caused by defects in nucleotide excision repair genes. Although individuals with CS and TTD are photosensitive like XP individuals, they do not have an increased frequency of skin cancers.[138,139] XP and CS can occur together in the same individual as the XP/CS complex; these individuals often have skin and eye findings of XP with the short stature, immature sexual development, retinopathy, and progressive neurologic degeneration of CS.[138] It is interesting that polymorphisms in the *XPD* gene are related to early onset of sporadic basal cell carcinoma, suggesting the importance of the NER pathway in BCC development.[140–142]

Genetic Testing and Treatment

Clinical molecular testing is available for *XPA* and *XPC* genes only.[138] Treatment of XP involves early recognition, strict avoidance of UV exposure of the skin and eyes, routine skin examinations for detection followed by complete excision of skin cancers, and neurologic follow-up if needed. High-dose oral isotretinoin has been shown to decrease numbers of skin cancers in individuals with multiple skin cancers, though toxicity limits its use.[138]

DYSKERATOSIS CONGENITA
History and Overview

Dyskeratosis congenita (DC) is a rare syndrome with an unknown true prevalence, but is thought to affect about 1 in 1 million individuals in North America.[143] DC is characterized by abnormal skin pigmentation, nail dystrophy, oral premalignant leuko-plakia, bone marrow failure, and a predisposition to cancer, particularly myelodyspla-sia, acute myeloid leukemia, and cutaneous squamous cell carcinoma of the head and neck. Other findings include ocular abnormalities such as epiphora, blepharitis, and abnormal eyelashes; hair findings including alopecia and premature graying; dental findings such as periodontal disease, decreased tooth root/crown ratio, and enlarged tooth pulp chambers; microcephaly; short stature; and esophageal stenosis, among others.[143,144] Approximately 90% of affected individuals develop bone marrow failure by age 30 years, which accounts for the majority of mortality.[145] Age of onset and disease severity can vary among affected individuals, unpredictably, even within the same family.

Genetics

Mutations in 6 genes, *TERC* (RNA subunit of telomerase), *TERT* (telomerase reverse transcriptase), *DKC1* (dyskerin), *NHP2* (nucleolar protein family A, member 2, or NOLA2), *NOP10* (nucleolar protein family A, member 3, or NOLA3), and *TINF2* (TRF1-interacting nuclear factor 2), encoding telomerase complex components, cause about 50% of cases of DC.[145,146] The mode of inheritance varies by gene, and X-linked, autosomal recessive, and autosomal dominant inheritance patterns have been described. These mutations uniformly result in short telomeres, which accumulate as cells divide and recruit DNA damage proteins that lead to apoptosis or cellular senescence that can lead to organ failure.[146] Three main types of DC can occur: classic DC, and cryptic and severe variants.[145] Cryptic variants include aplastic anemia, myelodysplasia, paroxysmal nocturnal hemoglobinuria, essential thrombocy-themia, and pulmonary fibrosis. Severe variants include Hoyeraal-Hreidarsson syndrome and Revesz syndrome. Because there is marked clinical and genetic heterogeneity of DC, most of these variants were only recognized as being associated with classic DC after their underlying mutations were identified.[145] The link between short telomeres, cellular senescence, and malignancy may be present in sporadic cancers as well as in DC.[147–149]

Genetic Testing and Treatment

Leukocyte telomere length testing by automated multicolor flow cytometry fluores-cence in situ hybridization should be used in individuals with suspected DC; findings of DC include telomeres less than the first percentile for age in 3 to 4 of 6 cell types examined.[143,150] In these individuals, genetic testing should be considered.[143] Management of DC includes routine screening for malignancies by gynecologists, otolaryngologists, dermatologists, and dentists, and annual pulmonary function testing.[143] Treatment of bone marrow failure and/or leukemia may include hematopoi-etic stem cell transplant, but there is a higher mortality associated with use in DC than in other bone marrow failure syndromes.[145] Other treatments include androgen therapy.[143,151]

HEREDITARY MELANOMA
History and Overview

The incidence of cutaneous malignant melanoma (CMM), which occurs in a familial setting and sporadically, continues to increase and is the fifth and sixth most common cancer in the United States in men and women, respectively.[152,153] Unlike the other inherited genodermatoses discussed there is no distinctive, prodromic, or diagnostic phenotype of familial melanoma. Melanoma is heterogeneous and etiologically complex. The interaction of genetic, host, and environmental factors contributes to the development of CMM in melanoma-prone families and in sporadic cases. UV radiation is the main environmental risk factor for CMM, and data suggest that intense intermittent sun exposure at any age impacts on risk more than total lifetime exposure.[154] Phenotypic host factors, such as the presence and number of benign and dysplastic nevi, blond or red hair color, light eye color, freckling, and skin sensitivity to the sun, are also associated with increased risk of CMM. Within melanoma-prone families, these environmental and host factors are often shared. Norris, Clark, and Lynch were among the first to describe the occurrence of high rates of melanoma in certain families.[155–157] Approximately 5% to 12% of CMM cases occur in individuals with one or more affected first-degree relatives.[158] Within melanoma-prone families, CMM lesions are typically thinner, are diagnosed at a younger age, and there is a higher frequency of multiple primary melanomas (MPMs), compared with nonfamilial melanoma cases; however, lesion histology, prognosis, and survival are similar.[158,159]

Genetics

CDKN2A/CDK4

Two high-risk melanoma susceptibility genes have been identified: *CDKN2A* (cyclin-dependent kinase inhibitor 2A) and *CDK4* (cyclin-dependent kinase 4).[160–163] The inheritance pattern for both genes is autosomal dominant. *CDKN2A*, located on chromosome 9p21, is a tumor suppressor gene encoding 2 proteins, p16 and p14ARF, involved in cell cycle control maintenance. The p16 protein inhibits CDK4-mediated phosphorylation of the retinoblastoma protein (Rb), thus regulating G1-phase exit, and the p14ARF protein mediates cell cycle arrest through the p53 pathway.[164] *CDK4*, on chromosome 12q14, functions as an oncogene in the retinoblastoma pathway. Comparison of families with *CDKN2A* and *CDK4* mutations demonstrated similar age at diagnosis, number of CMMs, and number of nevi.[165] However, germline mutations in CDK4 are rare and, to date, reported in only about 10 families.[166–168] Germline mutations in *CDKN2A* account for about 20% to 50% of families with 3 or more members affected with CMM.[169,170] The frequency of detectable mutations increases as the number of CMM cases in a family increases; in families with only 2 affected members, the frequency of detectable *CDKN2A* mutations is less than 5%, whereas in families with greater than 6 affected members, the frequency of detectable *CDKN2A* mutations is more than 50%.[158,171] Similarly, in individuals with MPM, the percentage of detectable *CDKN2A* mutations increases from 10% in those with no family history of CMM to greater than 30% in those with 3 or more relatives with CMM.[158,171]

Studies suggest an association between *CDKN2A* and cancers other than melanoma, contributing to mortality within melanoma-prone families. In melanoma-prone families with *CDKN2A* mutations there is an increased risk of pancreatic cancer, though accurate prediction of who will develop pancreatic cancer among *CDKN2A* mutation-positive individuals is currently impossible.[172,173] Neural system tumors may be associated with *CDKN2A* mutations affecting p14ARF protein.[173] Breast cancer is associated with *CDKN2A* mutations in a subset of families, mostly from Sweden.[174]

Because only about 20% to 40% of familial melanoma cases are accounted for by *CDKN2A* and *CDK4* mutations, other genetic factors increase CMM risk within families. There is evidence of other high-penetrance loci on chromosomes 1p22 and 1p36, but the causal genes have not yet been identified.[175,176]

Variations in penetrance

Although *CDKN2A* mutations confer a high risk of melanoma, not all individuals with *CDKN2A* mutations within melanoma-prone families develop melanoma, suggesting incomplete penetrance. A large family-based study of *CKDN2A* mutation carriers from Europe, Australia, and the United States demonstrated that penetrance estimates varied with age as well as geographic location and reflected local incidence rates of CMM in each population.[177] Penetrance estimates in population-based studies in several geographic regions are lower than those from family-based studies.[178–180] Other characteristics also differ among mutation carriers even within one family, including age at CMM diagnosis, the presence and number of dysplastic nevi, the number of CMMs, and cosegregation of pancreatic cancer.

Other melanoma susceptibility genes and modifier genes
Low-penetrance melanoma susceptibility genes are also associated with sporadic and familial melanoma; several of these were identified by candidate gene approaches and/or genome-wide association studies. These genes include the melanocortin-1 receptor (*MC1R*) gene, tyrosinase (*TYR*), agouti signaling protein (*ASIP*), tyrosinase-related protein 1 (*TYRP1*), solute-carrier family 45, member 2 (*SLC45A2*), all of which are associated with pigmentation factors and melanoma; and methylthioadenosine phosphorylase (*MTAP*), near *CDKN2A*, and phospholipase A2, group VI (*PLA2G6*), which are associated with nevi and melanoma.[181–187] *MC1R* variants were found to modify the penetrance of *CDKN2A* mutations in melanoma-prone families, suggesting that gene-gene interactions may also contribute to increased CMM risk in melanoma-prone families.[188–191]

Genetic Testing

Commercial genetic testing is available to identify *CDKN2A* and *CDK4* mutations, and referral for genetic evaluation may be considered for individuals with 3 or more primary melanomas or families with at least 1 melanoma and 2 or more melanoma or pancreatic cancer cases among first- or second-degree relatives.[192] However, the frequency of detecting mutations is low even among high-risk individuals.[193] It is important to identify individuals at high risk, including those from melanoma-prone families, who would benefit from routine skin examinations to detect melanomas early, when they are easily cured.

ACKNOWLEDGMENTS

The authors thank Dilys Parry for her careful review of the manuscript.

REFERENCES

1. Binkley GW, Johnson HH Jr. Epithelioma adenoides cysticum: basal cell nevi, agenesis of the corpus callosum and dental cysts: a clinical and autopsy study. AMA Arch Derm Syphilol 1951;63(1):73–84.
2. Howell JB, Caro MR. The basal-cell nevus: its relationship to multiple cutaneous cancers and associated anomalies of development. AMA Arch Derm 1959; 79(1):67–77 [discussion: 77–80].
3. Gorlin RJ, Goltz RW. Multiple nevoid basal-cell epithelioma, jaw cysts and bifid rib. A syndrome. N Engl J Med 1960;262:908–12.
4. Farndon PA, Del Mastro RG, Evans DGR, et al. Location of gene for Gorlin syndrome. Lancet 1992;339:581–2.
5. Evans DG, Farndon PA. Nevoid basal cell carcinoma syndrome. In: Pagon RA, Bird TC, Dolan CR, et al, editors. GeneReviews. Seattle (WA): University of Washington; 2008.

6. Kimonis VE, Goldstein AM, Pastakia B, et al. Clinical manifestations in 105 persons with nevoid basal cell carcinoma syndrome. Am J Med Genet 1997; 69(3):299–308.
7. Chidambaram A, Goldstein AM, Gailani MR, et al. Mutations in the human homologue of the Drosophila patched gene in Caucasian and African-American nevoid basal cell carcinoma syndrome patients. Cancer Res 1996;56(20): 4599–601.
8. Wicking C, Shanley S, Smyth I, et al. Most germ-line mutations in the nevoid basal cell carcinoma syndrome lead to a premature termination of the PATCHED protein, and no genotype-phenotype correlations are evident. Am J Hum Genet 1997;60(1):21–6.
9. Boutet N, Bignon YJ, Drouin-Garraud V, et al. Spectrum of PTCH1 mutations in French patients with Gorlin syndrome. J Invest Dermatol 2003;121(3):478–81.
10. Smyth I, Wicking C, Wainwright B, et al. The effects of splice site mutations in patients with naevoid basal cell carcinoma syndrome. Hum Genet 1998; 102(5):598–601.
11. Gorlin RJ. Nevoid basal cell carcinoma (Gorlin) syndrome. Genet Med 2004; 6(6):530–9.
12. Anderson DE, Taylor WB, Falls HF, et al. The nevoid basal cell carcinoma syndrome. Am J Hum Genet 1967;19(1):12–22.
13. Gailani MR, Bale AE. Developmental genes and cancer: role of patched in basal cell carcinoma of the skin. J Natl Cancer Inst 1997;89(15):1103–9.
14. Levanat S, Gorlin RJ, Fallet S, et al. A two-hit model for developmental defects in Gorlin syndrome. Nat Genet 1996;12(1):85–7.
15. Guarneri B, Borgia F, Cannavò SP, et al. Multiple familial basal cell carcinomas including a case of segmental manifestation. Dermatology 2000;200(4): 299–302.
16. Fan Z, Li J, Du J, et al. A missense mutation in PTCH2 underlies dominantly inherited NBCCS in a Chinese family. J Med Genet 2008;45(5):303–8.
17. Pastorino L, Ghiorzo P, Nasti S, et al. Identification of a SUFU germline mutation in a family with Gorlin syndrome. Am J Med Genet A 2009;149A(7):1539–43.
18. Johnson RL, Rothman AL, Xie J, et al. Human homolog of patched, a candidate gene for the basal cell nevus syndrome. Science 1996;272(5268):1668–71.
19. Hahn H, Wicking C, Zaphiropoulous PG, et al. Mutations of the human homolog of Drosophila patched in the nevoid basal cell carcinoma syndrome. Cell 1996; 85(6):841–51.
20. Taipale J, Cooper MK, Maiti T, et al. Patched acts catalytically to suppress the activity of Smoothened. Nature 2002;418(6900):892–7.
21. Ingham PW, McMahon AP. Hedgehog signaling in animal development: paradigms and principles. Genes Dev 2001;15(23):3059–87.
22. Xie J, Murone M, Luoh SM, et al. Activating Smoothened mutations in sporadic basal-cell carcinoma. Nature 1998;391(6662):90–2.
23. Gailani MR, Ståhle-Bäckdahl M, Leffell DJ, et al. The role of the human homologue of Drosophila patched in sporadic basal cell carcinomas. Nat Genet 1996;14(1):78–81.
24. Taylor MD, Liu L, Raffel C, et al. Mutations in SUFU predispose to medulloblastoma. Nat Genet 2002;31(3):306–10.
25. Dong J, Gailani MR, Pomeroy SL, et al. Identification of PATCHED mutations in medulloblastomas by direct sequencing. Hum Mutat 2000;16(1):89–90.
26. Gu XM, Zhao HS, Sun LS, et al. PTCH mutations in sporadic and Gorlin-syndrome-related odontogenic keratocysts. J Dent Res 2006;85(9):859–63.

27. Le Brun Keris Y, Jouk PS, Saada-Sebag G, et al. Prenatal manifestation in a family affected by nevoid basal cell carcinoma syndrome. Eur J Med Genet 2008;51(5):472–8.
28. Gilchrest BA, Brightman LA, Thiele JJ, et al. Photodynamic therapy for patients with Basal cell nevus syndrome. Dermatol Surg 2009;35(10):1576–81.
29. Tang JY, Aszterbaum M, Athar M, et al. Basal cell carcinoma chemoprevention with nonsteroidal anti-inflammatory drugs in genetically predisposed PTCH1+/− humans and mice. Cancer Prev Res (Phila Pa) 2010;3:25–34.
30. Berman DM, Karhadkar SS, Hallahan AR, et al. Medulloblastoma growth inhibition by hedgehog pathway blockade. Science 2002;297(5586):1559–61.
31. Rudin CM, Hann CL, Laterra J, et al. Treatment of medulloblastoma with hedgehog pathway inhibitor GDC-0449. N Engl J Med 2009;361(12):1173–8.
32. Von Hoff DD, LoRusso PM, Rudin CM, et al. Inhibition of the hedgehog pathway in advanced basal-cell carcinoma. N Engl J Med 2009;361(12):1164–72.
33. Reynolds RM, Browning GG, Nawroz I, et al. Von Recklinghausen's neurofibromatosis: neurofibromatosis type 1. Lancet 2003;361(9368):1552–4.
34. Boyd KP, Korf BR, Theos A. Neurofibromatosis type 1. J Am Acad Dermatol 2009;61(1):1–14.
35. Williams VC, Lucas J, Babcock MA, et al. Neurofibromatosis type 1 revisited. Pediatrics 2009;123(1):124–33.
36. Ferner RE. Neurofibromatosis 1. Eur J Hum Genet 2007;15(2):131–8.
37. Zvulunov A, Barak Y, Metzker A. Juvenile xanthogranuloma, neurofibromatosis, and juvenile chronic myelogenous leukemia. World statistical analysis. Arch Dermatol 1995;131(8):904–8.
38. Rosser T, Packer RJ. Neurofibromas in children with neurofibromatosis 1. J Child Neurol 2002;17(8):585–91.
39. Savar A, Cestari DM. Neurofibromatosis type I: genetics and clinical manifestations. Semin Ophthalmol 2008;23(1):45–51.
40. Stewart DR, Cogan JD, Kramer MR, et al. Is pulmonary arterial hypertension in neurofibromatosis type 1 secondary to a plexogenic arteriopathy? Chest 2007; 132(3):798–808.
41. Perren A, Wiesli P, Schmid S, et al. Pancreatic endocrine tumors are a rare manifestation of the neurofibromatosis type 1 phenotype: molecular analysis of a malignant insulinoma in a NF-1 patient. Am J Surg Pathol 2006;30(8): 1047–51.
42. Ferner RE, Huson SM, Thomas N, et al. Guidelines for the diagnosis and management of individuals with neurofibromatosis 1. J Med Genet 2007;44(2): 81–8.
43. Brems H, Park C, Maertens O, et al. Glomus tumors in neurofibromatosis type 1: genetic, functional, and clinical evidence of a novel association. Cancer Res 2009;69(18):7393–401.
44. Stocker KM, Baizer L, Coston T, et al. Regulated expression of neurofibromin in migrating neural crest cells of avian embryos. J Neurobiol 1995;27(4):535–52.
45. Daston MM, Scrable H, Nordlund M, et al. The protein product of the neurofibromatosis type 1 gene is expressed at highest abundance in neurons, Schwann cells, and oligodendrocytes. Neuron 1992;8(3):415–28.
46. Colman SD, Williams CA, Wallace MR. Benign neurofibromas in type 1 neurofibromatosis (NF1) show somatic deletions of the NF1 gene. Nat Genet 1995; 11(1):90–2.
47. Khosravi-Far R, Der CJ. The Ras signal transduction pathway. Cancer Metastasis Rev 1994;13(1):67–89.

48. Theos A, Korf BR, American College of Physicians, American Physiological Society. Pathophysiology of neurofibromatosis type 1. Ann Intern Med 2006; 144(11):842–9.

49. Brems H, Chmara M, Sahbatou M, et al. Germline loss-of-function mutations in SPRED1 cause a neurofibromatosis 1-like phenotype. Nat Genet 2007;39(9): 1120–6.

50. Messiaen LM, Callens T, Mortier G, et al. Exhaustive mutation analysis of the NF1 gene allows identification of 95% of mutations and reveals a high frequency of unusual splicing defects. Hum Mutat 2000;15(6):541–55.

51. Ruggieri M, Huson SM. The clinical and diagnostic implications of mosaicism in the neurofibromatoses. Neurology 2001;56(11):1433–43.

52. Vandenbroucke I, van Doorn R, Callens T, et al. Genetic and clinical mosaicism in a patient with neurofibromatosis type 1. Hum Genet 2004;114(3):284–90.

53. Leppig KA, Kaplan P, Viskochil D, et al. Familial neurofibromatosis 1 microdeletions: cosegregation with distinct facial phenotype and early onset of cutaneous neurofibromata. Am J Med Genet 1997;73(2):197–204.

54. De Raedt T, Brems H, Wolkenstein P, et al. Elevated risk for MPNST in NF1 microdeletion patients. Am J Hum Genet 2003;72(5):1288–92.

55. Upadhyaya M, Huson SM, Davies M, et al. An absence of cutaneous neurofibromas associated with a 3-bp inframe deletion in exon 17 of the NF1 gene (c.2970-2972 delAAT): evidence of a clinically significant NF1 genotype-phenotype correlation. Am J Hum Genet 2007;80(1):140–51.

56. Gupta A, Cohen BH, Ruggieri P, et al. Phase I study of thalidomide for the treatment of plexiform neurofibroma in neurofibromatosis 1. Neurology 2003;60(1): 130–2.

57. Widemann BC, Salzer WL, Arceci RJ, et al. Phase I trial and pharmacokinetic study of the farnesyltransferase inhibitor tipifarnib in children with refractory solid tumors or neurofibromatosis type I and plexiform neurofibromas. Clin Oncol 2006;24(3):507–16.

58. Rosner M, Hanneder M, Siegel N, et al. The mTOR pathway and its role in human genetic diseases. Mutat Res 2008;659(3):284–92.

59. Bhola P, Banerjee S, Mukherjee J, et al. Preclinical in vivo evaluation of rapamycin in human malignant peripheral nerve sheath explant xenograft. Int J Cancer 2010;126(2):563–71.

60. Rouleau GA, Wertelecki W, Haines JL, et al. Genetic linkage of bilateral acoustic neurofibromatosis to a DNA marker on chromosome 22. Nature 1987;329(6136): 246–8.

61. Seizinger BR, Rouleau GA, Ozelius LJ, et al. Genetic linkage of von Recklinghausen neurofibromatosis to the nerve growth factor receptor gene. Cell 1987;49(5):589–94.

62. National Institutes of Health Consensus Development Conference Statement: neurofibromatosis. Bethesda, Md., USA, July 13-15, 1987. Neurofibromatosis 1988;1(3):172–8.

63. Evans DG, Huson SM, Donnai D, et al. A genetic study of type 2 neurofibromatosis in the United Kingdom. I. Prevalence, mutation rate, fitness, and confirmation of maternal transmission effect on severity. J Med Genet 1992;29(12):841–6.

64. Asthagiri AR, Parry DM, Butman JA, et al. Neurofibromatosis type 2. Lancet 2009;373(9679):1974–86.

65. Wiestler OD, von Siebenthal K, Schmitt HP, et al. Distribution and immunoreactivity of cerebral micro-hamartomas in bilateral acoustic neurofibromatosis (neurofibromatosis 2). Acta Neuropathol 1989;79(2):137–43.

66. Bosch MM, Boltshauser E, Harpes P, et al. Ophthalmologic findings and long-term course in patients with neurofibromatosis type 2. Am J Ophthalmol 2006; 141(6):1068–77.
67. Landau K, Dossetor FM, Hoyt WF, et al. Retinal hamartoma in neurofibromatosis 2. Arch Ophthalmol 1990;108(3):328–9.
68. Evans DG, Huson SM, Donnai D, et al. A clinical study of type 2 neurofibromatosis. Q J Med 1992;84(304):603–18.
69. Mautner VF, Lindenau M, Baser ME, et al. Skin abnormalities in neurofibromatosis 2. Arch Dermatol 1997;133(12):1539–43.
70. Martuza RL, Eldridge R. Neurofibromatosis 2 (bilateral acoustic neurofibromatosis). N Engl J Med 1988;318(11):684–8.
71. Parry DM, Eldridge R, Kaiser-Kupfer MI, et al. Neurofibromatosis 2 (NF2): clinical characteristics of 63 affected individuals and clinical evidence for heterogeneity. Am J Med Genet 1994;52(4):450–61.
72. Evans DGR, Huson SM, Donnai D, et al. A genetic study of type 2 neurofibromatosis in the United Kingdom. II. Guidelines for genetic counselling. J Med Genet 1992;29:847–52.
73. Evans DG, Moran A, King A, et al. Incidence of vestibular schwannoma and neurofibromatosis 2 in the North West of England over a 10-year period: higher incidence than previously thought. Otol Neurotol 2005;26(1):93–7.
74. Evans DG. Neurofibromatosis 2. In: Pagon RA, Bird TC, Dolan CR, et al, editors. GeneReviews. Seattle (WA): University of Washington; 2009.
75. Baser ME, Friedman JM, Aeschliman D, et al. Predictors of the risk of mortality in neurofibromatosis 2. Am J Hum Genet 2002;71(4):715–23.
76. Parry DM, MacCollin MM, Kaiser-Kupfer MI, et al. Germ-line mutations in the neurofibromatosis 2 gene: correlations with disease severity and retinal abnormalities. Am J Hum Genet 1996;59(3):529–39.
77. Evans DG, Trueman L, Wallace A, et al. Genotype/phenotype correlations in type 2 neurofibromatosis (NF2): evidence for more severe disease associated with truncating mutations. J Med Genet 1998;35(6):450–5.
78. Baser ME, Kuramoto L, Joe H, et al. Genotype-phenotype correlations for nervous system tumors in neurofibromatosis 2: a population-based study. Am J Hum Genet 2004;75(2):231–9.
79. Moyhuddin A, Baser ME, Watson C, et al. Somatic mosaicism in neurofibromatosis 2: prevalence and risk of disease transmission to offspring. J Med Genet 2003;40(6):459–63.
80. Evans DG, Baser ME, O'Reilly B, et al. Management of the patient and family with neurofibromatosis 2: a consensus conference statement. Br J Neurosurg 2005;19(1):5–12.
81. Larson JJ, van Loveren HR, Balko MG, et al. Evidence of meningioma infiltration into cranial nerves: clinical implications for cavernous sinus meningiomas. J Neurosurg 1995;83(4):596–9.
82. Couldwell WT, Fukushima T, Giannotta SL, et al. Petroclival meningiomas: surgical experience in 109 cases. J Neurosurg 1996;84(1):20–8.
83. James MF, Han S, Polizzano C, et al. NF2/merlin is a novel negative regulator of mTOR complex 1, and activation of mTORC1 is associated with meningioma and schwannoma growth. Mol Cell Biol 2009;29(15):4250–61.
84. Bourneville D. Sclérose tubéreuse des circonvolution cérébrales: idiotie et épidelpsie hemiplégique. Arch Neurol 1880;1:81–91.
85. Osborne JP, Fryer A, Webb D. Epidemiology of tuberous sclerosis. Ann N Y Acad Sci 1991;615:125–7.

86. Roach ES, Gomez MR, Northrup H. Tuberous sclerosis complex consensus conference: revised clinical diagnostic criteria. J Child Neurol 1998;13(12):624–8.
87. Curatolo P, Cusmai R, Cortesi F, et al. Neuropsychiatric aspects of tuberous sclerosis. Ann N Y Acad Sci 1991;615:8–16.
88. Curatolo P, Verdecchia M, Bombardieri R. Tuberous sclerosis complex: a review of neurological aspects. Eur J Paediatr Neurol 2002;6(1):15–23.
89. DiMario FJ Jr. Brain abnormalities in tuberous sclerosis complex. J Child Neurol 2004;19(9):650–7.
90. Luat AF, Makki M, Chugani HT. Neuroimaging in tuberous sclerosis complex. Curr Opin Neurol 2007;20(2):142–50.
91. Adriaensen ME, Schaefer-Prokop CM, Stijnen T, et al. Prevalence of subependymal giant cell tumors in patients with tuberous sclerosis and a review of the literature. Eur J Neurol 2009;16(6):691–6.
92. Curatolo P, Bombardieri R, Jozwiak S. Tuberous sclerosis. Lancet 2008; 372(9639):657–68.
93. Jóźwiak S, Goodman M, Lamm SH. Poor mental development in patients with tuberous sclerosis complex: clinical risk factors. Arch Neurol 1998;55(3):379–84.
94. Chou PC, Chang YJ. Prognostic factors for mental retardation in patients with tuberous sclerosis complex. Acta Neurol Taiwan 2004;13(1):10–3.
95. O'Callaghan FJ, Noakes MJ, Martyn CN, et al. An epidemiological study of renal pathology in tuberous sclerosis complex. BJU Int 2004;94(6):853–7.
96. El-Hashemite N, Zhang H, Henske EP, et al. Mutation in TSC2 and activation of mammalian target of rapamycin signalling pathway in renal angiomyolipoma. Lancet 2003;361(9366):1348–9.
97. Ewalt DH, Sheffield E, Sparagana SP, et al. Renal lesion growth in children with tuberous sclerosis complex. J Urol 1998;160(1):141–5.
98. Rakowski SK, Winterkorn EB, Paul E, et al. Renal manifestations of tuberous sclerosis complex: incidence, prognosis, and predictive factors. Kidney Int 2006;70(10):1777–82.
99. Tworetzky W, McElhinney DB, Margossian R, et al. Association between cardiac tumors and tuberous sclerosis in the fetus and neonate. Am J Cardiol 2003; 92(4):487–9.
100. Bader RS, Chitayat D, Kelly E, et al. Fetal rhabdomyoma: prenatal diagnosis, clinical outcome, and incidence of associated tuberous sclerosis complex. J Pediatr 2003;143(5):620–4.
101. Schwartz RA, Fernández G, Kotulska K, et al. Tuberous sclerosis complex: advances in diagnosis, genetics, and management. J Am Acad Dermatol 2007;57(2):189–202.
102. Hancock E, Osborne J. Lymphangioleiomyomatosis: a review of the literature. Respir Med 2002;96(1):1–6.
103. Rowley SA, O'Callaghan FJ, Osborne JP. Ophthalmic manifestations of tuberous sclerosis: a population based study. Br J Ophthalmol 2001;85(4):420–3.
104. Mlynarczyk G. Enamel pitting. A common sign of tuberous sclerosis. Ann N Y Acad Sci 1991;615:367–9.
105. Lygidakis NA, Lindenbaum RH. Oral fibromatosis in tuberous sclerosis. Oral Surg Oral Med Oral Pathol 1989;68(6):725–8.
106. Fitzpatrick TB, Szabó G, Hori Y, et al. White leaf-shaped macules. Earliest visible sign of tuberous sclerosis. Arch Dermatol 1968;98(1):1–6.
107. Jóźwiak S, Schwartz RA, Janniger CK, et al. Usefulness of diagnostic criteria of tuberous sclerosis complex in pediatric patients. J Child Neurol 2000;15(10): 652–9.

108. Bell SD, MacDonald DM. The prevalence of café-au-lait patches in tuberous sclerosis. Clin Exp Dermatol 1985;10(6):562–5.
109. Landau M, Krafchik BR. The diagnostic value of café-au-lait macules. J Am Acad Dermatol 1999;40(6 Pt 1):877–90.
110. van Slegtenhorst M, Nellist M, Nagelkerken B, et al. Interaction between hamartin and tuberin, the TSC1 and TSC2 gene products. Hum Mol Genet 1998;7(6): 1053–7.
111. Kwiatkowski DJ. Tuberous sclerosis: from tubers to mTOR. Ann Hum Genet 2003;67(Pt 1):87–96.
112. Tee AR, Manning BD, Roux PP, et al. Tuberous sclerosis complex gene products, Tuberin and Hamartin, control mTOR signaling by acting as a GTPase-activating protein complex toward Rheb. Curr Biol 2003;13(15):1259–68.
113. Inoki K, Guan KL. Tuberous sclerosis complex, implication from a rare genetic disease to common cancer treatment. Hum Mol Genet 2009;18(R1):R94–100.
114. Gao X, Pan D. TSC1 and TSC2 tumor suppressors antagonize insulin signaling in cell growth. Genes Dev 2001;15(11):1383–92.
115. Tapon N, Ito N, Dickson BJ, et al. The Drosophila tuberous sclerosis complex gene homologs restrict cell growth and cell proliferation. Cell 2001;105(3): 345–55.
116. Potter CJ, Huang H, Xu T. Drosophila Tsc1 functions with Tsc2 to antagonize insulin signaling in regulating cell growth, cell proliferation, and organ size. Cell 2001;105(3):357–68.
117. Napolioni V, Curatolo P. Genetics and molecular biology of tuberous sclerosis complex. Curr Genomics 2008;9(7):475–87.
118. Dabora SL, Jozwiak S, Franz DN, et al. Mutational analysis in a cohort of 224 tuberous sclerosis patients indicates increased severity of TSC2, compared with TSC1, disease in multiple organs. Am J Hum Genet 2001;68(1):64–80.
119. Jones AC, Shyamsundar MM, Thomas MW, et al. Comprehensive mutation analysis of TSC1 and TSC2-and phenotypic correlations in 150 families with tuberous sclerosis. Am J Hum Genet 1999;64(5):1305–15.
120. Sancak O, Nellist M, Goedbloed M, et al. Mutational analysis of the TSC1 and TSC2 genes in a diagnostic setting: genotype-phenotype correlations and comparison of diagnostic DNA techniques in tuberous sclerosis complex. Eur J Hum Genet 2005;13(6):731–41.
121. Northrup H, Au KS. Tuberous sclerosis complex. In: Pagon RA, Bird TC, Dolan CR, et al, editors. GeneReviews. Seattle (WA): University of Washington; 2009.
122. Khare L, Strizheva GD, Bailey JN, et al. A novel missense mutation in the GTPase activating protein homology region of TSC2 in 2 large families with tuberous sclerosis complex. J Med Genet 2001;38:347–9.
123. Jansen AC, Sancak O, D'Agostino MD, et al. Unusually mild tuberous sclerosis phenotype is associated with TSC2 R905Q mutation. Ann Neurol 2006;60: 528–39.
124. Brook-Carter PT, Peral B, Ward CJ, et al. Deletion of the TSC2 and PKD1 genes associated with severe infantile polycystic kidney disease—a contiguous gene syndrome. Nat Genet 1994;8(4):328–32.
125. Sampson JR, Maheshwar MM, Aspinwall R, et al. Renal cystic disease in tuberous sclerosis: role of the polycystic kidney disease 1 gene. Am J Hum Genet 1997;61(4):843–51.
126. Lendvay TS, Marshall FF. The tuberous sclerosis complex and its highly variable manifestations. J Urol 2003;169(5):1635–42.

127. Roach ES, DiMario FJ, Kandt RS, et al. Tuberous Sclerosis Consensus Conference: recommendations for diagnostic evaluation. National Tuberous Sclerosis Association. J Child Neurol 1999;14(6):401–7.
128. Hancock E, Osborne JP. Vigabatrin in the treatment of infantile spasms in tuberous sclerosis: literature review. J Child Neurol 1999;14(2):71–4.
129. Jambaqué I, Chiron C, Dumas C, et al. Mental and behavioural outcome of infantile epilepsy treated by vigabatrin in tuberous sclerosis patients. Epilepsy Res 2000;38(2-3):151–60.
130. Kenerson HL, Aicher LD, True LD, et al. Activated mammalian target of rapamycin pathway in the pathogenesis of tuberous sclerosis complex renal tumors. Cancer Res 2002;62:5645–50.
131. Zeng LH, Xu L, Gutmann DH, et al. Rapamycin prevents epilepsy in a mouse model of tuberous sclerosis complex. Ann Neurol 2008;63(4):444–53.
132. Rauktys A, Lee N, Lee L, et al. Topical rapamycin inhibits tuberous sclerosis tumor growth in a nude mouse model. BMC Dermatol 2008;8:1.
133. Franz DN, Leonard J, Tudor C, et al. Rapamycin causes regression of astrocytomas in tuberous sclerosis complex. Ann Neurol 2006;59(3):490–8.
134. Wienecke R, Fackler I, Linsenmaier U, et al. Antitumoral activity of rapamycin in renal angiomyolipoma associated with tuberous sclerosis complex. Am J Kidney Dis 2006;48(3):e27–9.
135. Bissler JJ, McCormack FX, Young LR, et al. Sirolimus for angiomyolipoma in tuberous sclerosis complex or lymphangioleiomyomatosis. N Engl J Med 2008;358(2):140–51.
136. Kraemer KH, Lee MM, Scotto J. Xeroderma pigmentosum. Cutaneous, ocular, and neurologic abnormalities in 830 published cases. Arch Dermatol 1987;123(2):241–50.
137. Kraemer KH, Lee MM, Andrews AD, et al. The role of sunlight and DNA repair in melanoma and nonmelanoma skin cancer. The xeroderma pigmentosum paradigm. Arch Dermatol 1994;130(8):1018–21.
138. Kraemer KH. Xeroderma pigmentosum. In: Pagon RA, Bird TC, Dolan CR, et al, editors. GeneReviews. Seattle (WA): University of Washington; 2008.
139. Kraemer KH, Patronas NJ, Schiffmann R, et al. Xeroderma pigmentosum, trichothiodystrophy and Cockayne syndrome: a complex genotype-phenotype relationship. Neuroscience 2007;145(4):1388–96.
140. Suárez-Martínez EB, Ruiz A, Matías J, et al. Early-onset of sporadic basal-cell carcinoma: germline mutations in the TP53, PTCH, and XPD genes. P R Health Sci J 2007;26(4):349–54.
141. Lovatt T, Alldersea J, Lear JT, et al. Polymorphism in the nuclear excision repair gene ERCC2/XPD: association between an exon 6-exon 10 haplotype and susceptibility to cutaneous basal cell carcinoma. Hum Mutat 2005;25(4):353–9.
142. Dybdahl M, Vogel U, Frentz G, et al. Polymorphisms in the DNA repair gene XPD: correlations with risk and age at onset of basal cell carcinoma. Cancer Epidemiol Biomarkers Prev 1999;8(1):77–81.
143. Savage SA. Dyskeratosis congenita. In: Pagon RA, Bird TC, Dolan CR, et al, editors. GeneReviews. Seattle (WA): University of Washington; 2009.
144. Savage SA, Alter BP. The role of telomere biology in bone marrow failure and other disorders. Mech Ageing Dev 2008;129:35–47.
145. Walne AJ, Dokal I. Advances in the understanding of dyskeratosis congenita. Br J Haematol 2009;145(2):164–72.
146. Armanios M. Syndromes of telomere shortening. Annu Rev Genomics Hum Genet 2009;10:45–61.

147. Savage SA, Chanock SJ, Lissowska J, et al. Genetic variation in five genes important in telomere biology and risk for breast cancer. Br J Cancer 2007; 97(6):832–6.

148. Rafnar T, Sulem P, Stacey SN, et al. Sequence variants at the TERT-CLPTM1L locus associate with many cancer types. Nat Genet 2009;41(2):221–7.

149. Hosgood HD 3rd, Cawthon R, He X, et al. Genetic variation in telomere mainte-nance genes, telomere length, and lung cancer susceptibility. Lung Cancer 2009;66(2):157–61.

150. Alter BP, Baerlocher GM, Savage SA, et al. Very short telomere length by flow fluorescence in situ hybridization identifies patients with dyskeratosis congenita. Blood 2007;110:1439–47.

151. Savage SA, Alter BP. Dyskeratosis congenita. Hematol Oncol Clin North Am 2009;23(2):215–31.

152. Tucker MA. Melanoma epidemiology. Hematol Oncol Clin North Am 2009;23(3): 383–95, vii.

153. Jemal A, Siegel R, Ward E, et al. Cancer statistics, 2009. CA Cancer J Clin 2009; 59(4):225–49.

154. Gruber SB, Armstrong BK. Cutaneous and ocular melanoma. In: Schottenfeld D, Fraumeni JF Jr, editors. Cancer epidemiology and prevention. 3rd edition. New York: Oxford University Press; 2006. p. 1196–229.

155. McLead RG, Davis NC, Sober AJ. A history of melanoma: from Hunter to Clark. In: Balch CM, Houghton A, Sober AJ, et al, editors. Cutaneous melanoma. 4th edition. St Louis (MO): Quality Medical Publishing Inc; 2003. p. 1–12.

156. Clark WH Jr, Reimer RR, Greene M, et al. Origin of familial malignant melanomas from heritable melanocytic lesions. 'The B-K mole syndrome'. Arch Dermatol 1978;114(5):732–8.

157. Lynch HT, Frichot BC 3rd, Lynch JF. Familial atypical multiple mole-melanoma syndrome. J Med Genet 1978;15(5):352–6.

158. Goldstein AM, Tucker MA. Familial melanoma and its management. In: Eeles RA, Easton DF, Ponder BAJ, et al, editors. Genetic predisposition to cancer. London: Edward Arnold Publishers Ltd; 2004. p. 352–9.

159. Florell SR, Boucher KM, Garibotti G, et al. Population-based analysis of prog-nostic factors and survival in familial melanoma. J Clin Oncol 2005;23(28): 7168–77.

160. Hussussian CJ, Struewing JP, Goldstein AM, et al. Germline p16 mutations in familial melanoma. Nat Genet 1994;8(1):15–21.

161. Kamb A, Gruis NA, Weaver-Feldhaus J, et al. A cell cycle regulator poten-tially involved in genesis of many tumor types. Science 1994;264(5157): 436–40.

162. Ranade K, Hussussian CJ, Sikorski RS, et al. Mutations associated with familial melanoma impair p16INK4 function. Nat Genet 1995;10(1):114–6.

163. Zuo L, Weger J, Yang Q, et al. Germline mutations in the p16INK4a binding domain of CDK4 in familial melanoma. Nat Genet 1996;12(1):97–9.

164. Hayward NK. Genetics of melanoma predisposition. Oncogene 2003;22(20): 3053–62.

165. Goldstein AM, Struewing JP, Chidambaram A, et al. Genotype-phenotype rela-tionships in U.S. melanoma-prone families with CDKN2A and CDK4 mutations. J Natl Cancer Inst 2000;92(12):1006–10.

166. Soufir N, Avril MF, Chompret A, et al. Prevalence of p16 and CDK4 germline mutations in 48 melanoma-prone families in France. The French Familial Mela-noma Study Group. Hum Mol Genet 1998;7(2):209–16.

167. Molven A, Grimstvedt MB, Steine SJ, et al. A large Norwegian family with inherited malignant melanoma, multiple atypical nevi, and CDK4 mutation. Genes Chromosomes Cancer 2005;44(1):10–8.
168. Helsing P, Nymoen DA, Ariansen S, et al. Population-based prevalence of CDKN2A and CDK4 mutations in patients with multiple primary melanomas. Genes Chromosomes Cancer 2008;47(2):175–84.
169. Goldstein AM. Familial melanoma, pancreatic cancer and germline CDKN2A mutations. Hum Mutat 2004;23(6):630.
170. Eliason MJ, Larson AA, Florell SR, et al. Population-based prevalence of CDKN2A mutations in Utah melanoma families. J Invest Dermatol 2006; 126(3):660–6.
171. Kefford RF, Newton Bishop JA, Bergman W, et al. Counseling and DNA testing for individuals perceived to be genetically predisposed to melanoma: a consensus statement of the melanoma genetics consortium. J Clin Oncol 1999;17(10):3245–51.
172. Goldstein AM, Chan M, Harland M, et al. Features associated with germline CDKN2A mutations: a GenoMEL study of melanoma-prone families from three continents. J Med Genet 2007;44(2):99–106.
173. Goldstein AM, Chan M, Harland M, et al. High-risk melanoma susceptibility genes and pancreatic cancer, neural system tumors, and uveal melanoma across GenoMEL. Cancer Res 2006;66(20):9818–28.
174. Borg A, Sandberg T, Nilsson K, et al. High frequency of multiple melanomas and breast and pancreas carcinomas in CDKN2A mutation-positive melanoma families. J Natl Cancer Inst 2000;92(15):1260–6.
175. Gillanders E, Juo SH, Holland EA, et al. Localization of a novel melanoma susceptibility locus to 1p22. Am J Hum Genet 2003;73:301–13.
176. Hussein MR, Roggero E, Tuthill RJ, et al. Identification of novel deletion loci at 1p36 and 9p22-21 in melanocytic dysplastic nevi and cutaneous malignant melanomas. Arch Dermatol 2003;139(6):816–7.
177. Bishop DT, Demenais F, Goldstein AM, et al. Geographical variation in the penetrance of CDKN2A mutations for melanoma. J Natl Cancer Inst 2002;94(12): 894–903.
178. Begg CB, Orlow I, Hummer AJ, et al. Lifetime risk of melanoma in CDKN2A mutation carriers in a population-based sample. J Natl Cancer Inst 2005; 97(20):1507–15.
179. Orlow I, Begg CB, Cotignola J, et al. CDKN2A germline mutations in individuals with cutaneous malignant melanoma. J Invest Dermatol 2007;127(5): 1234–43.
180. Goldstein AM, Stacey SN, Olafsson JH, et al. CDKN2A mutations and melanoma risk in the Icelandic population. J Med Genet 2008;45(5):284–9.
181. Gerstenblith MR, Goldstein AM, Fargnoli MC, et al. Comprehensive evaluation of allele frequency differences of MC1R variants across populations. Hum Mutat 2007;28(5):495–505.
182. Rees JL. Genetics of hair and skin color. Annu Rev Genet 2003;37:67–90.
183. Raimondi S, Sera F, Gandini S, et al. MC1R variants, melanoma and red hair color phenotype: a meta-analysis. Int J Cancer 2008;122(12):2753–60.
184. Gudbjartsson DF, Sulem P, Stacey SN, et al. ASIP and TYR pigmentation variants associate with cutaneous melanoma and basal cell carcinoma. Nat Genet 2008;40(7):886–91.
185. Brown KM, Macgregor S, Montgomery GW, et al. Common sequence variants on 20q11.22 confer melanoma susceptibility. Nat Genet 2008;40(7):838–40.

186. Falchi M, Bataille V, Hayward NK, et al. Genome-wide association study identifies variants at 9p21 and 22q13 associated with development of cutaneous nevi. Nat Genet 2009;41(8):915–9.

187. Bishop DT, Demenais F, Iles MM, et al. Genome-wide association study identifies three loci associated with melanoma risk. Nat Genet 2009;41(8):920–5.

188. Chaudru V, Laud K, Avril MF, et al. Melanocortin-1 receptor (MC1R) gene variants and dysplastic nevi modify penetrance of CDKN2A mutations in French melanoma-prone pedigrees. Cancer Epidemiol Biomarkers Prev 2005;14(10): 2384–90.

189. Box NF, Duffy DL, Chen W, et al. MC1R genotype modifies risk of melanoma in families segregating CDKN2A mutations. Am J Hum Genet 2001;69(4):765–73.

190. Goldstein AM, Landi MT, Tsang S, et al. Association of MC1R variants and risk of melanoma in melanoma-prone families with CDKN2A mutations. Cancer Epidemiol Biomarkers Prev 2005;14(9):2208–12.

191. van der Velden PA, Sandkuijl LA, Bergman W, et al. Melanocortin-1 receptor variant R151C modifies melanoma risk in Dutch families with melanoma. Am J Hum Genet 2001;69(4):774–9.

192. Leachman SA, Carucci J, Kohlmann W, et al. Selection criteria for genetic assessment of patients with familial melanoma. J Am Acad Dermatol 2009; 61(4):677, e1–14.

193. Kefford R, Bishop JN, Tucker M, et al. Genetic testing for melanoma. Lancet Oncol 2002;3(11):653–4.

Endocrine Cancer Predisposition Syndromes: Hereditary Paraganglioma, Multiple Endocrine Neoplasia Type 1, Multiple Endocrine Neoplasia Type 2, and Hereditary Thyroid Cancer

Wendy S. Rubinstein, MD, PhD[a,b,*]

KEYWORDS

- Paraganglioma • Pheochromocytoma • Neoplasia
- Primary hyperparathyroidism • Medullary thyroid carcinoma
- C-cell hyperplasia • Genomic imprinting • Tumor

The hereditary paraganglioma, MEN1, MEN2, and hereditary thyroid cancer syndromes overlap to some extent, but all are clinically discernable and genetically distinct. The first 3 syndromes have been well characterized in the past 10 to 15 years following identification of their molecular underpinnings, and genetic testing plays an indispensable role in clinical management in children and adults. The physician who recognizes these syndromes and uses a multidisciplinary team approach can take advantage of valuable opportunities for early and presymptomatic diagnosis, reduction of morbidity and mortality, and avoidance of surgical misadventures. Hereditary paraganglioma is a fascinating syndrome with parent-of-origin effects and gene-environment interactions that indicate a stamp placed on the human genome by natural selection, and the syndrome sheds light on the role of mitochondria and energy

[a] Department of Medicine, University of Chicago Pritzker School of Medicine, Chicago, IL 60637, USA
[b] Division of Medical Genetics, NorthShore University HealthSystem, Evanston, IL 60201, USA
* Center for Medical Genetics, 1000 Central Street, 620, Evanston, IL 60201.
E-mail address: wrubinstein@northshore.org

Hematol Oncol Clin N Am 24 (2010) 907–937
doi:10.1016/j.hoc.2010.06.008
0889-8588/10/$ – see front matter © 2010 Elsevier Inc. All rights reserved.

metabolism in cancer. MEN1 probably has the widest pleiotropy of any hereditary cancer syndrome. MEN2 is notable for remarkably precise genotype-phenotype correlations at the level of the codon that determine timing of surgical prevention. This article delineates the clinical presentation and practical management issues and summarizes the history, gene discovery, and molecular insights for each syndrome.

The clinical recognition and description of multiple endocrine neoplasia (MEN) and its subtypes began in the 1900s.[1] The importance of managing patients and families in the context of multidisciplinary teams including genetics professionals cannot be overemphasized for MEN type 1, MEN type 2, and hereditary paraganglioma syndromes.[2–4]

HEREDITARY PARAGANGLIOMA SYNDROME

The 1933 report by Chase[5] of carotid body tumors diagnosed in 2 sisters in their 20s, 1 of whom had bilateral disease, coupled with a report in the same year of paragangliomas in 3 sisters and several publications in the following decades,[6] shed light on the hereditary nature of paragangliomas, at least in some cases. Autosomal dominant inheritance was suggested in 1949 and in subsequently reported pedigrees.[6,7] A review of 88 familial and 835 nonfamilial carotid body tumor cases in the literature showed a high rate of bilateral disease in familial (31.8%) versus sporadic (4.4% cases), and an equal sex distribution in familial cases, consistent with autosomal dominant inheritance.[8] A medical record review of 222 carotid body tumors at 12 medical centers in the United States suggested the existence of a multiple primary tumor syndrome in familial cases that manifested bilateral disease, other extra-adrenal paragangliomas, and earlier age of onset.[9] Efforts then concentrated on the collection of families for linkage mapping,[10–15] culminating in the discovery of the first hereditary paraganglioma gene, *SDHD*,[16] and candidate gene analyses soon followed,[17,18] leading more recently to predictive clinical genetic testing, a better understanding of genotype-phenotype relationships and gene-environment interactions, and important insights into the role of mitochondrial metabolism in cancer and the mechanism of parent-of-origin effects seen in the PGL1 and PGL2 syndromes.

Nonchromaffin paragangliomas are rare, occurring in about 1:30,000 to 1:100,000 individuals in the general population.[19] Carotid body tumors are associated with conditions of low oxygen tension, such as emphysema, living at high altitude, and cyanotic congenital heart disease, and cluster in low-altitude countries.[20,21]

Pathology, Anatomy, and Biochemistry

Pheochromocytomas and extra-adrenal paragangliomas are tumors derived from neural crest tissues or organs, termed paraganglia. Classification is based on anatomic considerations; lesions cannot be distinguished using histologic features. The term pheochromocytoma is reserved by the World Health Organization (WHO) for tumors that arise from chromaffin cells of the adrenal medulla, a prototypical sympathetic nervous system paraganglion.[22] Extra-adrenal paragangliomas derive from either the sympathetic nervous system or the parasympathetic nervous system. The term extra-adrenal pheochromocytoma is imprecise.

The sympathetic nervous system includes the organ of Zuckerkandl (located at the origin of the inferior mesenteric artery and involved in fetal and newborn catecholamine metabolism) as well as chromaffin cells clustered in the paravertebral chain, aortic bifurcation, kidney, liver hila, bladder, and mediastinum. The parasympathetic nervous system is distributed from the middle ear and skull base to the pelvic floor, and includes the carotid body, a tiny organ located at the carotid bifurcation, which is the major oxygen sensor. Sympathetic extra-adrenal paragangliomas are often hormonally active. Parasympathetic extra-adrenal paragangliomas are usually located in the head and neck, and only about 1% are hormonally active.[6]

Terminology for head and neck paragangliomas is varied and includes chemodectoma, carotid body, jugular, vagal, tympanic tumor, and glomus tumor. Pheochromocytomas (of the adrenal medulla) often have an adrenergic profile, whereas extra-adrenal paragangliomas (when active) typically have a noradrenergic profile. Pheochromocytomas are more typical of MEN2A, MEN2B, von Hippel-Lindau syndrome (VHL) (particularly type 2), and neurofibromatosis type 1 (NF1) than hereditary paraganglioma syndromes, but overlap exists. For example, head and neck paragangliomas are an occasional feature of MEN2, VHL, and NF1, and the hereditary paraganglioma syndromes can manifest sympathetic extra-adrenal paragangliomas and pheochromocytomas. Hereditary nonchromaffin paragangliomas are slow-growing, highly vascularized tumors, most of which are benign. The WHO defines malignancy for pheochromocytomas and extra-adrenal paragangliomas not by local invasion but as metastatic spread to distal sites (which are typically devoid of paraganglionic tissue; generally bone, liver, and lung) or clearly identifiable lymph nodes.[23] Adequately resected MEN2 pheochromocytomas do not typically recur, whereas SDHB-related tumors have about a 50% rate of metastasis.

Inheritance and Genetics

Paraganglioma families typically have an autosomal dominant pattern with age-dependent penetrance. In certain linkage groups, individuals manifesting disease inherit the trait solely through the paternal lineage, suggestive of maternal imprinting.[24] The PGL1 (SDHD) and PGL2 loci both show parent-of-origin effects consistent with maternal imprinting. Parent-of-origin effects are shown in **Fig. 1**, and have important implications for screening. A single case of an affected offspring following maternal transmission of an SDHD mutation has been reported.[25] The PGL3 (SDHC) and PGL4 (SDHB) loci follow classic autosomal dominant inheritance for tumor predisposition.

Early linkage studies mapped the PGL1 gene (later shown to be SDHD) to 11q23-qter,[10–12] PGL2 (SDHAF2/SDH5) to 11q13,[13,14] and PGL3 (SDHC) to 1q21-q23.[15] PGL4 (SDHB) maps to 1p36.1-p35. Baysal and colleagues[16] identified the first paraganglioma gene in PGL1 kindreds as SDHD, which encodes the D subunit of heterotetrameric succinate dehydrogenase (SDH; mitochondrial complex II) enzyme complex, a component of the respiratory chain and the Krebs cycle. Following this discovery, the other SDH gene subunits became prime candidates for the other genetic loci. Mutations in SDHC occur in PGL3 families[17] and mutations in SDHB in PGL4 families.[18] However, the A subunit of SDH maps to chromosome 5p15, not to the remaining PGL2 locus at 11q13. SDHA mutations are one cause of Leigh syndrome, infantile subacute necrotizing encephalopathy. SDHAF2/SDH5 assignment to the PGL2 locus was accomplished in yeast models[26] and maps to 11q13, the PGL2 locus.

Clinical Presentation and Diagnosis

Paragangliomas of the head and neck typically present as slowly growing masses that can be asymptomatic for years or even decades.[6] On careful questioning or

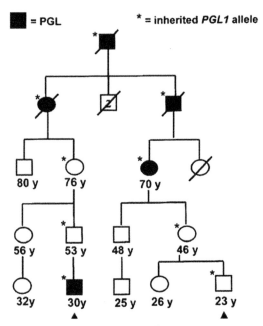

Fig. 1. Parent-of-origin effect in *SDHD*. *From* Drovdlic CM, Myers EN, Peters JA, et al. Proportion of heritable paraganglioma cases and associated clinical characteristics. Laryngoscope 2001;111:1823; with permission.

evaluation, what may seem to be an isolated case can lead to unmasking of a family history of neck mass or other related growth. About 10% of patients present with cranial nerve palsy, most commonly involving the vagal nerve. Left untreated, about 75% of patients develop cranial nerve palsies, providing the potential for presymptomatic diagnosis, intervention, and prevention of serious morbidity. Symptoms include tinnitus, hearing loss, hoarseness, vocal cord paralysis, cough, aspiration, dysphagia, pharyngeal fullness, facial paralysis, problems moving the tongue, or pain. Vagal paragangliomas are located behind the ramus of the mandible and can project into the oropharynx.[6] Magnetic resonance imaging (MRI) is diagnostic based on tumor vascularity and location, characterizes lesions for surgical planning, and assesses multifocality. Incisional biopsy of the highly vascular head and neck paragangliomas that are intimate with neurovascular structures is dangerous, usually unnecessary for diagnosis, and should be avoided; however, when a radiologic diagnosis is unclear, ultrasound-guided fine-needle aspiration can be used.[6]

Pheochromocytomas and functional extra-adrenal paragangliomas may present with the classic triad of episodic headache, diaphoresis, and tachycardia, or with other symptoms. More typically, the classic triad is not seen.[27] Persistent hypertension and normotension are also consistent with the diagnosis of a functional chromaffin cell tumor. Diagnosis of pheochromocytoma can be performed through biochemical testing and localization by imaging.[27,28] Biochemical testing entails measurement of either 24-hour urine catecholamines and metanephrines or fractionated plasma-free metanephrines; the rationale for choosing one rather than the other has been discussed.[27,28]

Genotype-Phenotype Correlations, Penetrance, and Expressivity

SDHD and *SDHB* mutations are more often associated with a positive family history than *SDHC* mutations.[19] *SDHC* mutation carriers have a lower risk of pheochromocytoma, multifocality, and malignant transformation.[29] The median age of onset for *SDHC* is slightly higher than for *SDHD* and *SDHB* and the earliest tumor reported in *SDHC* is at 13 years of age.[19] Age at diagnosis of the first tumor often occurs by age 10 years for *SDHB* (earliest reported age, 7 years) and penetrance is 25% by age 20 years. Age less than 10 years for a first tumor is rarer, but not unknown for *SDHD* (earliest reported age, 5 years) and penetrance is 15% by age 20 years.[19] The predominant phenotype for *SDHB* is extra-adrenal paraganglioma, and renal cell carcinoma is an important sign of *SDHB*.[19] *SDHB* is associated with a 41% prevalence of malignant tumors, which may be related to a trend toward malignancy in extra-adrenal paragangliomas.[19] The more severe phenotype of *SDHB* may be related to its role as part of the catalytic complex.[30] Carriers with nonsense/splicing mutations developed symptoms 8.5 years earlier than missense mutation carriers, and a trend was seen toward pheochromocytoma development with nonsense mutations.[31] Altitude correlates with tumor type.[31] Mutations in the 5′ portion of the *SDHD* gene are correlated with pheochromocytoma, whereas 3′ mutations are associated with head and neck paragangliomas.[32]

Several reports indicate that renal cell carcinoma is a component tumor for *SDHB*[19,30,33] and renal oncocytoma has also been reported.[19] Thyroid cancer,[9] in particular the papillary type,[30] might be part of the *SDH* gene spectrum, but this is not well established. In a large fraction of cases, the Carney-Stratakis syndrome (dyad) of paragangliomas and gastrointestinal stromal tumors (GIST) can be attributed to germline *SDHD*, *SDHB*, and *SDHC* mutations.[19] *SDHD* and *SDHB* germline mutations or variants have been found in patients with a Cowden syndrome–like presentation negative for *PTEN* mutations.[34] In these patients, the tumor spectrum seems to include breast, papillary thyroid, and renal cancers.

Diagnostic Criteria for Molecular Genetic Testing

There is an emerging consensus of opinion that all patients with a single head and neck paraganglioma,[35,36] extra-adrenal paraganglioma,[37] or nonsyndromic pheochromocytoma[38] should undergo molecular genetic testing. Although classic red flags for hereditary cancer still apply, the difficulty arises in using these features to accurately distinguish truly sporadic (ie, non–germline mutated) cases of head and neck paragangliomas from single tumors that have a hereditary basis. Functional paragangliomas that seem to be sporadic have a ~12% rate of mutation detection rate when testing *VHL*, *RET*, *SDHD*, and *SDHB*,[37] and nonsyndromic pheochromocytoma has a 24% mutation detection rate for *RET*, *VHL*, *SDHD*, and *SDHB*,[38] with *SDHD*[39] and *SDHB* as important contributors.

Regarding single head and neck paragangliomas, individuals with any hereditary features should undergo a genetic workup; that would include any individual with bilateral or multifocal head and neck paragangliomas, a single extra-adrenal paraganglioma in combination with a pheochromocytoma, or early-onset disease. Male gender can be considered an indication for testing. Sporadic head and neck paragangliomas occur more commonly in women, and a large study of head and neck paragangliomas found a 53% mutation detection rate for *SDHD*, *SDHB*, and *SDHC* testing in men.[40] Malignant paraganglioma is also suggestive of a genetic cause,[40] and the prevalence of an underlying *SDHB* mutation is not affect by a syndromic presentation or positive family history.[41]

Some studies have demonstrated a high genetic contribution to seemingly sporadic extra-adrenal paragangliomas, indicating that there would be many missed cases. Parent-of-origin effects and reduced penetrance contribute to a low specificity of family history, which may be compounded by lack of family history information, unrecognized disease in relatives, and lifelong hereditary risk that extends into the diagnosis age range of sporadic tumors. A decade ago, common wisdom held that only about 10% of head and neck paragangliomas (outside the Netherlands, where the rate is much higher because of founder mutations) had a genetic cause, but soon after the identification of the SDH genes a significantly higher hereditary proportion was better appreciated.[30,42,43] SDHD, SDHB, and SDHC mutations contribute to 9.5% of apparently sporadic, 71.4% of multiple cases, and 87.8% of familial head and neck paragangliomas.[19] A genetic workup should thus be considered for most, if not all, head and neck paragangliomas[35,36] and all malignant pheochromocytomas and extra-adrenal paragangliomas.[41]

Differential Diagnosis

The VHL, MEN2, and NF1 syndromes each have anecdotal reports of head and neck paragangliomas. Paraganglioma, gastric stromal tumor, and pulmonary chondroma comprise the Carney triad, which has an unknown genetic basis.[44] NF1 should be recognizable as a genodermatosis, and VHL and MEN2 are usually evident based on family history or clinical features. After exclusion of SDH genes, only about 0.5% of patients with head and neck paragangliomas have VHL mutations, whereas RET and NF1 mutations are rarer still, suggesting that VHL and RET testing could be foregone.[45]

Patients with a single nonsyndromic pheochromocytoma or extra-adrenal paraganglioma can be stratified for testing (eg, SDH gene testing for head and neck paraganglioma); SDHB initially for thoracic-retroperitoneal paraganglioma, and VHL/SDHB/RET algorithms for pheochromocytoma.[36] Renal cell carcinoma in combination with an extra-adrenal paraganglioma could suggest VHL, but, in the absence of other VHL features in the proband and family, SDHB testing could first be considered.

Diagnostics

DNA sequence analysis and deletion/duplication analysis are available on a clinical basis for SDHD, SDHB, and SDHC, but not SDHAF2/SDH5. The proportion of mutation types has been well summarized[19]; about 3% to 7% comprise large deletions that require analysis by multiplex ligation-dependent probe amplification (MLPA) or similar methods. Sensitivity of molecular genetic testing is probably about 70% to 90%. A study employing SDHB immunohistochemical (IHC) staining in 220 pheochromocytomas and paragangliomas showed that 6 tumors were SDHB IHC negative among 53 tumors without any detectable germline mutation, and 5 of the 6 cases had syndromic features. In the larger series, 102 tumors had detectable SDH mutations. This suggests a mutation detection rate of about 94% (102/108) for SDH gene testing using DNA sequencing and MLPA methodologies.

Because testing for numerous genes for head and neck paragangliomas is costly ($2700 for SDHD, SDHB, and SDHC in the United States); prioritization of genetic testing should be based on first-step predictors of positive family history, preceding pheochromocytoma, multiple tumors, malignant tumors, age 40 years or younger, and male gender which have a predicted sensitivity of 92% and predicted specificity of 94%.[40] An approach to case stratification using IHC staining of SDHB in formalin-fixed paraffin-embedded pheochromocytomas and paragangliomas, analogous to tumor testing of mismatch repair proteins to identify Lynch syndrome, has also been presented.[46]

Prognosis and Management

Treatment of head and neck paragangliomas is mainly surgical, but watchful waiting or radiation therapy may be the best approach for certain tumors such as slowly growing vagal and jugular fossa paragangliomas in older patients in whom surgery may be problematic. Because multicentricity is common, debility from cranial neuropathy is greatly magnified, thus all patients, including those with a single tumor, must undergo preoperative MRI of the head and neck, which also guides surgical planning.[6] It is particularly important to spare at least 1 vagal nerve and its laryngeal branches. Although functional head and neck paragangliomas are rare, preoperative biochemical screening for catecholamines and metanephrines is strongly advised to avoid the catastrophic cardiovascular collapse that can be precipitated by surgery. Biochemical screening also assesses unrecognized or asymptomatic pheochromocytomas and functioning extra-adrenal paragangliomas that occur at significant rates with all of the *SDH* syndromes.

For patients with pheochromocytomas and extra-adrenal paragangliomas, preoperative achievement of β-adrenergic blockade and maintenance of adequate volume status, as well as intraoperative monitoring and surgical approaches, are detailed elsewhere.[4,27,47] Surgical treatment of pheochromocytoma is usually curative, but follow-up testing is needed. Pheochromocytomas and extra-adrenal paragangliomas have an overall 5% to 15% rate of malignancy, but the risk of extra-adrenal paragangliomas and malignancy is higher in *SDHB* carriers.[41] *SDHB* mutation has been found to be an independent predictor of mortality for malignant pheochromocytoma or extra-adrenal paraganglioma (relative risk 2.7).[41] It has been suggested that *SDHB* testing be performed in all patients with malignant pheochromocytomas, and that carriers be more aggressively managed using a combination of surgery, metabolic radiotherapy (eg, ^{131}I-labeled *m*-iodobenzylguanidine or radioactive somatostatin analogues) with consideration of chemotherapy.[41] Further details on diagnosis, localization, and treatment have been summarized elsewhere.[48,49]

There has been no consensus conference outlining screening recommendations for the hereditary paraganglioma syndromes. One regimen is for head and neck MRI every 2 years beginning at age 16 years, along with urinary screening for pheochromocytoma every 2 years.[50] Another[30] recommends annual MRI of the neck, thorax, and abdomen/pelvis with [[18F]]fluorodopa or [[18F]]fluorodopamine positron emission tomography ([18F] DOPA PET) as a possible alternative, coupled with screening for catecholamines and metanephrines. Scans can also be performed with [111]indium pentetreotide scintigraphy, a somatostatin analogue that binds to somatostatin type 2 receptors usually present in paragangliomas, coupled to a radioisotope.[51] This method can detect small (5–10 mm) lesions with high accuracy. [18F] DOPA PET has higher sensitivity than MRI for lesions of less than 1 cm, and whole-body screening is a possible advantage, especially for *SDHB* carriers.[51] The 3.4% prevalence of renal malignancy in *SDHB*[19] opens the possibility for screening, particularly in families with this presentation. Age of onset may extend to less than 10 years, especially for *SDHB*. Genetic testing has been recommended to begin as early as age 5 to 10 years in *SDH* families, with annual screening in mutation carriers.[52] The later age of onset seen across case series of *SDHC* carriers[19] suggests that genetic testing and screening could be delayed.

Genetic Function and Genomic Imprinting

Mitochondrial complex II, the only complex in the respiratory chain completely encoded by nuclear genes, is a tetrameric protein encoded by 3 paraganglioma genes, *SDHD*, *SDHB*, and *SDHC*, and a fourth gene, *SDHA*, which is a cause of Leigh syndrome.[53] The recently discovered paraganglioma gene, *SDHAF2/SDH5*, is required for flavination of the complex, as shown in yeast.[26] Downregulation of SDH results in induction of the hypoxic pathway, and *SDH* has been proposed as an oxygen sensor, perhaps through the production of reactive oxygen species.[54,55] PGL1 (*SDHD*) and, apparently, PGL2 (*SDHAF2/SDH5*) kindreds both show parent-of-origin effects, whereby carrier offspring of carrier fathers, but not carrier mothers, manifest disease with age-dependent penetrance liabilities. This observation was noted before linkage or cloning of the underlying genes[10,14,24] and has held true with more direct evidence from mutational analysis,[56] save for 1 reported exception.[25]

The molecular basis of this parent-of-origin effect remains uncertain but models have been proposed.[16,53,56,57] One possibility is that the *SDHD* gene is not imprinted, but that selective somatic loss of the maternal wild-type *SDHD* allele is driven by loss of gene(s) at 11p15 that undergo imprinting. This would constitute a single hit, leaving only paternally imprinted 11p15 gene(s) that are in phase with paternally inherited *SDHD* mutations, thereby mimicking *SDHD* imprinting.[57] If PGL2 is more convincingly shown to have a parent-of-origin effect, the same mechanism could be used to explain this effect given its location on chromosome 11.[57]

The role of these genes in neoplasia is also being studied. *SDHD* was the first tumor suppressor gene identified that encodes a protein involved in mitochondrial metabolism. A second example of a tumor suppressor gene with a role in mitochondrial metabolism is the fumarate hydratase (*FH*) gene.[58] Cancer cells may gain a selective advantage by diverting glucose away from energy production and toward the production of macromolecules used to generate fatty acids, nonessential amino acids, and nucleotides[59] (consistent with the Warburg effect first observed in 1924).

MEN1
History

Wermer[60] reported the familial aggregation of pituitary tumors, multiple islet cell adenomas, diffuse parathyroid hyperplasia, and peptic ulcer disease, combinations of which had previously been reported only in individual patients. Separately, Zollinger and Ellison[61] reported an association of primary peptic ulcerations of the jejunum and other unusual locations, unremitting gastric acid secretion, and non–insulin producing pancreatic islet cell tumors. Later, these clinical presentations were recognized as representing a spectrum of disease common to 1 syndrome,[62] MEN1.

MEN1 is rare, occurring in up to 1 in 25,000 individuals based on autopsy data, although biochemical data suggest a prevalence closer to 10 to 175 per 100,000 individuals.[63] Inheritance is autosomal dominant with equal sex distribution. MEN1 typically becomes clinically apparent in the 30s and 40s, usually as a result of symptomatic primary hyperparathyroidism. The syndrome is occasionally manifested in childhood and the diagnosis is sometimes delayed until later adulthood.

Clinical Characteristics

MEN1 is characterized by an autosomal dominant predisposition to develop endocrine tumors of the parathyroids, gastroenteropancreatic (GEP) tract, and pituitary, as well as carcinoid tumors, adrenocortical tumors, specific nonendocrine tumors, and particular skin manifestations. About 25 unique growths are associated with the syndrome, many of which are hormonally active, resulting in a plethora of clinical features. Parathyroid hyperplasia is the most common manifestation, and primary hyperparathyroidism is usually the heralding feature of MEN1. Primary hyperparathyroidism emerges in the early 20s, about 30 years earlier than sporadic hyperparathyroidism, and penetrance is 80% to 100% by age 40 years.[64,65] Tumors of the anterior pituitary occur in 10% to 60% of cases,[64] including prolactinomas (the most common), other functional growths secreting growth hormone, TSH, and adrenocorticotropic hormone (ACTH), as well as nonfunctional pituitary tumors.

GEP tumors are synonymous with neuroendocrine tumors, as per the WHO,[66] and develop from endocrine cells in the pancreatic islets and the duodenal and gastric mucosa. Islet cell tumors are typically well differentiated and most are nonfunctioning tumors that nonetheless have malignant potential and pose crucial diagnostic and treatment dilemmas that are discussed later. Functioning islet cell tumors include gastrinomas (a cause of hypergastrinism, known as Zollinger-Ellison syndrome[61]), which affect about 50% of individuals; insulinomas, which affect 10% to 35% of MEN1 patients; glucaconomas; somatostatinomas; VIPomas; and GRFomas. Rarely, endocrine GEP tumors arise in other foregut locations including the first jejunal loop or biliary tract.[67]

MEN1 carcinoid tumors (also neuroendocrine tumors as per the WHO classification[66]) arise mainly in the foregut. Most MEN1 carcinoids are nonfunctional and thus do not result in the carcinoid syndrome.[65] Gastric carcinoids affect about 10% of MEN1 patients; bronchial and thymic carcinoids each affect about 2% of carriers.[65] Adrenocortical tumors affect 20% to 40% of carriers but only rarely are functional.[65] Malignant adrenocortical carcinomas are rare.[65] Central nervous system tumors include meningiomas and, rarely, ependymomas.

Skin manifestations affect most MEN1 carriers and include facial angiofibromas, collagenomas, café au lait macules, as well as lipomas of the skin and viscera.[65]

Neuroendocrine tumors have been distinguished from neuroendocrine carcinoma.[66] The neuroendocrine tumors derive from the system of disseminated neuroendocrine cells, which have been termed clear cells or APUD cells (APUDomas), reflecting their underlying biochemistry of amine precursor uptake and decarboxylation, and many of these tumors are still referred to as carcinoids.[66] Many, but not all, sporadic carcinoids produce serotonin, which leads to the carcinoid syndrome (flushing, diarrhea, valvular heart lesions, abdominal cramping, and other symptoms) and the noninterchangeability of these terms has led to some confusion. MEN1 carcinoids rarely produce the carcinoid syndrome.

Familial MEN1 is defined as at least 1 MEN1 case plus at least 1 first-degree relative with at least 1 of the 3 main endocrine manifestations.[64] In the Netherlands, 5 categories are used: (1) parathyroid hyperplasia or adenomas; (2) neuroendocrine tumor of the pancreas (pancreatic endocrine tumor); (3) neuroendocrine tumor of the gastrointestinal tract, thymus, or bronchus; (4) pituitary abnormalities; and (5) adrenal hyperplasia or adenomas.[68] In this schema, patients who meet at least 3 of 5 criteria have MEN1, and patients in an MEN1 family are affected if they have manifested at least 1 of the features.

Specific Clinical Manifestations of MEN1

The penetrance of hyperparathyroidism in MEN1 carriers, usually detected by increased calcium levels, is generally cited as approaching 100% by age 50 years.[64] This has been interpreted to mean that lack of primary hyperparathyroidism by middle adulthood rules out a diagnosis of MEN1 and obviates further assessment. However, lower penetrance has been documented, for example, in a regional study that found hyperparathyroidism in only 73% of MEN1 patients by age 50 years and 83% by age 70 years.[69]

Gastrinoma is diagnosed by high serum gastrin and increased gastric acid output. Patients may present with severe peptic ulcer disease and its complications. Penetrance is about 50% by age 50 years, and patients generally have multiple, small tumors with a high rate of metastasis.[65] The classic presentation of glucagonoma includes skin rash, glucose intolerance, and hypoaminoacidemia. Insulinomas are associated with intractable hypoglycemia that can elicit a catecholamine response and cause neurologic symptoms.

Pituitary tumors

MEN1 pituitary tumors involve the anterior pituitary and are typically larger than sporadic pituitary tumors. Macroadenoma is seen in 85% of MEN1 cases, compared with 42% of sporadic cases.[70] Multiple pituitary tumors can occur but are not common for MEN1. The usual age of onset for MEN1 pituitary disease is 30 to 35 years, similar to sporadic pituitary tumors, with a similar hormone profile (prolactin [62%], growth hormone [9%], ACTH [4%], cosecreting tumors most commonly with prolactin [10%], and nonsecreting tumors [15%]).[70] The Burin variant of MEN1, seen in several Newfoundland Canadian families, includes a combination of primary hyperparathyroidism, high penetrance of prolactinoma, and low penetrance of gastrinoma.[71]

Carcinoid tumors

Familial clustering of carcinoid tumors has been reported in some families, but germline MEN1 mutations are not evident with this presentation.[70] Although most sporadic carcinoids arise in the midgut or hindgut, MEN1-associated carcinoids usually arise in the foregut, an atypical location[70] that should prompt an MEN1 evaluation. In contrast to sporadic carcinoids, most MEN1 carcinoids are nonfunctional and are not associated with the carcinoid syndrome. The pathologic classification of most gastric carcinoids is type 2 gastric enterochromaffin–like cell carcinoids.

MEN1-related thymic carcinoids have a male predominance[72] and account for about a quarter of all thymic carcinoids. In contrast, bronchial carcinoids have a female predominance. MEN1-related thymic carcinoids have a penetrance of about 2.6% by age 40 years,[72,73] are insidious, are not associated with Cushing or carcinoid syndrome, can be detected with octreotide scanning, and seem to be more clinically aggressive than sporadic thymic carcinoids.[73] There is evidence for clustering of thymic carcinoid in close relatives,[72,73] and for an association between smoking and thoracic carcinoids.[74]

Skin manifestations

Skin manifestations include collagenomas[75] and multiple facial angiofibromas,[76] similar to those seen in tuberous sclerosis but in different locations (ie, the upper lip and vermillion border of the lip), locations that are usually spared in tuberous sclerosis.[65] Collagenomas (72%), café au lait macules (38%), lipomas (34%), confettilike hypopigmented macules (6%), and multiple gingival papules (6%) were seen in this series.[76]

Differential Diagnosis

Primary hyperparathyroidism is seen in 2% to 4% of the general population.[77] The genetic differential diagnosis of familial hyperparathyroidism includes MEN1, MEN2, familial isolated hyperparathyroidism, familial hypocalciuric hypercalcemia, and the hyperparathyroidism-jaw tumor syndrome.[78] Multiglandular parathyroid involvement is typical of MEN1 and familial isolated hyperparathyroidism, whereas sporadic hyperparathyroidism typically exhibits parathyroid adenoma. Hyperparathyroidism is the most common presenting feature of MEN1 and occurs about 3 decades earlier than sporadic cases, at about age 20 to 25 years.[64] However, diagnosis of hyperparathyroidism in MEN1 can be delayed,[69] perhaps through inadequate family history taking, unfamiliarity with the syndrome, or splintered care among subspecialists.

MEN1 mutations are found in about 23% of familial isolated hyperparathyroidism, but the genetic basis in most families remains unexplained.[79] The differential diagnosis also includes an overlap syndrome termed MEN4 (Online Mendelian Inheritance in Man [OMIM] 610755), involving pituitary adenomas with acromegaly and parathyroid hyperplasia caused by germline *CDKN1B* (p27Kip1) mutation.[80] However this seems to be a rare cause of mutation-negative MEN1 families.[81,82] About 20% to 30% of patients with the Zollinger-Ellison syndrome have MEN1. The percentage of patients with GRFomas who have MEN1 is high, about 33%, whereas patients with other pancreatic neuroendocrine tumors constitute less than 15%.[83] Infertility may be part of the homozygous (or compound heterozygous) MEN1 state.[84]

Genetics

MEN1 was mapped via genetic linkage studies to 11q13,[85–87] with further narrowing of the candidate region using closely linked markers[88] and haplotype analysis in affected families.[89] No evidence of locus heterogeneity was found. Tumor tissue studies showing loss of heterozygosity at 11q13 in malignancies from MEN1 patients, such as insulinomas and parathyroid tumors, and in sporadic MEN1-associated tumors such as gastrinomas, provided additional mapping data.[85,87,90,91] Murine and human comparative mapping analysis[92] also contributed toward MEN1 gene localization. Further fine-scale mapping, including high-resolution radiation hybrid mapping,[93,94] led to the ability to perform highly accurate predictive testing using linkage markers, opening the door for the first time to avoidance of invasive biochemical testing for noncarriers.[95]

A precisely ordered transcript map for the 2.8-Mb region containing the MEN1 locus was created,[96] providing 33 additional gene candidates. In 1997, Chandrasekharappa and colleagues[97] reported the positional cloning of the MEN1 gene. Independent confirmation was provided by the European Consortium on MEN1.[98] Additional large studies of unrelated MEN1 probands[71,99–101] identified a variety of *MENIN* mutations in most, but not all, families with MEN1, a prevalence of truncating mutations consistent with tumor suppressor activity, commonly observed absence of germline mutations in familial hyperparathyroidism[71,100] and familial acromegaly,[100] occasional de novo germline mutations,[71,100] and lack of genotype-phenotype correlations.[99,101,102] A compilation of 1336 mutations reported as of 2008 confirmed a general lack of genotype-phenotype correlations (familial isolated hyperparathyroidism and the Burin MEN1 variant are notable exceptions), and reported that more than 70% are truncating mutations that are generally distributed across the genomic sequence.[103]

Diagnostics

Molecular genetic testing for MEN1

Genetic testing is recommended in several situations[64]: diagnostic testing in individuals who meet clinical criteria for sporadic or familial MEN1 or in individuals who do not meet formal criteria but are suspicious for MEN1, and presymptomatic or confirmatory testing in relatives of a known MEN1 mutation carrier. Presymptomatic carriers should undergo age-appropriate screening, whereas those without a familial mutation (and their children) can avoid expensive, potentially distressing lifelong screening. MEN1 genetic testing is appropriate in children because it clarifies whether screening is needed. Prenatal diagnosis is feasible in families with a known mutation.

Sensitivity of DNA sequencing is about 70% to 90% in probands with familial MEN1 syndrome. Analysis of gene deletions and gross rearrangements, detectable through gene dosage methods or Southern blot analysis, adds an additional sensitivity of about 1% to 3%. The rate of positive genetic test results falls off to about 65% in simplex cases without familial features, and is fewer still for those with single MEN1-related features. A clinical laboratory-based study found a ~70% rate of detectable mutations in cases with parathyroid and islet cell tumors (irrespective of family history).[104] A lower mutation detection rate of 25% was found in cases with parathyroid and pituitary tumors (without pancreatic islet cell tumors); among 10 such sporadic cases (both tumors in a single individual; positive family history not reported), no mutations were found. The mutation detection rate was lowest for parathyroid-only cases. MEN1 mutations are identified in 20% to 25% of familial isolated hyperparathyroidism and seem to be more commonly associated with missense mutations than in classically affected MEN1 kindreds.[105,106]

At least 10% of MEN1 cases are believed to arise de novo.[65] Somatic mosaicism may explain the lower mutation detection rate seen in some index cases with multiple MEN1 tumors but no family history of MEN1.[104] As in neurofibromatosis type 2, a germline mutation in de novo cases can be missed on leukocyte DNA analysis but, in theory, may be detectable in tumor analysis and in offspring.[107]

Preoperative recognition of MEN1 significantly reduces the rate of surgical failures for parathyroidectomy.[108] A preoperative 6-question panel was superior to chart-based clinical history for identifying such patients who were often young, male, and found to have parathyroid hyperplasia at the time of surgery.[109] Prophylactic thymectomy can be planned at the same time only if the MEN1 syndrome is recognized preoperatively; however, not all authorities agree on the addition of this surgery to parathyroidectomy.[108,110] A sustained successful postsurgical outcome requires astute recognition of the syndrome and prospective screening.[111] A retrospective study of 1838 members of 34 MEN1 kindreds found that almost half of deaths in carriers were MEN1 related, chiefly from malignancies, occurring at an earlier median age of 47 years,[112] with other risks of premature death documented in other studies,[113,114] whereas a Finnish historical study[115] showed no differences in age of death for obligate heterozygotes compared with controls. The effect of presymptomatic genetic diagnosis relies heavily on clinical interventions, which are continuously developing. Nonetheless, the effect of genetic screening in those without the familial mutation cannot be overemphasized, because those individuals (and their offspring) can forgo burdensome screening tests.

Screening

The systematic evaluation of asymptomatic children who carry MEN1 mutations reveals a high prevalence of MEN1 growths, including primary hyperparathyroidism, nonfunctioning pancreatic neuroendocrine tumors, and pituitary microadenomas.[116] MEN1 carriers have occasionally been clinically affected as children; for example, a 5 year old with a pituitary macroadenoma secreting prolactin and growth hormone, insulinoma at age 5 years, parathyroid adenoma with hyperparathyroidism at age 8 years,[70,116] and thymic NET at age 16 years.[72] MEN1-related mortality in childhood is believed to be low, and screening is aimed at reducing morbidity. The age at which to initiate screening is based on earliest observation of the relevant disease manifestation. Annual biochemical testing with serum calcium and parathyroid hormone should be initiated by age 8 years.[64] Beginning at age 5 years, individuals should undergo annual prolactin and insulin growth factor (IGF)-I testing, and head MRI every 3 years. Beginning at age 5 years, individuals should undergo fasting glucose and insulin levels. Beginning at age 20 years, testing should be done annually for chromogranin-A, glucagon, and proinsulin. Imaging should be done every 3 years using ^{111}In-diethylenetriaminepentaacetic acid (DTPA) octreotide scan, computerized tomography (CT), or MRI. Beginning at age 20 years, annual biochemical testing should include gastrin level measurements. If gastrin levels are high, gastric acid output should be measured. Secretin-stimulated gastrin testing is measured if gastrin or gastric acid output is high. No biochemical testing is available for early detection of carcinoid tumors. CT is recommended every 3 years to screen for foregut carcinoid.[64] Octreotide scanning can detect thymic carcinoids and has been suggested for MEN1 carriers, along with chest CT or MRI.[73] Clustering within families suggests that particular attention should be paid to screening in these kindreds.[72]

The surgical approach to treating MEN1 primary hyperparathyroidism is subtotal parathyroidectomy or total parathyroidectomy with nondominant forearm autotransplantation of parathyroid tissue (or cryopreservation for subsequent autografting). Cervical thymectomy may be performed concurrently as a prophylactic surgery. The surgical management of gastrinoma has been controversial.[117] Surgery for patients with sporadic and MEN1-associated Zollinger-Ellison syndrome can reduce the rate of hepatic metastasis, implying a survival benefit.[118] There is now evidence that long-term survival in MEN1 patients with gastrinoma can be improved through surgery.[117] Remaining controversies about the potential for cure and the role of the Whipple procedure are well described.[119] Surgery is curative for most insulinomas, chiefly through enucleation but also distal pancreatectomy or pancreaticoduodenectomy for large or malignant tumors.[119] Medical management of other functional, non–Zollinger-Ellison syndrome tumors is available (eg, somatostatin analogues such as octreotide and peptide receptor radionuclide therapy).[120] These tumors merit surgical exploration and can frequently be cured.[118] Prophylactic thymectomy during subtotal or total parathyroidectomy has been proposed as a way to reduce the risk of developing thymic carcinoid, particularly given its aggressive nature, and to reduce the risks of recurrent hyperparathyroidism following surgery.[73] Avoidance of tobacco smoking and exposure to secondhand smoke is a practical approach given the suggestion that thymic carcinoid may be smoking related.[74] There is no consensus on how to treat MEN1-related adrenal cortical tumors, but functional tumors should be resected.[64]

Gene Function

The MEN1 gene has long been recognized as a tumor suppressor gene based on loss of the wild-type allele in MEN1-related tumors and the autosomal dominant tumor predisposition pattern seen in families. The MEN1 gene product, menin, is a nuclear protein with tumor suppressor functions and also plays a role in maintaining DNA stability and gene regulation.[121,122] Menin has the unique property of promoting oncogenesis in the hematopoietic lineage but suppressing tumorigenesis in the endocrine lineage.[123]

MEN2
History

Syndromic descriptions of MEN2 were reported in the 1960s, involving pheochromocytoma and medullary thyroid carcinoma (MTC).[124,125] A dozen cases of mucosal neuroma syndrome, now known as MEN type 2B, had been reported at that time. MEN2 has an estimated prevalence of roughly 2.5 per 100,000. One of the major manifestations, MTC, accounts for about 5% of thyroid carcinomas.[126]

Clinical Characteristics and Classification

MEN2 encompasses 3 syndromes, MEN2A, MEN2B, and familial medullary thyroid cancer (FMTC). All are autosomal dominant disorders and attributable to germline mutations in the *RET* gene. The MEN2A syndrome (initially called Sipple syndrome), accounts for more than 75% of MEN2 and is characterized by MTC affecting 90% of adult mutation carriers, pheochromocytoma in 50%, and primary parathyroid hyperplasia in 20% to 30%.[64] MEN2B (initially called mucosal neuroma syndrome or Wagenmann-Froboese syndrome[127]) is characterized by very early-onset, clinically aggressive MTC, pheochromocytoma, but not primary parathyroid hyperplasia. MEN2B patients show a Marfanoid habitus and manifest mucosal neuromas of the lips and tongue as well as intestinal ganglioneuromas. FMTC is similar to MEN2A with a narrowed expressivity limited to MTC only.

Diagnostic Criteria

The diagnostic criteria for MEN2A are the presence of MTC, pheochromocytoma, and primary hyperparathyroidism and a germline *RET* gene mutation. The mutation detection rate is about 95%, thus few families present a diagnostic dilemma when fewer than 3 clinical features are present. In cases in which only 1 or 2 clinical features are present, the diagnosis can be made either when a first-degree relative shows MEN2A features or a *RET* mutation is identified. At a minimum, the diagnosis can be made when 2 clinical features are present, even when an autosomal dominant pattern is not evident and a *RET* mutation has not been demonstrated.[128]

FMTC is, by definition, phenotypically limited to MTC,[129] but the phenotype could emerge over time and overlap with MEN2A, especially in small families. The penetrance of MTC in FMTC may be lower, and the age of onset higher, than in MEN2A. Stringent criteria are applied so as not to misconstrue an MEN2A family for an FMTC family, thereby missing opportunities to manage pheochromocytoma. FMTC may be diagnosed when there are more than 10 carriers in the kindred, multiple carriers, or affected members more than 50 years of age, and an adequate medical history has been elicited, particularly in older members.[64]

Specific Clinical Manifestations of MEN2

MTC is the first clinical manifestation in most MEN2 kindreds because of its high penetrance and typically early age of onset.[64] All patients with MEN2 develop diffuse, premalignant C-cell hyperplasia involving the parafollicular cells of the thyroid, which are of neural crest origin. Not all C-cell hyperplasia is caused by germline *RET* mutations.[130] About 15% of patients present with aggressive MTCs that are associated with hoarseness, dysphagia, and shortness of breath.[131] Ectopic production of ACTH and Cushing syndrome is occasionally seen.[131] Distant metastatic spread to liver, lung, and bone is seen in 12% to 15% of patients and is associated with diarrhea and facial flushing caused by calcitonin production. Patients with MEN2B may have gastrointestinal dysmotility from intestinal ganglioneuromatosis, which can be compounded by calcitonin and other humoral factors produced by MTC.[64] About 50% of MEN2A and MEN2B patients develop pheochromocytoma. Bilateral disease is common, but extra-adrenal paragangliomas and metastatic pheochromocytoma are rare in MEN2. Diffuse medullary disease of the adrenals is typical of MEN2 and less common in VHL disease. A genotype-phenotype correlation is seen between mutations in specific codons and age-dependent penetrance of pheochromocytoma, which can be used to guide screening recommendations.[132]

Patients with MEN2A have a 20% to 30% lifetime penetrance of multiglandular parathyroid hyperplasia, and there is a close association with mutations in codon 634.[133] MEN2A carriers have a milder form of primary hyperparathyroidism than MEN1 carriers.[64] The clinical presentation of primary hyperparathyroidism was discussed earlier.

Rare kindreds with MEN2A or FMTC develop cutaneous lichen amyloidosis, involving keratin (not calcitonin) deposition.[134,135] The association is seen with mutations in codon 634, involving about a third of such patients. A neurologic pruritis of the upper back can begin in infancy and can precede (and may be causative of) cutaneous lichen amyloidosis.[136]

Hirschsprung disease

Hirschsprung disease involves a congenital absence of enteric innervation, which can vary in the amount of terminal bowel that is affected. MEN2A and FMTC may be seen in association with Hirschsprung disease.[137] Almost half of familial Hirschsprung disease is attributable to inactivating mutations in the RET proto-oncogene (90% per linkage studies) and up to a third of sporadic Hirschsprung disease is caused by somatic RET mutations.[64,138] RET mutations are more highly penetrant for Hirschsprung disease in men than women.[139]

Mutations in exon 10 (including activating mutations) are typical of MEN2-associated Hirschsprung disease.[128] The C620 mutation, known as the Janus mutation (the Roman god of doorways looking in both directions), accounts for only 12% of mutations associated with MTC, but 50% of germline RET mutations seen in Hirschsprung disease.[138] Exon 10 RET mutation analysis is indicated for all individuals with Hirschsprung disease,[64,128] particularly because a high rate of de novo RET mutation is seen in sporadic cases of Hirschsprung disease.[139] Patients who have Hirschsprung disease with MEN2 should be managed accordingly.[140]

Papillary thyroid cancer

The observation of papillary thyroid cancer in 9% of patients with mutations in RET exons 13 and 14 has been interpreted as being due to chance.[128] Somatic rearrangements that align the RET tyrosine kinase domain with other genes, creating chimeric oncogenes, are found in about 40% of cases of papillary thyroid carcinoma.[141]

Genetics

Most MTC cases are nonhereditary, unilateral, unicentric malignancies. The range of germline RET mutations reported for apparently sporadic MTC cases varies widely from approximately 5% based on direct testing[142-144] to about 25% using family history–based assessments.[130] The importance of identifying all MEN2-associated MTC cases for optimal patient and family management has led to a recommendation to offer pre- and post-test genetic counseling and genetic testing for RET mutations to all patients with MTC.[128]

Somatic RET mutations, particularly M918T, are seen in about half of sporadic MTCs. Rare germline sequence variants may also contribute to the development of sporadic MTC.[145] The NTRK1 gene encodes a tyrosine kinase nerve growth factor receptor and is expressed in MTCs. Like RET, NTRK1 is involved in gene rearrangements resulting in fusion genes that are commonly seen in papillary thyroid carcinomas. Mutational analysis of NTRK1 in sporadic MTC revealed sequence variants that were also present in the germline, suggesting that NTRK1 may be a low-penetrance gene for MTC.[146]

Germline homozygous RET mutations have been reported and are thus compatible with development.[147,148] About 50% of MEN2B cases arise de novo, whereas closer to 5% of MEN2A cases are de novo.[144,149] Not all physical manifestations of MEN2B may be present in infants, so a high level of suspicion must be maintained to recognize the syndrome and to accomplish early prophylactic total thyroidectomy.[150]

After many years of unfruitful linkage studies with chromosome 20p12 as the suspected MEN2 locus, linkage to *RBP3* (now positioned at 10q11.2) was found.[151] Linkage studies continued to narrow the critical region [152–155] and the data indicated lack of genetic heterogeneity of MEN2A, MEN2B, and familial MTC.[156,157] Mulligan and colleagues[158] recognized the *RET* proto-oncogene, a tyrosine kinase receptor gene that maps to the critical MEN2 region, as a viable candidate gene and demonstrated missense mutations in multiple distinct MEN2A families, with a recurrent mutation involving a cysteine residue.

Diagnostics

Diagnosis of MTC is accomplished with fine-needle aspiration biopsy of a solitary thyroid nodule, or biopsy of a dominant nodule within a multinodular goiter. Diagnostic accuracy is improved by IHC staining positivity for calcitonin, carcinoembryonic antigen (CEA), and amyloid, and negative staining for thyroglobulin.[131] Basal or calcium-stimulated calcitonin measurement (which has replaced pentagastrin stimulation in the United States) and CEA serum levels are preoperatively assessed and correlate with tumor size, postoperative normalization, curative potential of surgery, and risk of metastatic disease.[159,160] In cases with local lymph node involvement or high preoperative basal calcitonin levels, more extensive imaging is warranted.[128] The diagnostic workup of pheochromocytoma and hyperparathyroidism were discussed earlier.

The calcitonin C-cell stimulation test was the mainstay of screening for MTC in MEN2 carriers in the past, but this role has largely been replaced by genetic testing followed by prophylactic thyroidectomy at crucial ages as determined by specific mutation.[161,162] The C-cell stimulation test remains important in the occasional family in which a mutation cannot be discerned. Calcitonin monitoring continues to play a role in management after prophylactic thyroidectomy or treatment of MTC.

Molecular genetic testing for MEN2

RET testing is indicated for all cases of MTC, as part of the genetic evaluation of pheochromocytoma, to diagnose MEN2B, and for presymptomatic diagnosis and management in families with MEN2 syndromes and a known *RET* mutation. Linkage analysis is an option for families with an unidentifiable *RET* mutation and may have an accuracy of ~95%.[163] Preimplantation genetic diagnosis has been performed for MEN2A.[164]

Genetic testing for *RET* mutations is recommended to proceed in stepwise fashion based on the high rate of exon 10 or 11 mutation in MEN2A and characteristically affected codons in MEN2B.[128,165,166] The mutation detection rate is about 95% for MEN2A families, with codon 634 cys mutations accounting for about 84% of families. The mutation detection rate is 88% for FMTC families,[165,166] found in exons 10, 11, 13, and 14, and most often involving codons 609, 611, 618, 620, and 634. About 95% of MEN2B cases are caused by an M918T mutation in exon 16.[167,168] Additional MEN2B mutations are A883F as well as 2 mutations, V804M and Y806C, acting in cis.[169]

Surgical Recommendations Applicable to Mutation Carriers

Total thyroidectomy with central cervical lymph node dissection is the recommended surgical procedure for MEN2 carriers.[128,131] Earlier age at surgery results in less chance of recurrence, but there have been differing opinions about the optimal timing of surgery. Genotype-phenotype correlations in MEN2 are strong both in terms of being mutation-specific and highly predictive of age of MTC onset, which makes genotyping an indispensable tool in planning the age of prophylactic surgery on an individual basis.[128,131,161]

An approach put forth by the National Comprehensive Cancer Network[128,131] is to stratify risk by genotype into the following categories, and to time surgery accordingly.

MEN2B mutation carriers at codons 883, 918, or 922 are the highest-risk patients and should have surgery during the first year of life. Surgery at a later date is less likely to be curative. Carriers with mutations in codons 634, 630, and 609 are high-risk patients (MEN2A phenotype) and should undergo surgery between the ages of 2 and 4 years. Intermediate risk is seen with mutations in codons 611, 620, and 891 (MEN2A), and an atypical MEN2B is seen with mutations in codon 804; surgery is recommended by 6 years of age. Low risk is seen with codon 768, 790, and 791 mutations. The determination for prophylactic thyroidectomy can be made by serial C-cell stimulation testing. In the absence of an identifiable mutation, clinical judgment is needed.

Incident cases of medullary thyroid cancer are managed as per the American Thyroid Association guidelines,[128] with total thyroidectomy with central lymph node dissection as the only curative approach, mandatory for MEN2 carriers (further neck dissection is determined by evidence of lateral lymph node involvement). The likelihood of MEN2 in a patient with MTC is so high that thyroidectomy is indicated for all patients with MTC. Likewise, a preoperative biochemical evaluation for pheochromocytoma is required for all patients with MTC, which would require biochemical management and resection before thyroid surgery.[170,171]

Careful preoperative pharmacologic management for pheochromocytoma is essential.[27] In the case of a unilateral MEN2-related pheochromocytoma, unilateral cortical-sparing adrenalectomy using a laparascopic approach is preferable to bilateral adrenalectomy.[47,64] Although the risk of bilateral pheochromocytoma in MEN2 is high, the risk of death from Addisonian crisis in a patient dependent on corticosteroids may outweigh the risk of death from a second pheochromocytoma. However, in the case of bilateral pheochromocytoma coupled with diffuse medullary disease (more typical of MEN2 than VHL), bilateral adrenalectomy is preferred.

Surgical management for patients with MEN2A with primary hyperparathyroidism is similar for patients with MEN1, even if multiglandular involvement is not evident.[172]

Prognosis of hereditary MTC is probably similar to that of sporadic MTC when age is taken into account. Postoperative calcitonin doubling time was an independent predictor of survival in a multivariate analysis and might outperform clinical staging.[173] MTC in MEN2B carriers is known for its aggressiveness, and chances for cure with surgery are much lower than in MEN2A carriers or sporadic cases. This emphasizes the need for clinical recognition of MEN2B (a problem compounded by a high de novo rate) and early prophylactic surgery.[150]

Effect of genetic screening on clinical outcome

Screening for early disease manifestations in families with MEN2 done before the ability to perform genetic testing showed that recognition improved dramatically compared with clinical symptoms.[174] Serum calcitonin testing coupled with prophylactic surgery led to a dramatic reduction in primary tumor size, bilateral MTC, and rate of lymph node metastasis.[161] Genetic testing now facilitates presymptomatic diagnosis and prevention, which is tailored to the specific genotype.[161] With these advances, life expectancy has improved in MEN2 carriers, probably at least as much from effective pheochromocytoma management as from surgical prophylaxis of MTC and improved MTC management.[64] The use of DNA-based testing to guide management is also cost-effective.[175]

Screening Recommendations Applicable to Known or Highly Likely Mutation Carriers

Codon-specific risks and age of onset have been described for pheochromocytoma.[132,176] It has been suggested that annual screening for pheochromocytoma may be warranted, beginning at age 10 years, for carriers of mutations in codons

918, 634, and 630. Carriers with mutations at other codons could initiate screening at age 20 years.[132] In addition, because a hypertensive crisis can be precipitated by pregnancy, labor, or delivery, biochemical screening for pheochromocytoma should be done for all *RET* mutation carriers early in pregnancy.[64]

Genetics

The rearranged during transfection (*RET*) proto-oncogene encodes a receptor tyrosine kinase that functions in the differentiation of neural crest tissues such as thyroid parafollicular C-cells, adrenal medulla, and parathyroid chief cells. *RET* also controls the survival, proliferation, differentiation, and migration of the enteric nervous system progenitor cells.[138] The extracellular domain of *RET* contains 4 calcium-dependent cell adhesion (cadherin)–like domains and a cysteine-rich domain that influences tertiary structure and ligand-induced dimerization of 2 *RET* molecules.[177] The transmembrane domain of *RET* (codons 636–657) enhances noncovalent receptor-receptor interactions. The intracellular domain has a juxtamembrane region and 2 tyrosine kinase subdomains that control several signal transduction cascades.[177] Activation of *RET* is accomplished through dimerization and autophosphorylation.

In MEN2A, *RET* proto-oncogene mutations are typically missense mutations, commonly involving cysteine residues at codons 515, 609, 611, 618, 620, 630, and 634 (or the addition of cysteine at codons 533, 606, or 631), which lead to constitutive gain of function. Gain-of-function mutations also occur in the transmembrane domain (eg, codon 649), the intracellular tyrosine kinase domain involving the adenosine triphosphate binding site (codons 768, 790, 791, 804, and 891), and at the intracellular catalytic core (codon 918).[177] In contrast, most Hirschsprung disease involves loss of function *RET* mutations, resulting in haploinsufficiency, or promoter mutations.[138]

HEREDITARY THYROID CANCER
Introduction

The genetic basis of familial nonmedullary thyroid cancer (FNMTC) is less well understood than for MTC (as discussed earlier). Epidemiologic studies suggest the existence of susceptibility genes for FNMTC, which is supported by reports of large kindreds with FNMTC, and linkage studies indicating the existence of specific predisposition genes. In rare instances, direct analysis suggests specific genetic causes, but the full scope of FNMTC is yet to be fully elucidated.

Thyroid cancer accounts for about 1% of malignancies, with an annual incidence of about 37,200 (10,000 men and 27,200 women) and 1630 deaths each year in the United States.[178] The major histopathologic subtypes are papillary carcinoma (including follicular variant of papillary carcinoma), follicular carcinoma (including Hurthle cell carcinoma), medullary carcinoma, and undifferentiated (anaplastic) carcinoma. Nonmedullary thyroid carcinomas (NMTCs) originate from thyroid epithelial cells, encompassing the papillary, follicular, and undifferentiated histopathologic subtypes.

The incidence of thyroid cancer, primarily papillary carcinoma, seems to be increasing, possibly as a result of increased diagnostic scrutiny.[179] Women are disproportionately affected, accounting for 60% to 75% of thyroid cancer cases among the various histopathologic subtypes.[180]

Ionizing radiation is an established risk factor for thyroid cancer, as noted in survivors of the Hiroshima and Nagasaki atomic bombs and the Chernobyl nuclear accident in 1986.[181] In the past, exposures in the United States occurred from nuclear weapons testing and therapeutic uses (acne, adenoid enlargement, tinea capitis, thymic enlargement). Some iatrogenic exposures remain relevant; for example, thyroid cancer is the second most common solid tumor observed following mantle irradiation in childhood for Hodgkin disease (breast cancer is the most common).[182] A history of prior head and neck irradiation may account for about 9% of incident thyroid cancers.[183] Reported risk factors for thyroid cancer also include a history of benign thyroid nodules or goiter.[183]

Familial Risk

As with most malignancies, a family history of thyroid cancer poses a risk factor for developing thyroid cancer.[183] For example, pedigree analysis of 339 unselected patients diagnosed with NMTC and 319 unaffected ethnically matched controls found an incidence rate ratio of 10.3 in relatives of patients who have cancer, compared with controls (95% confidence interval, 2.2–47.6).[184] FNMTC cases were all papillary thyroid cancers. Other studies that primarily addressed family history as a risk factor for NMTC have found a magnitude of risk in the 8- to 11-fold range.[184–187]

Genetic Syndromes Involving NMTC

Familial studies of NMTC have assessed whether specific cancers are observed in excess, thus potentially delineating FNMTC syndromes, but few clear patterns have emerged. A relationship between breast and thyroid cancer has been suggested by epidemiologic data. However, a study examining family history of probands with double primary breast and thyroid cancer ascertained from population- and hospital-based registries did not bear out this connection.[188]

Cancer predisposition syndromes with NMTC a nonpredominant feature

Syndromes with NMTC as a component tumor where nonthyroidal tumors predominate include Cowden syndrome (multiple hamartoma syndrome, *PTEN*, OMIM 158350), familial adenomatous polyposis (FAP; *APC* OMIM 175100), the Carney complex type 1 (Carney complex type 1 *PRKAR1a*, OMIM 160980, and Carney complex type 1 with an unknown gene at chromosomal locus 2p16, OMIM 605244), McCune-Albright syndrome (*GNAS1* mosaic, OMIM 174800), and Werner syndrome (*WRN*, OMIM 277700).

Most recognized syndromes including NMTC are inherited in an autosomal dominant pattern (which could reflect ascertainment bias). Follicular thyroid carcinoma is the predominant histopathologic subtype in Cowden syndrome, along with multicentric follicular adenomas, adenomatous nodules, and microadenomas.[189] Double primary breast and thyroid cancer cases do not seem to be caused by *PTEN* mutations to any appreciable extent,[188] but ascertainment from high-risk clinics could be higher than from population- and hospital-based registries. Papillary thyroid carcinoma is an extracolonic manifestation of FAP syndrome. The lifetime risk in *APC* mutation carriers is about 2% to 12%; young female carriers face about a 160-fold increased risk.[190] Most cases present as bilateral and multifocal cancer, and the rare cribriform-morular variant is suggestive of FAP.[190] Multiple thyroid nodules, primarily follicular, are seen in up to 75% of individuals with the Carney complex, and papillary or follicular thyroid cancer may occur.[191] NMTC has been reported for MEN2 and the hereditary paraganglioma syndromes but is not a well-established feature of either.[9,30,128] A *PTEN* mutation–negative, Cowden syndrome–like presentation for mitochondrial dysfunction, possibly involving thyroid cancer, has been observed.[34] Thyroid carcinoma is also a feature of Werner syndrome and McCune-Albright syndrome.[192]

FNMTC syndromes

FNMTC accounts for about 6% of patients with papillary thyroid carcinomas[184] and 10.5% of patients with follicular cell origin thyroid carcinomas.[190] Hereditary features that indicate FNMTC include 3 or more affected relatives in a kindred, early-onset disease, or cancer in men (female predilection is generally observed). Reports of such kindreds bolstered the notion that FNMTC susceptibility genes exist.[193,194]

The main clues enabling the discovery of putative susceptibility genes have come from linkage analyses of large FNMTC kindreds. Evidence of linkage has been reported for the following syndromes and chromosomal loci. Familial papillary thyroid carcinoma (OMIM 188550) has been mapped to several genetic loci. Evidence for linkage to chromosome 14q31 was reported in a large family with multinodular goiter and papillary thyroid cancer (MNG1; OMIM 138800)[195] but probably accounts for a small proportion of FNMTC.[195,196] A family with oxyphilic tumors (notable for granular eosinophilic cytoplasm and mitochondria) was linked to chromosome 19p13.2 and the gene named TCO (thyroid tumors with cell oxyphilia) or TCO1 (OMIM 603386).[197] Evidence for linkage of FNMTC without oxyphilia (papillary type) to chromosome 19p13.2 was also reported, but most FNMTC families did not map to this locus.[196] A large family with papillary thyroid carcinoma, thyroid nodules, and multifocal papillary renal neoplasia demonstrated linkage to chromosome 1q21 (PTCPRN, PRN1, OMIM 605642).[198] In addition, an FNMTC susceptibility gene was mapped to 2q21 in families with papillary thyroid cancer, stratified by the presence of the follicular variant of PTC (NMTC1, OMIM 606240).[199]

Treatment of FNMTC

Multifocality and association with multiple benign nodules is characteristic of FNMTC. Disease recurrence is more likely and shorter disease-free survival is seen in FNMTC patients. These features have raised the possibility of favoring aggressive initial treatment with total thyroidectomy and careful follow-up.[189,200] The delineation of the individual syndromes is not yet mature enough to specify the role of prophylactic thyroidectomy. Likewise, thyroid ultrasound might be useful, but the prevalence of thyroid nodules in various FNMTC syndromes leaves open questions about diagnostic accuracy for malignant disease. Clinical genetic testing is not available for these syndromes and most FNMTC remains unexplained by known loci. With additional gene discovery and definition of FNMTC syndromes, the ability to perform presymptomatic diagnosis would enable tailoring of management in at-risk relatives and reduction of screening measures in noncarriers.

REFERENCES

1. Thakker RV. Multiple endocrine neoplasia–syndromes of the twentieth century. J Clin Endocrinol Metab 1998;83:2617–20.
2. Alexakis N, Connor S, Ghaneh P, et al. Hereditary pancreatic endocrine tumours. Pancreatology 2004;4:417–33.
3. Moore FD, Dluhy RG. Prophylactic thyroidectomy in MEN-2A–a stitch in time? N Engl J Med 2005;353:1162–4.
4. Neumann HP, Eng C. The approach to the patient with paraganglioma. J Clin Endocrinol Metab 2009;94:2677–83.
5. Chase WH. Familial and bilateral tumours of the carotid body. J Pathol Bacteriol 1933;36:1–12.
6. van der Mey AG, Jansen JC, van Baalen JM. Management of carotid body tumors. Otolaryngol Clin North Am 2001;34:907–24, vi.

7. Kroll AJ, Alexander B, Cochios F, et al. Hereditary deficiencies of clotting factors vii and x associated with carotid-body tumors. N Engl J Med 1964;270:6–13.
8. Grufferman S, Gillman MW, Pasternak LR, et al. Familial carotid body tumors: case report and epidemiologic review. Cancer 1980;46:2116–22.
9. Parry DM, Li FP, Strong LC, et al. Carotid body tumors in humans: genetics and epidemiology. J Natl Cancer Inst 1982;68:573–8.
10. Heutink P, van der Mey AG, Sandkuijl LA, et al. A gene subject to genomic imprinting and responsible for hereditary paragangliomas maps to chromosome 11q23-qter. Hum Mol Genet 1992;1:7–10.
11. Baysal BE, Farr JE, Rubinstein WS, et al. Fine mapping of an imprinted gene for familial nonchromaffin paragangliomas, on chromosome 11q23. Am J Hum Genet 1997;60:121–32.
12. Baysal BE, van Schothorst EM, Farr JE, et al. Repositioning the hereditary paraganglioma critical region on chromosome band 11q23. Hum Genet 1999;104: 219–25.
13. Mariman EC, van Beersum SE, Cremers CW, et al. Analysis of a second family with hereditary non-chromaffin paragangliomas locates the underlying gene at the proximal region of chromosome 11q. Hum Genet 1993;91: 357–61.
14. Mariman EC, van Beersum SE, Cremers CW, et al. Fine mapping of a putatively imprinted gene for familial non-chromaffin paragangliomas to chromosome 11q13.1: evidence for genetic heterogeneity. Hum Genet 1995;95:56–62.
15. Niemann S, Becker-Follmann J, Nurnberg G, et al. Assignment of PGL3 to chromosome 1 (q21–q23) in a family with autosomal dominant non-chromaffin paraganglioma. Am J Med Genet 2001;98:32–6.
16. Baysal BE, Ferrell RE, Willett-Brozick JE, et al. Mutations in SDHD, a mitochondrial complex II gene, in hereditary paraganglioma. Science 2000;287: 848–51.
17. Niemann S, Muller U. Mutations in SDHC cause autosomal dominant paraganglioma, type 3. Nat Genet 2000;26:268–70.
18. Astuti D, Latif F, Dallol A, et al. Gene mutations in the succinate dehydrogenase subunit SDHB cause susceptibility to familial pheochromocytoma and to familial paraganglioma. Am J Hum Genet 2001;69:49–54.
19. Pasini B, Stratakis CA. SDH mutations in tumorigenesis and inherited endocrine tumours: lesson from the phaeochromocytoma–paraganglioma syndromes. J Intern Med 2009;266:19–42.
20. Nissenblatt MJ. Cyanotic heart disease: "low altitude" risk for carotid body tumor? Johns Hopkins Med J 1978;142:18–22.
21. van Schothorst EM, Jansen JC, Grooters E, et al. Founder effect at PGL1 in hereditary head and neck paraganglioma families from the Netherlands. Am J Hum Genet 1998;63:468–73.
22. Tischler AS. Pheochromocytoma and extra-adrenal paraganglioma: updates. Arch Pathol Lab Med 2008;132:1272–84.
23. Goldstein RE, O'Neill JA Jr, Holcomb GW III, et al. Clinical experience over 48 years with pheochromocytoma. Ann Surg 1999;229:755–64.
24. van der Mey AG, Maaswinkel-Mooy PD, Cornelisse CJ, et al. Genomic imprinting in hereditary glomus tumours: evidence for new genetic theory. Lancet 1989;2:1291–4.
25. Pigny P, Vincent A, Cardot BC, et al. Paraganglioma after maternal transmission of a succinate dehydrogenase gene mutation. J Clin Endocrinol Metab 2008;93: 1609–15.

26. Hao HX, Khalimonchuk O, Schraders M, et al. SDH5, a gene required for flavination of succinate dehydrogenase, is mutated in paraganglioma. Science 2009;325:1139–42.

27. Joynt KE, Moslehi JJ, Baughman KL. Paragangliomas: etiology, presentation, and management. Cardiol Rev 2009;17:159–64.

28. Pacak K, Eisenhofer G, Ahlman H, et al. Pheochromocytoma: recommendations for clinical practice from the First International Symposium. October 2005. Nat Clin Pract Endocrinol Metab 2007;3:92–102.

29. Schiavi F, Boedeker CC, Bausch B, et al. Predictors and prevalence of paraganglioma syndrome associated with mutations of the SDHC gene. JAMA 2005; 294:2057–63.

30. Neumann HP, Pawlu C, Peczkowska M, et al. Distinct clinical features of paraganglioma syndromes associated with SDHB and SDHD gene mutations. JAMA 2004;292:943–51.

31. Astrom K, Cohen JE, Willett-Brozick JE, et al. Altitude is a phenotypic modifier in hereditary paraganglioma type 1: evidence for an oxygen-sensing defect. Hum Genet 2003;113:228–37.

32. Eng C, Kiuru M, Fernandez MJ, et al. A role for mitochondrial enzymes in inherited neoplasia and beyond. Nat Rev Cancer 2003;3:193–202.

33. Vanharanta S, Buchta M, McWhinney SR, et al. Early-onset renal cell carcinoma as a novel extraparaganglial component of SDHB-associated heritable paraganglioma. Am J Hum Genet 2004;74:153–9.

34. Ni Y, Zbuk KM, Sadler T, et al. Germline mutations and variants in the succinate dehydrogenase genes in Cowden and Cowden-like syndromes. Am J Hum Genet 2008;83:261–8.

35. Boedeker CC, Neumann HP, Offergeld C, et al. Clinical features of paraganglioma syndromes. Skull Base 2009;19:17–25.

36. Cascon A, Lopez-Jimenez E, Landa I, et al. Rationalization of genetic testing in patients with apparently sporadic pheochromocytoma/paraganglioma. Horm Metab Res 2009;41:672–5.

37. Amar L, Bertherat J, Baudin E, et al. Genetic testing in pheochromocytoma or functional paraganglioma. J Clin Oncol 2005;23:8812–8.

38. Neumann HP, Bausch B, McWhinney SR, et al. Germ-line mutations in nonsyndromic pheochromocytoma. N Engl J Med 2002;346:1459–66.

39. Gimm O, Armanios M, Dziema H, et al. Somatic and occult germ-line mutations in SDHD, a mitochondrial complex II gene, in nonfamilial pheochromocytoma. Cancer Res 2000;60:6822–5.

40. Neumann HP, Erlic Z, Boedeker CC, et al. Clinical predictors for germline mutations in head and neck paraganglioma patients: cost reduction strategy in genetic diagnostic process as fall-out. Cancer Res 2009;69:3650–6.

41. Amar L, Baudin E, Burnichon N, et al. Succinate dehydrogenase B gene mutations predict survival in patients with malignant pheochromocytomas or paragangliomas. J Clin Endocrinol Metab 2007;92:3822–8.

42. Drovdlic CM, Myers EN, Peters JA, et al. Proportion of heritable paraganglioma cases and associated clinical characteristics. Laryngoscope 2001;111:1822–7.

43. Baysal BE, Willett-Brozick JE, Lawrence EC, et al. Prevalence of SDHB, SDHC, and SDHD germline mutations in clinic patients with head and neck paragangliomas. J Med Genet 2002;39:178–83.

44. Stratakis CA, Carney JA. The triad of paragangliomas, gastric stromal tumours and pulmonary chondromas (Carney triad), and the dyad of paragangliomas

and gastric stromal sarcomas (Carney-Stratakis syndrome): molecular genetics and clinical implications. J Intern Med 2009;266:43–52.

45. Boedeker CC, Erlic Z, Richard S, et al. Head and neck paragangliomas in von Hippel–Lindau disease and multiple endocrine neoplasia type 2. J Clin Endocrinol Metab 2009;94:1938–44.

46. van Nederveen FH, Gaal J, Favier J, et al. An immunohistochemical procedure to detect patients with paraganglioma and phaeochromocytoma with germline SDHB, SDHC, or SDHD gene mutations: a retrospective and prospective analysis. Lancet Oncol 2009;10:764–71.

47. Walz MK, Alesina PF, Wenger FA, et al. Laparoscopic and retroperitoneoscopic treatment of pheochromocytomas and retroperitoneal paragangliomas: results of 161 tumors in 126 patients. World J Surg 2006;30:899–908.

48. Eisenhofer G, Siegert G, Kotzerke J, et al. Current progress and future challenges in the biochemical diagnosis and treatment of pheochromocytomas and paragangliomas. Horm Metab Res 2008;40:329–37.

49. Mittendorf EA, Evans DB, Lee JE, et al. Pheochromocytoma: advances in genetics, diagnosis, localization, and treatment. Hematol Oncol Clin North Am 2007;21:509–25.

50. McCaffrey TV, Meyer FB, Michels VV, et al. Familial paragangliomas of the head and neck. Arch Otolaryngol Head Neck Surg 1994;120:1211–6.

51. Myssiorek D, Ferlito A, Silver CE, et al. Screening for familial paragangliomas. Oral Oncol 2008;44:532–7.

52. Renard L, Godfraind C, Boon LM, et al. A novel mutation in the SDHD gene in a family with inherited paragangliomas–implications of genetic diagnosis for follow up and treatment. Head Neck 2003;25:146–51.

53. Baysal BE, Rubinstein WS, Taschner PE. Phenotypic dichotomy in mitochondrial complex II genetic disorders. J Mol Med 2001;79:495–503.

54. Baysal BE. A phenotypic perspective on mammalian oxygen sensor candidates. Ann N Y Acad Sci 2006;1073:221–33.

55. Baysal BE. Clinical and molecular progress in hereditary paraganglioma. J Med Genet 2008;45:689–94.

56. Baysal BE. Genomic imprinting and environment in hereditary paraganglioma. Am J Med Genet C Semin Med Genet 2004;129C:85–90.

57. Hensen EF, Jordanova ES, van M, et al. Somatic loss of maternal chromosome 11 causes parent-of-origin-dependent inheritance in SDHD-linked paraganglioma and phaeochromocytoma families. Oncogene 2004;23:4076–83.

58. Tomlinson IP, Alam NA, Rowan AJ, et al. Germline mutations in FH predispose to dominantly inherited uterine fibroids, skin leiomyomata and papillary renal cell cancer. Nat Genet 2002;30:406–10.

59. Vander Heiden MG, Cantley LC, Thompson CB. Understanding the Warburg effect: the metabolic requirements of cell proliferation. Science 2009;324:1029–33.

60. Wermer P. Genetic aspects of adenomatosis of endocrine glands. Am J Med 1954;16:363–71.

61. Zollinger RM, Ellison EH. Primary peptic ulcerations of the jejunum associated with islet cell tumors of the pancreas. Ann Surg 1955;142:709–23.

62. Lulu DJ, Corcoran TE, Andre M. Familial endocrine adenomatosis with associated Zollinger–Ellison syndrome. Wermer's syndrome. Am J Surg 1968;115:695–701.

63. Marx SJ. Multiple endocrine neoplasia type 1. In: Vogelstein B, Kinzler K, editors. The genetic basis of human cancer. New York: McGraw-Hill; 2002. p. 475–9.

64. Brandi ML, Gagel RF, Angeli A, et al. Guidelines for diagnosis and therapy of MEN type 1 and type 2. J Clin Endocrinol Metab 2001;86:5658–71.
65. Schussheim DH, Skarulis MC, Agarwal SK, et al. Multiple endocrine neoplasia type 1: new clinical and basic findings. Trends Endocrinol Metab 2001;12: 173–8.
66. Kloppel G, Perren A, Heitz PU. The gastroenteropancreatic neuroendocrine cell system and its tumors: the WHO classification. Ann N Y Acad Sci 2004;1014: 13–27.
67. Tonelli F, Fratini G, Falchetti A, et al. Surgery for gastroenteropancreatic tumours in multiple endocrine neoplasia type 1: review and personal experience. J Intern Med 2005;257:38–49.
68. Pieterman CR, Schreinemakers JM, Koppeschaar HP, et al. Multiple endocrine neoplasia type 1 (MEN1): its manifestations and effect of genetic screening on clinical outcome. Clin Endocrinol (Oxf) 2009;70:575–81.
69. Carty SE, Helm AK, Amico JA, et al. The variable penetrance and spectrum of manifestations of multiple endocrine neoplasia type 1. Surgery 1998;124: 1106–13.
70. Agarwal SK, Ozawa A, Mateo CM, et al. The MEN1 gene and pituitary tumours. Horm Res 2009;71(Suppl 2):131–8.
71. Agarwal SK, Kester MB, Debelenko LV, et al. Germline mutations of the MEN1 gene in familial multiple endocrine neoplasia type 1 and related states. Hum Mol Genet 1997;6:1169–75.
72. Goudet P, Murat A, Cardot-Bauters C, et al. Thymic neuroendocrine tumors in multiple endocrine neoplasia type 1: a comparative study on 21 cases among a series of 761 MEN1 from the GTE (Groupe des Tumeurs Endocrines). World J Surg 2009;33:1197–207.
73. Teh BT, Zedenius J, Kytola S, et al. Thymic carcinoids in multiple endocrine neoplasia type 1. Ann Surg 1998;228:99–105.
74. Wilkinson S, Teh BT, Davey KR, et al. Cause of death in multiple endocrine neoplasia type 1. Arch Surg 1993;128:683–90.
75. Witchel SF, Ranganathan S, Kilpatrick M, et al. Reverse referral: from pathology to endocrinology. Endocr Pathol 2009;20:78–83.
76. Darling TN, Skarulis MC, Steinberg SM, et al. Multiple facial angiofibromas and collagenomas in patients with multiple endocrine neoplasia type 1. Arch Dermatol 1997;133:853–7.
77. Marx SJ. Multiple endocrine neoplasia type 1. In: Scriver CR, Beaudet AL, Sly WS, et al, editors. The metabolic and molecular bases of inherited disease. 8th edition. New York: McGraw-Hill; 2001. p. 943–66.
78. Falchetti A, Marini F, Giusti F, et al. DNA-based test: when and why to apply it to primary hyperparathyroidism clinical phenotypes. J Intern Med 2009;266: 69–83.
79. Warner J, Epstein M, Sweet A, et al. Genetic testing in familial isolated hyperparathyroidism: unexpected results and their implications. J Med Genet 2004; 41:155–60.
80. Pellegata NS, Quintanilla-Martinez L, Siggelkow H, et al. Germ-line mutations in p27Kip1 cause a multiple endocrine neoplasia syndrome in rats and humans. Proc Natl Acad Sci U S A 2006;103:15558–63.
81. Igreja S, Chahal HS, Akker SA, et al. Assessment of p27 (cyclin-dependent kinase inhibitor 1B) and aryl hydrocarbon receptor-interacting protein (AIP) genes in multiple endocrine neoplasia (MEN1) syndrome patients without any detectable MEN1 gene mutations. Clin Endocrinol (Oxf) 2009;70:259–64.

82. Owens M, Stals K, Ellard S, et al. Germline mutations in the CDKN1B gene encoding p27 Kip1 are a rare cause of multiple endocrine neoplasia type 1. Clin Endocrinol (Oxf) 2009;70:499–500.
83. Jensen RT. Pancreatic neuroendocrine tumors: overview of recent advances and diagnosis. J Gastrointest Surg 2006;10:324–6.
84. Brandi ML, Weber G, Svensson A, et al. Homozygotes for the autosomal dominant neoplasia syndrome MEN1. Am J Hum Genet 1993;53:1167–72.
85. Larsson C, Skogseid B, Oberg K, et al. Multiple endocrine neoplasia type 1 gene maps to chromosome 11 and is lost in insulinoma. Nature 1988;332:85–7.
86. Bale SJ, Bale AE, Stewart K, et al. Linkage analysis of multiple endocrine neoplasia type 1 with INT2 and other markers on chromosome 11. Genomics 1989;4:320–2.
87. Thakker RV, Bouloux P, Wooding C, et al. Association of parathyroid tumors in multiple endocrine neoplasia type 1 with loss of alleles on chromosome 11. N Engl J Med 1989;321:218–24.
88. Nakamura Y, Larsson C, Julier C, et al. Localization of the genetic defect in multiple endocrine neoplasia type 1 within a small region of chromosome 11. Am J Hum Genet 1989;44:751–5.
89. Debelenko LV, Emmert-Buck MR, Manickam P, et al. Haplotype analysis defines a minimal interval for the multiple endocrine neoplasia type 1 (MEN1) gene. Cancer Res 1997;57:1039–42.
90. Friedman E, Sakaguchi K, Bale AE, et al. Clonality of parathyroid tumors in familial multiple endocrine neoplasia type 1. N Engl J Med 1989;321:213–8.
91. Bystrom C, Larsson C, Blomberg C, et al. Localization of the MEN1 gene to a small region within chromosome 11q13 by deletion mapping in tumors. Proc Natl Acad Sci U S A 1990;87:1968–72.
92. Rochelle JM, Watson ML, Oakey RJ, et al. A linkage map of mouse chromosome 19: definition of comparative mapping relationships with human chromosomes 10 and 11 including the MEN1 locus. Genomics 1992;14:26–31.
93. Richard CW III, Withers DA, Meeker TC, et al. A radiation hybrid map of the proximal long arm of human chromosome 11 containing the multiple endocrine neoplasia type 1 MEN-1 and bcl-1 disease loci. Am J Hum Genet 1991;49:1189–96.
94. Fujimori M, Wells SA Jr, Nakamura Y. Fine-scale mapping of the gene responsible for multiple endocrine neoplasia type 1 (MEN 1). Am J Hum Genet 1992;50:399–403.
95. Larsson C, Shepherd J, Nakamura Y, et al. Predictive testing for multiple endocrine neoplasia type 1 using DNA polymorphisms. J Clin Invest 1992;89:1344–9.
96. Guru SC, Olufemi SE, Manickam P, et al. A 2.8-Mb clone contig of the multiple endocrine neoplasia type 1 (MEN1) region at 11q13. Genomics 1997;42:436–45.
97. Chandrasekharappa SC, Guru SC, Manickam P, et al. Positional cloning of the gene for multiple endocrine neoplasia-type 1. Science 1997;276:404–7.
98. Lemmens I, Van de Ven WJ, Kas K, et al. Identification of the multiple endocrine neoplasia type 1 (MEN1) gene. The European Consortium on MEN1. Hum Mol Genet 1997;6:1177–83.
99. Giraud S, Zhang CX, Serova-Sinilnikova O, et al. Germ-line mutation analysis in patients with multiple endocrine neoplasia type 1 and related disorders. Am J Hum Genet 1998;63:455–67.
100. Teh BT, Kytola S, Farnebo F, et al. Mutation analysis of the MEN1 gene in multiple endocrine neoplasia type 1, familial acromegaly and familial isolated hyperparathyroidism. J Clin Endocrinol Metab 1998;83:2621–6.

101. Wautot V, Vercherat C, Lespinasse J, et al. Germline mutation profile of MEN1 in multiple endocrine neoplasia type 1: search for correlation between phenotype and the functional domains of the MEN1 protein. Hum Mutat 2002;20: 35–47.

102. Machens A, Schaaf L, Karges W, et al. Age-related penetrance of endocrine tumours in multiple endocrine neoplasia type 1 (MEN1): a multicentre study of 258 gene carriers. Clin Endocrinol (Oxf) 2007;67:613–22.

103. Lemos MC, Thakker RV. Multiple endocrine neoplasia type 1 (MEN1): analysis of 1336 mutations reported in the first decade following identification of the gene. Hum Mutat 2008;29:22–32.

104. Klein RD, Salih S, Bessoni J, et al. Clinical testing for multiple endocrine neoplasia type 1 in a DNA diagnostic laboratory. Genet Med 2005;7:131–8.

105. Pannett AA, Kennedy AM, Turner JJ, et al. Multiple endocrine neoplasia type 1 (MEN1) germline mutations in familial isolated primary hyperparathyroidism. Clin Endocrinol (Oxf) 2003;58:639–46.

106. Miedlich S, Lohmann T, Schneyer U, et al. Familial isolated primary hyperparathyroidism–a multiple endocrine neoplasia type 1 variant? Eur J Endocrinol 2001;145:155–60.

107. Evans DG, Ramsden RT, Shenton A, et al. Mosaicism in neurofibromatosis type 2: an update of risk based on uni/bilaterality of vestibular schwannoma at presentation and sensitive mutation analysis including multiple ligation-dependent probe amplification. J Med Genet 2007;44:424–8.

108. Tonelli F, Marcucci T, Fratini G, et al. Is total parathyroidectomy the treatment of choice for hyperparathyroidism in multiple endocrine neoplasia type 1? Ann Surg 2007;246:1075–82.

109. Yip L, Ogilvie JB, Challinor SM, et al. Identification of multiple endocrine neoplasia type 1 in patients with apparent sporadic primary hyperparathyroidism. Surgery 2008;144:1002–6.

110. Powell AC, Alexander HR, Pingpank JF, et al. The utility of routine transcervical thymectomy for multiple endocrine neoplasia 1-related hyperparathyroidism. Surgery 2008;144:878–83.

111. Yeung MJ, Pasieka JL. Gastrinomas: a historical perspective. J Surg Oncol 2009;100:425–33.

112. Doherty GM, Olson JA, Frisella MM, et al. Lethality of multiple endocrine neoplasia type I. World J Surg 1998;22:581–6.

113. Dean PG, van Heerden JA, Farley DR, et al. Are patients with multiple endocrine neoplasia type I prone to premature death? World J Surg 2000;24:1437–41.

114. Geerdink EA, van der Luijt RB, Lips CJ. Do patients with multiple endocrine neoplasia syndrome type 1 benefit from periodical screening? Eur J Endocrinol 2003;149:577–82.

115. Ebeling T, Vierimaa O, Kytola S, et al. Effect of multiple endocrine neoplasia type 1 (MEN1) gene mutations on premature mortality in familial MEN1 syndrome with founder mutations. J Clin Endocrinol Metab 2004;89:3392–6.

116. Newey PJ, Jeyabalan J, Walls GV, et al. Asymptomatic children with multiple endocrine neoplasia type 1 mutations may harbor nonfunctioning pancreatic neuroendocrine tumors. J Clin Endocrinol Metab 2009;94:3640–6.

117. Norton JA, Fraker DL, Alexander HR, et al. Surgery increases survival in patients with gastrinoma. Ann Surg 2006;244:410–9.

118. Norton JA, Alexander HR, Fraker DL, et al. Comparison of surgical results in patients with advanced and limited disease with multiple endocrine neoplasia type 1 and Zollinger–Ellison syndrome. Ann Surg 2001;234:495–505.

119. Norton JA, Fang TD, Jensen RT. Surgery for gastrinoma and insulinoma in multiple endocrine neoplasia type 1. J Natl Compr Canc Netw 2006;4:148–53.

120. Bushnell D. Therapy with radiolabeled somatostatin peptide analogs for metastatic neuroendocrine tumors. J Gastrointest Surg 2006;10:335–6.

121. Gracanin A, Dreijerink KM, van der Luijt RB, et al. Tissue selectivity in multiple endocrine neoplasia type 1-associated tumorigenesis. Cancer Res 2009;69:6371–4.

122. Dreijerink KM, Lips CJ, Timmers HT. Multiple endocrine neoplasia type 1: a chromatin writer's block. J Intern Med 2009;266:53–9.

123. Yokoyama A, Cleary ML. Menin critically links MLL proteins with LEDGF on cancer-associated target genes. Cancer Cell 2008;14:36–46.

124. Schimke RN, Hartmann WH. Familial amyloid-producing medullary thyroid carcinoma and pheochromocytoma. A distinct genetic entity. Ann Intern Med 1965;63:1027–39.

125. Steiner AL, Goodman AD, Powers SR. Study of a kindred with pheochromocytoma, medullary thyroid carcinoma, hyperparathyroidism and Cushing's disease: multiple endocrine neoplasia, type 2. Medicine (Baltimore) 1968;47:371–409.

126. Bergholm U, Adami HO, Telenius-Berg M, et al. Incidence of sporadic and familial medullary thyroid carcinoma in Sweden 1959 through 1981. A nationwide study in 126 patients. Swedish MCT Study Group. Acta Oncol 1990;29:9–15.

127. Morrison PJ, Nevin NC. Multiple endocrine neoplasia type 2B (mucosal neuroma syndrome, Wagenmann-Froboese syndrome). J Med Genet 1996;33:779–82.

128. Kloos RT, Eng C, Evans DB, et al. Medullary thyroid cancer: management guidelines of the American Thyroid Association. Thyroid 2009;19:565–612.

129. Farndon JR, Leight GS, Dilley WG, et al. Familial medullary thyroid carcinoma without associated endocrinopathies: a distinct clinical entity. Br J Surg 1986;73:278–81.

130. Ponder BAJ. Multiple endocrine neoplasia type 2. In: Vogelstein B, Kinzler KW, editors. The genetic basis of human cancer. New York: McGraw-Hill; 1998. p. 475–87.

131. Ogilvie JB, Kebebew E. Indication and timing of thyroid surgery for patients with hereditary medullary thyroid cancer syndromes. J Natl Compr Canc Netw 2006;4:139–47.

132. Machens A, Brauckhoff M, Holzhausen HJ, et al. Codon-specific development of pheochromocytoma in multiple endocrine neoplasia type 2. J Clin Endocrinol Metab 2005;90:3999–4003.

133. Schuffenecker I, Virally-Monod M, Brohet R, et al. Risk and penetrance of primary hyperparathyroidism in multiple endocrine neoplasia type 2A families with mutations at codon 634 of the RET proto-oncogene. Groupe D'etude des Tumeurs a Calcitonine. J Clin Endocrinol Metab 1998;83:487–91.

134. Nunziata V, Giannattasio R, di GG, et al. Hereditary localized pruritus in affected members of a kindred with multiple endocrine neoplasia type 2A Sipple's syndrome. Clin Endocrinol (Oxf) 1989;30:57–63.

135. Donovan DT, Levy ML, Furst EJ, et al. Familial cutaneous lichen amyloidosis in association with multiple endocrine neoplasia type 2A: a new variant. Henry Ford Hosp Med J 1989;37:147–50.

136. Verga U, Fugazzola L, Cambiaghi S, et al. Frequent association between MEN 2A and cutaneous lichen amyloidosis. Clin Endocrinol (Oxf) 2003;59:156–61.

137. Verdy M, Weber AM, Roy CC, et al. Hirschsprung's disease in a family with multiple endocrine neoplasia type 2. J Pediatr Gastroenterol Nutr 1982;1:603–7.

138. Moore SW, Zaahl MG. Multiple endocrine neoplasia syndromes, children, Hirschsprung's disease and RET. Pediatr Surg Int 2008;24:521–30.
139. Attie T, Pelet A, Edery P, et al. Diversity of RET proto-oncogene mutations in familial and sporadic Hirschsprung disease. Hum Mol Genet 1995;4:1381–6.
140. Eng C, Clayton D, Schuffenecker I, et al. The relationship between specific RET proto-oncogene mutations and disease phenotype in multiple endocrine neoplasia type 2. International RET Mutation Consortium analysis. JAMA 1996;276:1575–9.
141. Tallini G, Santoro M, Helie M, et al. RET/PTC oncogene activation defines a subset of papillary thyroid carcinomas lacking evidence of progression to poorly differentiated or undifferentiated tumor phenotypes. Clin Cancer Res 1998;4:287–94.
142. Eng C, Mulligan LM, Smith DP, et al. Low frequency of germline mutations in the RET proto-oncogene in patients with apparently sporadic medullary thyroid carcinoma. Clin Endocrinol (Oxf) 1995;43:123–7.
143. Bugalho MJ, Domingues R, Santos JR, et al. Mutation analysis of the RET proto-oncogene and early thyroidectomy: results of a Portuguese cancer centre. Surgery 2007;141:90–5.
144. Wohllk N, Cote GJ, Bugalho MM, et al. Relevance of RET proto-oncogene mutations in sporadic medullary thyroid carcinoma. J Clin Endocrinol Metab 1996;81:3740–5.
145. Gimm O, Neuberg DS, Marsh DJ, et al. Over-representation of a germline RET sequence variant in patients with sporadic medullary thyroid carcinoma and somatic RET codon 918 mutation. Oncogene 1999;18:1369–73.
146. Gimm O, Greco A, Hoang-Vu C, et al. Mutation analysis reveals novel sequence variants in NTRK1 in sporadic human medullary thyroid carcinoma. J Clin Endocrinol Metab 1999;84:2784–7.
147. Wu SL, Chang TC, Huang CN, et al. Germline RET proto-oncogene mutations in two Taiwanese families with multiple endocrine neoplasia type 2A. J Formos Med Assoc 1998;97:614–8.
148. Lesueur F, Cebrian A, Cranston A, et al. Germline homozygous mutations at codon 804 in the RET protooncogene in medullary thyroid carcinoma/multiple endocrine neoplasia type 2A patients. J Clin Endocrinol Metab 2005;90:3454–7.
149. Schuffenecker I, Ginet N, Goldgar D, et al. Prevalence and parental origin of de novo RET mutations in multiple endocrine neoplasia type 2A and familial medullary thyroid carcinoma. Le Groupe d'Etude des Tumeurs a Calcitonine. Am J Hum Genet 1997;60:233–7.
150. Wells SA Jr, Dilley WG, Farndon JA, et al. Early diagnosis and treatment of medullary thyroid carcinoma. Arch Intern Med 1985;145:1248–52.
151. Yamamoto M, Takai S, Miki T, et al. Close linkage of MEN2A with RBP3 locus in Japanese kindreds. Hum Genet 1989;82:287–8.
152. Narod SA, Sobol H, Nakamura Y, et al. Linkage analysis of hereditary thyroid carcinoma with and without pheochromocytoma. Hum Genet 1989;83:353–8.
153. Carson NL, Wu JS, Jackson CE, et al. The mutation for medullary thyroid carcinoma with parathyroid tumors (MTC with PTs) is closely linked to the centromeric region of chromosome 10. Am J Hum Genet 1990;47:946–51.
154. Narod SA, Sobol H, Schuffenecker I, et al. The gene for MEN 2A is tightly linked to the centromere of chromosome 10. Hum Genet 1991;86:529–30.
155. Gardner E, Papi L, Easton DF, et al. Genetic linkage studies map the multiple endocrine neoplasia type 2 loci to a small interval on chromosome 10q11.2. Hum Mol Genet 1993;2:241–6.

156. Lairmore TC, Howe JR, Korte JA, et al. Familial medullary thyroid carcinoma and multiple endocrine neoplasia type 2B map to the same region of chromosome 10 as multiple endocrine neoplasia type 2A. Genomics 1991;9:181–92.
157. Narod SA, Lavoue MF, Morgan K, et al. Genetic analysis of 24 French families with multiple endocrine neoplasia type 2A. Am J Hum Genet 1992;51:469–77.
158. Mulligan LM, Kwok JB, Healey CS, et al. Germ-line mutations of the RET proto-oncogene in multiple endocrine neoplasia type 2A. Nature 1993;363:458–60.
159. Cohen R, Campos JM, Salaun C, et al. Preoperative calcitonin levels are predictive of tumor size and postoperative calcitonin normalization in medullary thyroid carcinoma. Groupe d'Etudes des Tumeurs a Calcitonine (GETC). J Clin Endocrinol Metab 2000;85:919–22.
160. Machens A, Schneyer U, Holzhausen HJ, et al. Prospects of remission in medullary thyroid carcinoma according to basal calcitonin level. J Clin Endocrinol Metab 2005;90:2029–34.
161. Machens A, Dralle H. Genotype–phenotype based surgical concept of hereditary medullary thyroid carcinoma. World J Surg 2007;31:957–68.
162. Doyle P, Duren C, Nerlich K, et al. Potency and tolerance of calcitonin stimulation with high-dose calcium versus pentagastrin in normal adults. J Clin Endocrinol Metab 2009;94:2970–4.
163. Howe JR, Lairmore TC, Mishra SK, et al. Improved predictive test for MEN2, using flanking dinucleotide repeats and RFLPs. Am J Hum Genet 1992;51:1430–42.
164. Offit K, Sagi M, Hurley K. Preimplantation genetic diagnosis for cancer syndromes: a new challenge for preventive medicine. JAMA 2006;296:2727–30.
165. Mulligan LM, Eng C, Healey CS, et al. Specific mutations of the RET proto-oncogene are related to disease phenotype in MEN 2A and FMTC. Nat Genet 1994;6:70–4.
166. Mulligan LM, Marsh DJ, Robinson BG, et al. Genotype–phenotype correlation in multiple endocrine neoplasia type 2: report of the International RET Mutation Consortium. J Intern Med 1995;238:343–6.
167. Eng C, Smith DP, Mulligan LM, et al. Point mutation within the tyrosine kinase domain of the RET proto-oncogene in multiple endocrine neoplasia type 2B and related sporadic tumours. Hum Mol Genet 1994;3:237–41.
168. Carlson KM, Dou S, Chi D, et al. Single missense mutation in the tyrosine kinase catalytic domain of the RET protooncogene is associated with multiple endocrine neoplasia type 2B. Proc Natl Acad Sci U S A 1994;91:1579–83.
169. Miyauchi A, Futami H, Hai N, et al. Two germline missense mutations at codons 804 and 806 of the RET proto-oncogene in the same allele in a patient with multiple endocrine neoplasia type 2B without codon 918 mutation. Jpn J Cancer Res 1999;90:1–5.
170. Raue F, Frank-Raue K, Grauer A. Multiple endocrine neoplasia type 2. Clinical features and screening. Endocrinol Metab Clin North Am 1994;23:137–56.
171. Gagel RF, Robinson MF, Donovan DT, et al. Clinical review 44: medullary thyroid carcinoma: recent progress. J Clin Endocrinol Metab 1993;76:809–14.
172. Machens A, Dralle H. Parathyroid gland preservation in situ versus total parathyroidectomy with autotransplantation in patients at risk of MEN2A. Endocr J 2009; 56:633–6.
173. Barbet J, Campion L, Kraeber-Bodere F, et al. Prognostic impact of serum calcitonin and carcinoembryonic antigen doubling-times in patients with medullary thyroid carcinoma. J Clin Endocrinol Metab 2005;90:6077–84.
174. Easton DF, Ponder MA, Cummings T, et al. The clinical and screening age-at-onset distribution for the MEN-2 syndrome. Am J Hum Genet 1989;44:208–15.

175. Gilchrist DM, Morrish DW, Bridge PJ, et al. Cost analysis of DNA-based testing in a large Canadian family with multiple endocrine neoplasia type 2. Clin Genet 2004;66:349–52.

176. Yip L, Cote GJ, Shapiro SE, et al. Multiple endocrine neoplasia type 2: evaluation of the genotype–phenotype relationship. Arch Surg 2003;138:409–16.

177. Machens A, Lorenz K, Dralle H. Constitutive RET tyrosine kinase activation in hereditary medullary thyroid cancer: clinical opportunities. J Intern Med 2009; 266:114–25.

178. SEER cancer statistics review, 1975–2006. SEER Cancer Statistics Review, 1975-2006 [serial online]. Bethesda (MD): National Cancer Institute; 2009. Available at: http://seer.cancer.gov/csr/1975_2006/. Accessed December 24, 2009.

179. Davies L, Welch HG. Increasing incidence of thyroid cancer in the United States, 1973–2002. JAMA 2006;295:2164–7.

180. Hundahl SA, Fleming ID, Fremgen AM, et al. A National Cancer Data Base report on 53,856 cases of thyroid carcinoma treated in the U.S., 1985–1995 [see comments]. Cancer 1998;83:2638–48.

181. Antonelli A, Miccoli P, Derzhitski VE, et al. Epidemiologic and clinical evaluation of thyroid cancer in children from the Gomel region (Belarus). World J Surg 1996;20:867–71.

182. Bhatia S, Robison LL, Oberlin O, et al. Breast cancer and other second neoplasms after childhood Hodgkin's disease. N Engl J Med 1996;334:745–51.

183. Ron E, Kleinerman RA, Boice JD Jr, et al. A population-based case-control study of thyroid cancer. J Natl Cancer Inst 1987;79:1–12.

184. Pal T, Vogl FD, Chappuis PO, et al. Increased risk for nonmedullary thyroid cancer in the first degree relatives of prevalent cases of nonmedullary thyroid cancer: a hospital-based study. J Clin Endocrinol Metab 2001;86: 5307–12.

185. Goldgar DE, Easton DF, Cannon-Albright LA, et al. Systematic population-based assessment of cancer risk in first-degree relatives of cancer probands. J Natl Cancer Inst 1994;86:1600–8.

186. Hemminki K, Dong C. Familial relationships in thyroid cancer by histopathological type. Int J Cancer 2000;85:201–5.

187. Hemminki K, Eng C, Chen B. Familial risks for nonmedullary thyroid cancer. J Clin Endocrinol Metab 2005;90:5747–53.

188. Pal T, Hamel N, Vesprini D, et al. Double primary cancers of the breast and thyroid in women: molecular analysis and genetic implications. Fam Cancer 2001;1:17–24.

189. Harach HR, Soubeyran I, Brown A, et al. Thyroid pathologic findings in patients with Cowden disease. Ann Diagn Pathol 1999;3:331–40.

190. Nose V. Familial non-medullary thyroid carcinoma: an update. Endocr Pathol 2008;19:226–40.

191. Boikos SA, Stratakis CA. Carney complex: the first 20 years. Curr Opin Oncol 2007;19:24–9.

192. Collins MT, Sarlis NJ, Merino MJ, et al. Thyroid carcinoma in the McCune-Albright syndrome: contributory role of activating Gs alpha mutations. J Clin Endocrinol Metab 2003;88:4413–7.

193. Lote K, Andersen K, Nordal E, et al. Familial occurrence of papillary thyroid carcinoma. Cancer 1980;46:1291–7.

194. Burgess JR, Duffield A, Wilkinson SJ, et al. Two families with an autosomal dominant inheritance pattern for papillary carcinoma of the thyroid. J Clin Endocrinol Metab 1997;82:345–8.

195. Bignell GR, Canzian F, Shayeghi M, et al. Familial nontoxic multinodular thyroid goiter locus maps to chromosome 14q but does not account for familial nonmedullary thyroid cancer. Am J Hum Genet 1997;61:1123–30.
196. Bevan S, Pal T, Greenberg CR, et al. A comprehensive analysis of MNG1, TCO1, fPTC, PTEN, TSHR, and TRKA in familial nonmedullary thyroid cancer: confirmation of linkage to TCO1. J Clin Endocrinol Metab 2001;86:3701–4.
197. Canzian F, Amati P, Harach HR, et al. A gene predisposing to familial thyroid tumors with cell oxyphilia maps to chromosome 19p13.2. Am J Hum Genet 1998;63:1743–8.
198. Malchoff CD, Sarfarazi M, Tendler B, et al. Papillary thyroid carcinoma associated with papillary renal neoplasia: genetic linkage analysis of a distinct heritable tumor syndrome. J Clin Endocrinol Metab 2000;85:1758–64.
199. McKay JD, Lesueur F, Jonard L, et al. Localization of a susceptibility gene for familial nonmedullary thyroid carcinoma to chromosome 2q21. Am J Hum Genet 2001;69:440–6.
200. Grossman RF, Tu SH, Duh QY, et al. Familial nonmedullary thyroid cancer. An emerging entity that warrants aggressive treatment. Arch Surg 1995;130:892–7.

Heritability of Hematologic Malignancies: From Pedigrees to Genomics

Jane E. Churpek, MD[a], Kenan Onel, MD, PhD[b,c],*

KEYWORDS

• Familial • Leukemia • Lymphoma • Genetics • Genomics

It has long been recognized that there are several familial genetic syndromes, such as Lynch syndrome or hereditary breast and ovarian cancer syndrome, associated with a predisposition to solid tumors. Although not as well characterized, there also is an underlying heritable component to many hematologic malignances. Striking family pedigrees have been described in which multiple individuals are affected by leukemia or lymphoma, and hematologic malignancies are among the tumors associated with cancer predisposing syndromes such as Li-Fraumeni and ataxia telangiectasia (reviewed in Refs.[1,2]). Epidemiologic data also provide evidence for a heritable component to even seemingly sporadic cases of leukemia and lymphoma. Indeed, first-degree relatives of patients with leukemia are at a 2.5- to 6-fold increased risk of leukemia,[3,4] and first-degree relatives of patients with non-Hodgkin lymphoma (NHL) are at a 1.6- to 3.5-fold increased risk of NHL.[4,5]

Although these observations clearly demonstrate that there is an inherited component of risk for several hematologic malignancies, these genetic susceptibilities remain largely unknown. There is an extensive body of research characterizing the multitude of acquired recurrent genetic abnormalities in sporadic leukemia and lymphoma,

This work was supported by the Bear Necessities Pediatric Cancer Foundation (KO), the Cancer Research Foundation (KO), and NIH grants T32 CA009566-23 (JEC), HD0433871 (KO), and CA40046 (KO).

[a] Section of Hematology/Oncology, Department of Medicine, The University of Chicago, 5841 South Maryland Avenue, MC2115, Chicago, IL 60637, USA
[b] Section of Hematology/Oncology, Department of Pediatrics, The University of Chicago, 900 East 57th Street, Room 5140, Chicago, IL 60637, USA
[c] Familial Cancer Clinic, The University of Chicago, 900 East 57th Street, Room 5140, Chicago, IL 60637, USA
* Corresponding author. Section of Hematology/Oncology, Department of Pediatrics, The University of Chicago, 900 East 57th Street, Room 5140, Chicago, IL 60637.
E-mail address: konel@uchicago.edu

which have facilitated the classification of these diseases into prognostically and therapeutically important subgroups. Little is known, however, about the genetic abnormalities that predispose one toward their development and influence the subtype diagnosed in any given individual. Thus far, with few exceptions, attempts to identify the genetic factors underlying even highly familial hematologic malignancies have not been successful. Consequently, new strategies are necessary to unravel the heritability in these families.

This review describes what has been learned about the genetic contribution to hematologic malignancies through the study of both familial and sporadic disease. Furthermore, the authors highlight how the study of familial disease may inform the study of sporadic disease. Thus, the goal is to provide a comprehensive overview of our current understanding of the heritable component of hematologic malignancies in the genomics era. Although some of the genetic syndromes with which hematologic malignancies are already known to be associated are discussed in this review, a more comprehensive list is provided in **Table 1**.

CHRONIC LYMPHOCYTIC LEUKEMIA

As early as the 1920s, detailed reports were published describing familial clustering of chronic lymphocytic leukemia (CLL) cases and proposing a possible genetic basis to this disease.[6–8] Now, more than 200 familial CLL pedigrees have been identified.[9] The largest of these families comprises 222 individuals, of whom 10 have developed CLL, 1 has developed a T-cell NHL, and others have developed a variety of other cancers.[10] In a second family comprising 144 individuals, 11 have developed CLL.[11] The onset of CLL in these multiplex families is markedly younger than is observed in sporadic disease, with an average age at diagnosis of 56 years compared with 72 years for sporadic cases.[9] Several large epidemiologic studies undertaken in cohorts mainly comprised of individuals of European descent have confirmed that there is a heritable component of risk for CLL, demonstrating a 3- to 8.5-fold increased risk of CLL among first-degree relatives of probands.[4,12–14] In addition, indolent NHLs cosegregate with CLL in these families with lymphoplasmacytic lymphoma/Waldenstrom macroglobulinemia (4-fold risk) and hairy cell leukemia (3.3-fold risk) the most common.[12] Initially, it was believed that the inheritance of CLL in these large families was consistent with an autosomal dominant mode of inheritance with incomplete penetrance,[10,11] but in smaller families, consisting mostly of affected siblings, it was found to be more consistent with a recessive or other mode of inheritance.[7,11] Using DNA from multiple individuals within large multigenerational pedigrees, positional cloning techniques such as familial linkage mapping provided a logical method by which to uncover candidate CLL susceptibility genes. Consequently, both single-family and combined multifamily linkage studies were undertaken.

Neither of the 2 single-family studies undertaken was successful in identifying a single locus that was associated with disease, although several regions did emerge as interesting candidates. In the first study of 8 affected and 14 unaffected individuals from a single family, a locus at chromosome 14q24 achieved a suggestive nonparametric linkage (NPL) score of 2.24, and 3 other loci at 2q37, 4q35, and 11p15, achieved less significant NPL scores (0.3–2.07).[11] In the second study of 4 affected and 2 unaffected individuals in a smaller family, chromosome 9q achieved an NPL score of 0.96.[15] Multifamily studies, adding both genetic heterogeneity and a greater number of individuals for analysis, also identified numerous loci.[9,16–18] In the largest and most recent of these studies, more than 10,000 single nucleotide polymorphisms (SNPs) were genotyped in more than 400 affected individuals from 182 CLL pedigrees and 24 pedigrees showing cosegregation of CLL and B-cell lymphoproliferative disorders.[9] This study yielded evidence suggestive of linkage to 2q21.2 (maximum NPL 3.02, $P = .001$), linking 68% of families under a common recessive model of inheritance.[9]

Comparing all CLL linkage studies, however, no single locus was consistently identified from study to study.[9,16–18] In addition, none of the most significant loci identified in these studies corresponded to loci commonly somatically mutated in sporadic CLL, such as 13q14 (up to 55% of sporadic cases), 11q (17%–20%), 12q (16%–20%), 6q (2%–7%), and 17p (3%–5%).[19,20] Although pedigree data from family studies provide some evidence for Mendelian inheritance, no single locus has emerged to support a simple Mendelian inheritance pattern. Instead, the data suggest a model in which multiple common susceptibility alleles are co-inherited, each of which contributes only modestly to CLL susceptibility.

Identifying these risk variants is challenging. Multiple candidate gene studies, in which individual genes are investigated, based on their known involvement in biologically relevant pathways, such as B-cell differentiation, or based on their location within disease-associated regions identified in linkage or association studies, have been performed in an attempt to identify these risk variants. Overall, they have had limited success in identifying genetic variants accounting for a significant portion of CLL heritability. Some, however, have yielded insight into potentially disrupted pathways that merit further investigation.

One such candidate gene, initially identified through a familial linkage study, was DAPK1. In this study, Raval and colleagues[15] identified a common inherited haplotype on 9q in family members by linkage mapping. They selected DAPK1, which encodes a serine/threonine kinase that promotes apoptosis, for further investigation because they had previously shown that DAPK1 expression was commonly decreased in sporadic CLL by promoter hypermethylation. Consequently, they hypothesized that this gene was also involved in familial CLL. Indeed, in their familial CLL cases, they demonstrated decreased expression of DAPK1 by both genetic and epigenetic mechanisms. First, they identified a rare suppressor-region SNP, which was associated with a 70% decrease in gene transcription relative to wild-type.[15] Then, they demonstrated an even further attenuation of gene expression in affected family members by promoter hypermethylation-mediated gene silencing. These results are intriguing, as they not only identify a single gene potentially involved in both familial and sporadic cases but also highlight epigenetic modulation as one possible mechanism underlying the development of CLL. This adds to evidence from sporadic disease, in which aberrant methylation has been found in both promoters of individual genes and more globally at nonrandom sites within 4.8% of the CLL genome.[21,22]

In 2 other candidate gene studies undertaken in sporadically occurring CLL, investigators genotyped SNPs located in candidate cancer-related genes[23,24] and detected putative risk loci in genes that are members of the ATM-BRCA2-CHEK2 DNA damage response pathway,[24] as well as in genes involved in apoptosis (APAF1 and CASP8), immunoregulation (NOS2A, IL16, and CCR7), and cell cycle regulation (CCNH).[23] More than 900 candidate gene studies have been published on CLL. Despite the considerable effort involved in these investigations and these few intriguing results, most findings from candidate gene studies await replication in subsequent analyses. Thus, candidate gene studies have been largely unsuccessful in identifying sources of inherited genetic variation responsible for a significant portion of CLL risk.[25,26] This is not surprising as they are inherently limited to the investigation of genes and variants based on preexisting knowledge.

Genome-wide association studies (GWAS) are a recently developed method of undertaking an unbiased analysis of the entire genome to identify common

Table 1
Genetic syndromes featuring hematologic malignancies

Heme Malignancy	Pathway Disrupted	Syndrome	Inheritance Pattern	Gene Abnormality	Chromosomal Location	Risk of Heme Malignancy	References
AML	Tumor suppressor	Familial leukemia with CEBPA mutation	AD	*CEBPA*	19q13	Near 100%	152,162
		Familial platelet disorder	AD	*RUNX1*	21q22	MDS/AML: 50%[a]	152,158
		Neurofibromatosis, type I	AD	*NF1*	17q11	Myeloid: 500-fold JMML 224-fold	183
	DNA damage response	Li-Fraumeni	AD	*TP53* *CHK2*	17p13.1 22q12.1	4.8%[b]	184,185
	Telomere maintenance	Dyskeratosis congenita	X-linked R AD	*DKC1* *TERC* *TERT* *TNF2* *NHP2* *NOP10*	Xq28 3q26 5p15 14q12 5q35 15q14	MDS: >2000-fold (10%) AML: 200-fold (4%)	186
	Ribosome biogenesis	Shwachman-Diamond syndrome	AR	*SBDS*	7q11	10%–25%	153,187
		Diamond-Blackfan anemia	AD	*RPS19* *RPS17* *RPS24* *RPL11* *RPL35A*	19q13 15q 10q22-q23 1p36.1-p35 3q29-qter	4%	1
	DNA repair	Fanconi anemia	AR	*FANCA* *FANCC* *FANCD1 (BRCA2)* *FANCD2* *FANCE* *FANCF* *FANCG* *FANCI* *FANCJ*	16q24 9q22 13q12 3p26 6p22 11p15 9q13 15q26 17q22	650- to 868-fold (8%)	188

Category	Syndrome	Inheritance	Gene	Locus	Risk	Ref
		X-linked R	FANCL	2p16.1		
			FANCM	14q21.2		
			FANCN	16p12.2		
			FANCB	Xp22.2		
	Bloom syndrome	AR	BLM (RECQL3)	15q26.1	13%	189
	Werner	AR	RECQL2	8p12	Unknown	190
	Rothmund-Thomson	AR	RECQL4	8q24.3	Unknown	191
	Nijmegen breakage syndrome	AR	NBS1	8q21	1%–2%	192
Megakaryopoiesis	Congenital amegakaryocytic thrombocytopenia	AR	MPL	1p34	Unknown	193
Chromosome number	Down syndrome	Sporadic	Trisomy 21	Additional 21	M7 AML 400-fold TMPD 10%	2
Ras/MAPK pathway	Noonan syndrome	AD	PTPN11	12q24	Unknown	2,194
Other	Severe congenital neutropenia	AD	ELA2 (50%–60%)	19p13.3	10%	187,195
			GFI1	1p22		
			CSF3R	1p35-p34.3		
		AR	HAX1c	1q21.3		
			G6PC3	17q21.31		
		X-linked R	WAS	Xp11.23-11.22		
ALL						
Chromosome number	Down syndrome	Sporadic	Trisomy 21	Additional 21	ALL: 10-20-fold	196
Tumor suppressor	Neurofibromatosis, type I	AD	NF1	17q11	ALL: 5.4-fold	183
DNA damage response	Ataxia telangiectasia	AR	ATM	11q22.3	ALL, PLL, lymphoma (mostly T cell): 13%	197
	Li-Fraumeni	AD	TP53	17p13.1	4.8%b	184,185
			CHK2	22q12.1		
DNA repair	Bloom syndrome	AR	BLM (RECQL3)	15q26.1	13%	189
	Nijmegen breakage syndrome	AR	NBS1	8q21	3%–4%	192
Immune deficiency	Wiskott-Aldrich	X-linked R	WAS	Xp11.23	13%d	198
Ras/MAPK pathway	Noonan syndrome	AD	PTPN11	12q24	Unknown	2,194

(continued on next page)

Table 1
(continued)

Heme Malignancy	Pathway Disrupted	Syndrome	Inheritance Pattern	Gene Abnormality	Chromosomal Location	Risk of Heme Malignancy	References
HL	Apoptosis defect	ALPS	AD	APT1 (TNFRSF6)	10q24.1	50-fold	55
	DNA damage response	Li-Fraumeni	AD	TP53 CHK2	17p13.1 22q12.1	4.8%[b]	184,185
	DNA repair	Bloom syndrome	AR	BLM (RECQL3)	15q26.1	1%	189
	Immune deficiency	Immunodeficiency with hyper-IgM	X-linked R	CD40LG	Xq26	Unknown	2
NHL	Apoptosis defect	ALPS	AD	APT1 (TNFRSF6)	10q24.1	14-fold	55
	Tumor suppressor	Neurofibromatosis, type I	AD	NF1	17q11	NHL: 10-fold	183
	DNA damage response	Ataxia telangiectasia	AR	ATM	11q22.3	ALL, PLL, lymphoma (mostly T cell): 13%	197
	DNA repair	Bloom syndrome	AR	BLM (RECQL3)	15q26.1	13%	189
		Nijmegen breakage syndrome	AR	NBS1	8q21	29%	192
	Immune deficiency	Wiskott-Aldrich	X-linked R	WAS	Xp11.23	13%[d]	198
		Common variable immunodeficiency	AR and AD	TNFRSF13B and others	17p11.2	9%	2
		Severe combined immunodeficiency	AR	ADA	20q13.11	5%	199
		X-linked lymphoproliferative syndrome	X-linked	SAP (SH2D1A)	Xq25	20%	2
		Immunodeficiency with Hyper-IgM	X-linked R	CD40LG	Xq26	Unknown	2
CLL	DNA damage response	Li-Fraumeni	AD	TP53 CHK2	17p13.1 22q12.1	4.8%[b]	184,185

Abbreviations: AD, autosomal dominant; ALL, acute lymphoblastic leukemia; ALPS, autoimmune lymphoproliferative syndrome; AML, acute myelogenous leukemia; AR, autosomal recessive; CLL, chronic lymphocytic leukemia; HL, Hodgkin lymphoma; IgM, immunoglobulin M; JMML, juvenile myelomonocytic leukemia; MDS, myelodysplastic syndrome; NHL, non-Hodgkin lymphoma; PLL, prolymphocytic leukemia; TMPD, transient myeloproliferative disorder; X-linked R, X-linked recessive.

[a] Denotes the median incidence of MDS/AML in FPD/AML.
[b] Denotes incidence of all hematologic malignancies in Li-Fraumeni.
[c] Kostman syndrome is another name for severe congenital neutropenia with HAX1 mutations.
[d] Denotes incidence of all lymphoreticular malignancies in Wiskott-Aldrich.

susceptibility alleles associated with a complex disease. In GWAS, SNPs throughout the genome are genotyped in cases and controls. Although only a relatively small number of SNPs are actually genotyped using even the densest of currently available genotyping platforms, because of linkage disequilibrium (LD), these SNPs serve as tags to identify genomic regions containing disease-associated variation. These studies, however, require large numbers of ethnically similar cases and controls to attain sufficient power for the detection of this variation, as well as sophisticated statistical analyses to control for multiple testing and to assess the potentially confounding effects of unsuspected genetic or nongenetic factors. Furthermore, because the effect size of most disease-associated variants is frequently small, these studies are reliant on replication in an independent cohort for validation. Consequently, the role of GWAS has been largely limited to the study of sporadic CLL.

However, one GWAS undertaken in CLL was enriched for familial disease with 155 probands from multiplex families included among 517 CLL cases of European descent analyzed.[27] More than 350,000 SNPs were genotyped in these cases and in 1500 controls. Six susceptibility loci were identified and replicated in 2 separate case-control cohorts. Of these, one, located at 6p25.3 was in a gene involved in B-cell development and differentiation (*IRF4*), and another, located at 2q37.1, was near a gene regulating the immunologic response to viral infection (*SP140*). In both cases, the risk-associated SNP was correlated with decreased mRNA expression in Epstein-Barr virus (EBV)-transformed lymphocytes. None of the other 4 loci, 2q13, 11q24.1, 15q23, and 19q13.32, were associated with specific genes.

Recently, the investigation of microRNAs in cancer has engendered considerable excitement. MicroRNAs are 18 to 22 nucleotide single-stranded noncoding RNAs formed from a double stranded RNA precursor. They play a prominent role in the regulation of gene expression via multiple epigenetic mechanisms (reviewed in Ref.[28]). One mechanism by which microRNAs attenuate gene expression is by binding messenger RNAs through sequence complementarity and targeting them for degradation.[28] Because of its short length, a single microRNA often has homology to a variety of mRNAs, and is therefore able to control the expression of a network of genes by binding to multiple messenger RNAs. Altered expression of microRNAs through various mechanisms, including somatic mutation, has been implicated in the pathogenesis of multiple cancers, including CLL.[29]

To identify microRNAs involved in CLL pathogenesis, Calin and colleagues[30] examined the global microRNA expression profile of CLL cells from 94 patients and identified a signature containing 13 microRNAs, which differentiated patients with poor prognostic molecular markers (ZAP-70 expression and unmutated *IgV_H*) from those without these markers. In addition, a germline mutation was identified in 1 allele of the precursor to *miR-16-1* in 2 patients, including 1 with other family members with CLL and breast cancer. In both patients, a somatic mutation in the other allele was observed. This germline mutation in *pri-miR-16-1* was associated with decreased expression of both *miR-16-1* and *miR-15a*, which function as tumor suppressors in CLL by regulating the expression of many genes including the CLL-associated genes as *BCL-2* and *WT1*.[28,30] These 2 microRNAs are located at 13q14, the site most frequently deleted in sporadic disease, and were previously shown to be lost in most sporadic cases of CLL.[29,31] This evidence of microRNA deregulation in both sporadic and familial CLL gives further weight to their likely role in CLL pathogenesis.

Although suggestive, the positive associations identified through these varied techniques require replication in additional cohorts for validation. In addition, given the multiple loci identified from candidate gene, linkage, genome-wide association, and microRNA studies, the challenge now is to prioritize for further investigation and functional verification those associations that truly contribute to CLL risk. Ideally, as consistent genetic abnormalities and predispositions are identified, studies integrating genomics, bioinformatics, and molecular biology can be used to generate a network of independent and interacting susceptibility variants that together define the pathways associated with CLL risk.

For now, however, clinicians are limited in their ability to counsel families with CLL about the genetic basis of their disease. They can estimate the risk in family members for CLL to be between 3 and 8.5 times that of the general population.[4,12–14] Given that the lifetime risk of CLL development in the general population is low at 0.47% (http://seer.cancer.gov/statfacts/html/clyl.html), however, the overall risk for family members remains small. The same is true for risk of other indolent lymphomas in these families. Epidemiologic data suggest that the risk of solid tumors (in particular, breast, prostate, and gastrointestinal cancer) is also increased in relatives of patients with CLL[4,13] and in individuals with CLL. Multiple retrospective and observational studies have identified an overall 1.2- to 3-fold increased risk of second malignancies in patients with CLL, particularly lung and skin cancer, although a variety of tumor types have been reported, so these patients should follow routine cancer screening guidelines and be aware of this increased risk (reviewed in Ref.[32]).

Within a single family, clinicians may be able to identify specific individuals more likely to develop CLL than others through detection of a monoclonal B-cell lymphocytosis (MBL). MBL is a clonal population of B cells at low levels not meeting the criteria for overt CLL, and can now be detected by sensitive techniques such as flow cytometry. MBL is considered a precursor condition to CLL. MBL is found in 3.5% to 5% of normal individuals in the general population with an approximately 1.1% per year risk of overt CLL development,[33] but is found in up to 13.5% of healthy relatives of case with familial CLL, suggesting that these individuals may be at increased risk for CLL.[34] Although interesting, the risk of progression to CLL among these individuals remains unknown and, even if MBL is detected and monitored, thus far, there is no evidence that early intervention for asymptomatic individuals has an effect on overall survival.[35] Therefore, routine screening of relatives of CLL patients with MBL is currently not recommended, and they can be counseled that their risk of CLL and indolent NHL is low.[12]

HODGKIN LYMPHOMA

Classic Hodgkin lymphoma (HL) is morphologically characterized by clonal populations of neoplastic binucleated B cells, Reed-Sternberg cells, contained within a dense background of inflammatory cells. Antecedent exposure to EBV has been associated with the development of HL, especially the mixed cellularity subtype in children and older adults,[36] but data suggest that there is also a heritable component to HL susceptibility. Familial clustering of HL is rare, but multiplex families have been identified in population-based registries[14,37,38] and single or multi-institution case series.[39–41] From these studies, first-degree relatives of probands have a 2.6- to 4.9-fold increased risk of HL compared with the general population,[14,37,38] which increases further if the proband developed HL at less than 40 years of age.[37] Twin studies also suggest a genetic component to HL risk. In 1 study of 179 monozygotic (MZ) and 187 dizygotic (DZ) twin pairs followed for 14 years in which 1 twin had been diagnosed with HL, 10 cases of HL occurred in previously unaffected MZ twins, but none in previously unaffected DZ twins, resulting in an impressive 100-fold increased risk of HL in an MZ twin of a proband.[39] Most of these twin pairs were also concordant for HL subtype.[39]

Risk within these HL families is not evenly distributed. In particular, siblings and cousins of probands are at greatest risk. This risk has been observed in both population-based registry studies, in which it is estimated that there is a 4.3- to 6.2-fold increased risk for siblings compared with a 1.2- to 3.1-fold increased risk for parents or offspring of probands,[37,42] and in case series of multiplex families.[43] Among siblings, same sex sibs are at even greater risk. Of the affected sibling pairs reported in the literature, sex concordance has been observed in 80 of 120 sib pairs.[44] Based on data from population-based registries, the standardized incidence ratio is 8 for the brother of an affected brother and 11.8 for the sister of an affected sister, but only 1.37 for gender discordant sibling pairs.[42]

This strong sex concordance has led to the hypothesis that an HL predisposition gene may be located on the pseudoautosomal region (PAR) of the sex chromosomes, which if inherited without recombination from a carrier father, results in gender concordant affected offspring.[44,45] Evidence in support of this hypothesis includes (1) the finding that when gender was used as a covariate in a linkage study of 503 affected relatives from 112 HL families, a region in the PAR of the X chromosome was identified with a statistically significant logarithm of odds (LOD) score of 2.41[44]; (2) the co-occurrence of HL in 1 pair of sisters affected by Leri-Weill dyschondrosteosis, a disorder caused by microdeletions in SHOX, a homeobox gene located in the PAR[46]; and (3) the localization to the PAR of MIC2, which encodes CD99, a cell adhesion protein negatively regulated by EBV latent membrane protein 1 and, which when knocked down in B cells by expressing antisense CD99 mRNA, results in cells phenotypically similar to Reed-Sternberg cells.[47]

Other candidate genes have been proposed in familial HL, most of which are involved in immune modulation. The most extensively studied of these are the HLA region genes on chromosome 6, which have been associated with both sporadic and familial HL. Reed-Sternberg cells are antigen-presenting cells that express class II antigens, and, in EBV-positive HL, also express class I antigens.[48] It has been proposed that altered antigen presentation by the Reed-Sternberg cells could lead to activation of inflammatory cells and may underlie the inflammatory infiltrate characteristic of this disease (reviewed in Ref.[49]). Among both familial and sporadic HL, associations with multiple HLA class I and HLA class II alleles have been repeatedly reported, with A1, B5, B18, and DPB1*0301 the most consistently identified (reviewed in Ref.[49]). More recently, associations between specific HLA alleles and particular HL subtypes (eg, DRB1*1501-DQA1*0102-DQB1-0602 and nodular sclerosing HL[50,51]), and between specific HLA alleles and EBV status (eg, 2 HLA class I alleles near microsatellite markers D6S265 and D6S510 and EBV-positive HL[52]) have been reported. Despite these multiple associations, however, specific causative mutations have not been identified. This is largely because of strong LD within this vast region, containing more than 220 genes, which makes it difficult to distinguish disease-causing genetic variants from variants associated with disease by virtue of LD.

IL-6 and IL-12, 2 cytokines involved in immune system regulation, have also been implicated in HL risk, specifically among those developing HL as young adults. IL-6 has potent B-cell stimulatory properties and is secreted by Reed-Sternberg cells,[53] and IL-12 stimulates cell-mediated immune responses.[54] In HL twin pair studies, whereas inherited polymorphisms in IL-6 resulting in lower IL-6 blood levels were found to be protective against HL, polymorphisms in IL-12 resulting in lower IL-12 levels were associated with a nearly 3-fold increased risk of HL.[53,54]

Because HL is a component of inherited immunodeficiency syndromes, the genes underlying these disorders have also been assessed for association with HL (see **Table 1**). Perhaps the best studied is autoimmune lymphoproliferative syndrome

(ALPS, also known as Canale-Smith syndrome), an inherited disorder characterized by chronic lymphadenopathy, splenomegaly, autoimmunity, and a particularly high risk of HL (50-fold).[55] Individuals with ALPS are frequently found to have germline mutations in the *APT1* gene, encoding Fas, a cell surface receptor with a key role in initiating apoptosis in activated lymphocytes. In both in vitro and in mouse models, fas-mutant lymphocytes are resistant to fas-mediated apoptosis, which may result in inappropriate lymphocyte survival, enlarged lymphoid organs, and an increased risk of lymphoma.[55]

Investigation of the fas pathway in 10 families with familial lymphoma, of which 3 had familial HL, led to the identification of another defect in this pathway in 2 families. In affected individuals compared with healthy controls, protein levels of caspase 8, an apoptotic initiator downstream of fas, were decreased relative to cFlip, a downstream apoptosis inhibitor.[56] The mechanism accounting for this altered protein ratio was not identified nor was it determined if this defect was germline or acquired.[56] Nonetheless, these data suggest that further investigation of the association between HL and both the fas pathway and deregulated lymphocyte apoptosis is warranted.

An additional candidate gene, *KLHDC8B*, a gene with previously unknown function located at 3p21, was identified by the mapping of a constitutional reciprocal translocation involving chromosomes 2 and 3 in a family with multiple individuals with HL.[57] This translocation disrupted the 5′ portion of *KLHDC8B* and resulted in loss of gene expression. In addition, a heterozygous single nucleotide variant in the 5′ untranslated region of the same gene that led to decreased mRNA and protein levels was identified in 3 of 52 other multiplex HL families and was found to segregate with disease in the affected families. The protein was investigated and found to localize to the midbody of the cytoplasmic bridge linking dividing daughter cells during cytokinesis, and its depletion via RNA interference led to the formation of binucleated cells similar to HL's characteristic Reed-Sternberg cells.[57] The association between *KLHDC8B* and sporadic HL remains to be investigated.

In addition to these candidate gene studies, 1 group also undertook a genome-wide linkage study in HL families. They genotyped more than 1000 microsatellite markers in 254 individuals from 44 HL families and found evidence for linkage on chromosome 4p (peak LOD score 2.6, $P = .0002$), linking 43% of families under a recessive model.[43] Other regions with less significant evidence of linkage were identified on chromosomes 4q, 7, and 17. Only modest linkage was seen on chromosome 6 near the HLA region (maximum NPL score 2), suggesting a more limited association of HLA in this larger population of HL families.[43] Although all these studies have yielded some plausible candidate HL susceptibility genes, specific variants accounting for the increased risk of HL in these families have not yet been identified.

Clinically, there is limited information for HL families. They can, however, be counseled on the differing risks to specific family members so that those at the highest risk (ie, same sex sibs) can be closely followed. It must be kept in mind, however, that the lifetime risk of HL in the general population is estimated to be 0.24%.[37] Thus, the overall lifetime risk for HL, even in same sex sibs, remains low at 2% to 3%.[42] With regard to risk of other tumors, a small increased risk of NHL and CLL, as well as breast, ovarian, cervical, and brain tumors, was reported for relatives of individuals with HL in 1 population-based study[37]; these findings, however, await confirmation.

NHL

NHL encompasses a diverse group of more than 50 lymphomas with distinct morphologic, immunophenotypic, cytogenetic, genetic, and clinical features.[58] Diffuse large

B-cell lymphoma (DLBCL) and follicular lymphoma (FL) are the most common subtypes, accounting for 25% to 36% and 17% to 32% of NHL, respectively, in western countries.[59] Ideally, investigations into the cause of NHL would examine each subtype separately to identify environmental and genetic risk factors unique to each lymphoma. This has not been feasible, however, because of the relative rarity of many NHL subtypes. In addition, the changing NHL classification systems[58] have made it difficult to compare results from older and newer studies. The current World Health Organization classification system (2008), divides lymphoid neoplasms by cell of origin (eg, B vs T cell) and stage of lymphocyte development (precursor vs mature).[60] This groups plasma cell disorders and CLL (ie, small lymphocytic lymphoma) with other mature B-cell NHLs. However, this section focuses on evidence for inherited susceptibility to NHL, excluding CLL and plasma cell disorders, which are addressed separately.

Despite significant research, the cause of most NHLs remains unknown. Lifestyle risk factors and the possible contribution of chemical and other environmental exposures to risk have been studied extensively, but except for the well-recognized association between NHL and infectious agents such as EBV and human immunodeficiency virus (HIV), the results of these studies have been controversial.[61] That there is a heritable component to NHL is based on several observations. First, there are multiple reports of clustering of NHL with and without other types of hematopoietic malignancies in families (reviewed in Ref.[1,62]). Second, immigrants retain the NHL incidence patterns of their country of origin rather than adopting that of their new location.[63–65] Multiple large population-based studies, including a pooled analysis of 17 studies conducted in the United States and Europe, have identified a 1.5- to 3-fold increased risk of NHL in first-degree relatives of patients with NHL.[4,5,66,67] Other population-based studies, however, conducted in the United States and Iceland, did not confirm this increased risk,[14,38] and the results of twin studies to determine whether the MZ twin of an individual with NHL is at greater risk than the DZ twin have been conflicting.[39,68]

These inconsistencies are likely due in part to the heterogeneity of NHL itself. Risk factors almost certainly differ among different NHL subtypes, and both genetic risk factors and environmental exposures are also likely to differ among different ethnicities. To minimize disease heterogeneity, several large studies have assessed susceptibilities to the most common lymphoma subtypes. One large registry-based study from Sweden found a significantly increased risk of DLBCL in relatives of patients with DLBCL (relative risk [RR] 9.8), and an increased risk of FL (RR 4) and other indolent NHL (RR 2) among relatives of patients with FL.[69] The largest population-based study undertaken to date, in which more than 10,000 patients with NHL were compared with 11,000 controls by the International Lymphoma Epidemiology Consortium (InterLymph), examined the risk of specific NHL subtypes in relatives of patients with NHL and found an increased risk of DLBCL (odds ratio [OR] 1.4) and FL (OR 1.8) among those with a family history of NHL, which increased if the affected case was male (OR 2 and 2.2 for DLBCL and FL, respectively) and increased even further if the case was a brother (OR 2.7 and 2.6).[66] Relatives with a brother with NHL also had a statistically significant increased risk of marginal zone lymphoma (RR 6.1) and mantle cell lymphoma (RR 4.9).[66] However, a much smaller study did not find increased risks for any subtype among those with a family history of NHL.[70] These studies highlight the need for large numbers of cases to discover subtype- and population-specific risks.

Clues to the genetic basis of heritability in NHL have come from examining genetic syndromes with an increased risk of NHL. One such group of syndromes is caused by defects in DNA repair, and includes autosomal recessive disorders (gene defects noted in parentheses) such as ataxia telangiectasia (ATM), Bloom syndrome (BLM), Nijmegen breakage syndrome (NBS1),[1] and mismatch repair deficiency syndrome (MSH2, MLH1, MSH6, PMS2),[71] in which affected individuals have a striking propensity to develop lymphomas at an early age. In addition, individuals with 1 defective copy of some of these same genes may also be at increased risk of NHL, suggesting a dosage effect. Heterozygous carriers of the NBS1 657del5 mutation, the founder Nijmegen breakage syndrome mutation in Eastern Europeans, for example, were enriched among Polish adults and children with NHL[72,73] but not adults with NHL in the United States.[74] Heterozygous carriers of mismatch repair gene defects have hereditary nonpolyposis colon cancer (Lynch syndrome) and are at risk for development of multiple tumor types, especially colon cancer. An increased risk of lymphoma in these patients has been controversial,[75] but multiple reports of lymphoma in patients with Lynch syndrome exist, with 1 report suggesting that lymphoma in these patients is associated with an acquired inactivating mutation of the remaining wild-type copy of the mismatch repair gene.[76]

Genetic syndromes with defects in immune function are also associated with a significant risk of NHL. Individuals with common variable immunodeficiency caused by defects in CD40 signaling, severe combined immunodeficiency disease caused by adenosine deaminase defects, Wiskott-Aldrich syndrome caused by WASP defects, and 2 X-linked immunodeficiency syndromes (X-linked lymphoproliferative syndrome and X-linked immunodeficiency with normal or increased immunoglobulin M [IgM]) all have a propensity to develop lymphoma, which is often striking (eg, 18% of patients with Wiskott-Aldrich syndrome develop lymphoma).[1,75] In addition, patients with syndromes characterized by autoimmunity are also at risk. Individuals with ALPS are not only at risk for HL (50-fold increased risk) but they also have a 14-fold increased risk of NHL compared with the general population.[55] The increased risk of NHL in patients with sporadically occurring medical conditions characterized by autoimmunity such as rheumatoid arthritis (RR 1.5–3.9), systemic lupus erythematosus (RR 4.6–8.4), Sjogren syndrome (RR 5.1–18.8), and celiac disease (RR 2.1–9.1) provides further evidence that pathways involved in autoimmunity have a role in lymphomagenesis (reviewed in Ref.[61]).

These observations have suggested potential candidate pathways for investigation into associations with NHL. To screen the large number of genes involved in the multiple proposed pathways in the genomics era, many groups have undertaken association studies comparing the frequency of a large number of individual SNPs located in candidate genes in patients affected with NHL versus controls. To date, the most consistently replicated finding has been the association between SNPs in the inflammatory response pathway (TNF and LTA) and in the immunoregulatory gene, IL10, and NHL, in particular DLBCL.[77,78] The largest candidate gene association study in NHL was undertaken through the InterLymph Consortium and examined TNF family SNPs in more than 3500 cases and 4000 controls, mostly of European descent, pooled from 8 separate case-control studies.[79] This study found a statistically significant increased risk of NHL with SNPs in TNF (−308G>A, OR 1.19, $P = .005$) and IL10 (−3575 T>A, OR 1.11, $P = .037$) in the pooled analysis. These same SNPs were associated with an even greater risk of DLBCL (OR 1.33, $P = .00021$, and OR 1.22, $P = .006$, respectively). An SNP in LTA (252 A>G), which is in LD with the TNF −303G>A SNP in the HLA III region on chromosome 6p21, was also associated with an increased risk of NHL (for homozygous GG: OR 1.18, $P = .11$) and DLBCL (for homozygous GG: OR 1.47, $P = .001$).[79] These associations have been confirmed in other studies undertaken primarily in individuals of European descent,[78,80–83] strengthening the evidence that these regions are associated with increased risk for NHL.

Other candidate gene association studies have been performed looking at cell cycle, apoptosis, lymphocyte development, DNA repair, immune system regulation, metabolism (both 1 carbon and xenobiotics), hormone production, and oxidative stress pathways. A review of these studies is beyond the scope of this article (see Ref.[77] for an excellent review), but some of the more recently identified positive associations are highlighted here. For NHL as a group, associations with SNPs in or near several other genes within the TNF/NFκB pathway (NFKBIL1, FAS, IRF4, TNFSF13B, TANK, TNFSF7, and TNFRSF13C[78,84]), within lymphocyte development and immune system regulation (BCL6,[85,86] BCL2L11, PIM1, and BCL7A[86]), within apoptosis pathways (CASP1, CASP8, and CASP9[87]) and within innate immunity pathways (TLR10-TLR1-TLR6 gene cluster[88]) have been reported. In addition, a deletion polymorphism in a glutathione S-transferase (GSTT1*0), an enzyme involved in detoxification of reactive oxygen species, has been found to increase NHL and HL risk in those homozygous for this polymorphism in several studies (reviewed in Ref.[77]). Among specific NHL subtypes, associations have been identified for DLBCL (IL10, TNF, LTA as described, as well as BCL7A and PIM1[86]), FL (BCL2L11, BCL6,[86] FAS, TNFSF7,[78] TNFRSF5[89]), and marginal zone lymphoma (TLR4,[88] TNFRSF13C,[78] BCL6[86]).

Familial clustering of lymphoplasmacytic lymphoma/Waldenstrom macroglobulinemia (LPL/WM) has also been described. In these families, unaffected family members have a low-level IgM monoclonal gammopathy of unknown significance (MGUS), which is characterized by detection of a low-level monoclonal immunoglobulin in the serum without evidence of multiple myeloma (MM)-related end-organ dysfunction and less than 10% plasma cells in the bone marrow,[90] at a much higher rate than in the general population (3.2–6.3% vs 0.25–0.64%, respectively), suggesting that this may be a precursor condition.[91] A population-based case-control study from Sweden examining 2144 LPL/WM cases and more than 24,000 controls found a 20-fold increased risk of LPL/WM in first-degree relatives of cases.[92] In addition, relatives were at increased risk of NHL (RR 3), CLL (RR 3.4), and MGUS (RR 5), suggesting shared susceptibilities for these disorders. Relatives of LPL/WM patients were not at increased risk for MM, despite known associations between MGUS and MM.[92] A genome-wide linkage analysis performed on 11 LPL/WM families found evidence suggestive of linkage at 1q and 4q (NPL 2.5 and 3.1, respectively) and less strongly at 3q and 6q, which may suggest that these regions harbor susceptibility alleles for LPL/WM, as well as associated conditions such as CLL and MGUS.[93]

Clinically, genetic counseling is currently of limited value for NHL families. Detailed family and medical histories are essential, especially in children, to rule out any of the known genetic syndromes with a predisposition to NHL. For those families with specific subtypes of NHL, they can be counseled regarding subtype specific risks. For example, families with LPL/WM can be counseled about the increased risk of IgM MGUS and can be screened for this condition. If IgM MGUS is diagnosed, monitoring is necessary because of the increased risk for LPL/WM (1.5% per year).[91] The identification of highly penetrant NHL families may ultimately yield families large enough for linkage analysis. In addition, GWAS in NHL are currently underway, which will contribute significantly to our understanding of the heritable contribution to risk in NHL.

MM

MM is a malignant hematologic disorder characterized by anemia, destructive bony lesions, recurrent infections, and renal failure caused by the expansion of neoplastic plasma cells and the accumulation of the abnormal monoclonal immunoglobulins these cells produce. MGUS, a precursor condition to MM, has been identified in 3% to 6% of healthy adults more than 50 years of age (reviewed in Ref.[94]) and is associated with a 1% to 3% per year risk of progressing to overt MM.[95] Both MM and MGUS are twice as common in African Americans compared with whites and are less common in Asians. In all populations, these 2 conditions cosegregate in families.[94]

The cause of MM and MGUS remains unknown, but associations with both environmental exposures and genetic factors have been proposed. Studies have implicated specific exposures such as benzene-containing products, infections, and inflammatory and autoimmune disorders, with the latter possibly acting through chronic antigenic stimulation (reviewed in Ref.[96]). A genetic predisposition has been postulated based on clustering of MM and MGUS within families. Thus far, more than 100 such families of European descent have been reported.[96] In addition, several population-based case-control studies, including mostly individuals of European descent, have demonstrated an increased risk of MM in first-degree relatives of cases (RR 1.7–5.6),[97–100] and also of MGUS in relatives of patients with MM (RR 2–2.9) and MGUS (RR 2.8–3.3).[101,102] The only study examining racial differences in MM risk included 142 African American and 182 white patients with MM and found a greater risk of MM in relatives of African American MM probands (OR 17.4) than in relatives of white MM probands (OR 1.5), although these estimates were based on small numbers of cases.[98]

With little known about genetic factors contributing to MM susceptibility, several investigators have compiled familial case series[96,103–106] to assess possible inheritance patterns and disease phenotypes. Because of the rarity of familial MM, however, only a small number of families have been studied thus far, and results must be interpreted with caution.[103] In 1 study, for example, inheritance was assessed in 36 MM families, and an autosomal recessive pattern of inheritance was described.[104] In other reports, however, an autosomal dominant inheritance pattern was described, but these contained several much larger, multigenerational pedigrees.[96,103] There is little consistency in the disease phenotype observed in these studies, with some reporting a similar age of onset compared with sporadic MM patients[104] and others reporting both a younger age at diagnosis and even anticipation within families.[103,106] Virtually all reports, however, note the cosegregation of MM with a variety other cancers, both hematologic malignancies and solid tumors, within these families, suggesting a shared susceptibility (reviewed in Ref.[103]). Attempts to identify additional families are underway with the formation of a familial MM registry.[96]

Several population-based studies in the United States and Sweden have provided insight into familial risk in MM. First-degree relatives of individuals with MM are at a 2- to 6-fold increased risk of MM,[97–100] and there are some data to suggest that female relatives of patients with MM and relatives of female probands are at an even greater risk.[100] Familial susceptibility to other tumor types was also investigated. In 1 study of more than 30,000 first-degree relatives of 14,000 patients with MM in Sweden, these relatives were found to have a significantly increased risk of bladder cancer (RR 1.3), acute lymphoblastic leukemia (ALL) (RR 2.1), and prostate cancer (RR 1.1).[99] In an earlier study in which 239 patients with MM and 220 healthy controls self-reported family history of cancer, relatives of patients with MM were found to be at increased risk for prostate cancer (RR 3.1) and brain tumors (RR 6.61).[97] In addition, relatives of patients with MGUS were found to be at increased risk of bladder cancer (RR 1.4), spinal cord cancer (RR 3), and melanoma (RR 1.3).[107] In contrast to these population-based studies, in the few reports of MM multiplex pedigrees, it was reported that MM most frequently cosegregated with colon cancer, breast cancer, pancreatic cancer, leukemia, and lymphoma,[103] perhaps implicating MM as part of a cancer predisposition syndrome. Reports of MM in BRCA 1 and 2 carriers, and in those with hereditary CDKN2A mutations, known to cause hereditary melanoma and pancreatic cancer, provide some support for this hypothesis.[103]

With limited knowledge about the cause of MM and no linkage or association studies undertaken to date, it is not surprising that few strong candidate loci have emerged. One potential candidate locus is a heterozygous 200-bp deletion in a pseu-dogene, poly(ADP-ribose) polymerase-like gene (PADRP), on the long arm of chromo-some 13. This region is frequently deleted in sporadic MM as well as other B-cell malignancies, and portends a poor prognosis.[108] In 1 study of 54 African Americans with MM and MGUS and 37 African American controls, this deletion was found to be significantly associated with MM,[108] but these findings have not been replicated. Another group found that the hyperphosphorylation of paratarg-7, a protein without clear function that is an autoimmune target of MM/MGUS paraproteins, cosegregated with familial MM and MGUS.[109] This paratarg-7 variant appeared to be inherited in an autosomal dominant fashion and was estimated to confer nearly an 8-fold increased risk of MM/MGUS.

Thus far, the most biologically plausible candidates are members of the NF-kB pathway, which is known to be altered in MM and is the target of a new class of drugs used to treat MM, the proteosome inhibitors.[110] Keats and colleagues[110] analyzed samples from 42 patients with MM and 46 MM cell lines by high-density array comparative genomic hybridization, and another 125 patient samples and 44 MM cell lines by global gene expression profiling. They identified somatic mutations and corresponding alterations in expression in 10 different genes involved in the regulation of the noncanonical NF-kB pathway. Of these, inactivating mutations in TRAF3, a negative regulator of NF-kB signaling, were the most common, found in 13% of patients with MM examined. In addition, they demonstrated in another set of patient samples that those with decreased TRAF3 expression and concomitant activation of the NF-kB pathway were most likely to respond clinically to proteosome inhibitors.[110]

Clinically, there is limited information concerning genetic factors contributing to susceptibility in MM/MGUS families. Careful family histories may reveal patterns consistent with syndromes such as hereditary breast and ovarian cancer syndrome (BRCA1/2) or hereditary melanoma and pancreatic cancer (CDKN2A) that have been associated with MM (reviewed in Ref.[103]), which would require referral to a cancer risk specialist for further evaluation. In addition, a careful history may identify a large multigenerational pedigree with enough informative individuals for linkage anal-ysis. A familial MM registry has been created to further this goal.[96] Families can be counseled about the increased risk of MGUS, and offered screening to identify those at greatest risk of MM development. Family members should be encouraged to get recommended routine cancer screening examinations as they may have a greater propensity to develop cancer than the general population.

MYELOPROLIFERATIVE NEOPLASMS

The Philadelphia chromosome-negative myeloproliferative neoplasms (MPNs) are a heterogeneous group of disorders resulting from a defect in the hematopoietic stem cell that are characterized by clonal populations of mature-appearing blood cells, a propensity to thrombosis and bleeding, and an increased risk of leukemic transformation. These disorders include polycythemia vera (PV), essential thrombocythemia (ET), primary myelofibrosis (PMF) as well as several other rare disorders. For decades, little was known about the cause of MPNs, and, until recently, only a small number of case reports and case series describing families with multiple affected individuals[111–113] provided evidence for a possible heritable component to these disorders. The results of a linkage study in a cohort of familial MPN pedigrees undertaken to identify a disease locus did not provide support for suspected candidate loci such as 9p, 13q, and 20q, regions in which acquired deletions were common in MPNs, nor did they suggest that inherited mutations in biologically plausible candidates such as the thrombopoietin receptor gene and the erythropoietin receptor gene (MPL and EPOR) (LOD <−2)[113] were associated with familial MPN.

In 2005, several different groups reported the identification of a mutation in the Janus kinase 2 (JAK2) gene located on chromosome 9p in sporadic PV.[114–117] This exact same mutation, JAK2 V617F, was then shown to be present not only in patients with PV but also in most patients with MPN, occurring in 95% to 100% of patients with PV and nearly 50% of patients with ET and PMF.[117] This mutation affects the pseudo-kinase domain of the protein, which negatively regulates its tyrosine kinase domain through conformational interactions between these 2 domains.[118] It alters a key residue involved in this interaction, thereby providing a proliferative advantage to hematopoietic stem cells with this mutation (reviewed in Ref.[118]). The identification of this novel mutation allowed patients with MPN to be readily distinguished from those with myeloproliferative processes from other causes (eg, inherited erythrocytosis caused by EPOR mutations). As a result, the presence of this mutation was added as a major diagnostic criterion in the 2008 World Health Organization's updated diagnostic schemata for the MPNs.[119]

Following this discovery, a flurry of research has yielded insight into the functional consequences of this mutation and its implication for the MPN disorders. In vitro studies demonstrated that expression of JAK2 V617F in human hematopoietic progenitor cells resulted in the formation of erythroid colonies in the absence of growth factors, thus replicating the characteristic endogenous erythroid colony (EEC) phenotype of PV patients.[120] In addition, expression of this mutation in a mouse model resulted in a PV-like phenotype, suggesting that this mutation was a causative factor.[116]

Attempts to examine JAK2 in familial MPN led to efforts to identify such kindreds. The incidence of familial MPN was found to be much greater than had been suspected. In 1 study of 458 patients with apparently sporadic MPNs, for example, 35 were found to be members of multiplex MPN families.[121] From this study, it was estimated that the prevalence of familial disease was 8.7%, 5.9%, and 8.2% for PV, ET, and PMF respectively.[121] Likewise, in the only population-based study yet performed, investigators in Sweden found a 5- to 7-fold increased risk of MPN in first-degree relatives of patients with an MPN.[122] Multiple types of MPNs were observed in about 40% of these families, suggesting that they share a common predisposing genetic lesion.[121,123] The inheritance pattern in these families followed an autosomal dominant pattern with incomplete penetrance.[121,123]

JAK2 mutation analysis in these familial cases has led to several important observations. First, even among familial cases in which all affected family members shared the V617F mutation, this mutation was not identified in all tissues of affected individuals, indicating that it is an acquired and not an inherited mutation.[123,124] This was confirmed in other pedigrees, in which some individuals with MPN had the V617F mutation, but others did not.[123] Thus, the predisposing susceptibility loci are yet to be identified.[113,123] Indeed, studies in patients with sporadic MPN also indicate that the JAK2 V617F mutation is a late event occurring in the context of already established clonal hematopoiesis (reviewed in Ref.[118]). Furthermore, the mutation was found in some patients at surprisingly low levels (allelic burden <25%) for a supposed driving mutation, and was at times independently acquired in separate clones within an individual patient.[125] Overall, the incidence of the V617F mutation is similar in familial and sporadic MPNs, and is found in 55% to 75% of familial cases of PV versus 95% of sporadic cases, 75%–90% of familial cases of PMF versus 50% of sporadic cases, and 50%–69% of familial cases of ET versus 50% of sporadic cases.[117,123]

Although the *JAK2* V617F is not an inherited MPN-predisposing mutation, recently 3 separate studies all implicated germline *JAK2* variants in susceptibility to sporadic MPN. The first study identified a 4-SNP haplotype in 333 patients who preferentially acquired the V617F as opposed to 99 controls. It was associated with MPN irrespective of the presence or absence of the V617F mutation.[125] The second study identified a larger 14-SNP germline haplotype in *JAK2* containing some of the same SNPs as identified in the first study, and was associated with V617F-positive PV, ET, and PMF.[126] One haplotype, designated the 46/1 haplotype, preferentially acquired the V617F mutation. This study estimated that the 46/1 haplotype accounted for 28% of the population attributable risk. In 1 family, however, only 1 of 2 affected individuals examined had this haplotype, suggesting that it may not fully account for familial disease risk.[126] In the third study, a GWAS was undertaken in which more than 200,000 SNPs were genotyped in 217 individuals with MPN and 3000 controls.[127] A germline *JAK2* variant was identified that was associated with V617F-positive MPN, and accounted for 46% of the population attributable risk of MPN. This allele, however, was not associated with familial disease in any of the 25 kindreds examined.[127] Thus, many questions remain regarding the contribution of *JAK2* to different disease phenotypes and its role in the cause of MPN. Recently, acquired mutations in *TET2*, a putative tumor suppressor gene of unknown function located at 4q24 have been identified in 12% of sporadic MPN[128] and 20% of familial MPN,[129] but thus far no germline variants have been identified associated with either sporadic or familial disease.

Clinically, careful family histories are essential to uncover previously unsuspected cases of familial MPN. In these families, screening blood counts may be used to identify affected individuals at an early stage (ie, those with thrombocytosis or erythrocytosis) and could lead to interventions to prevent disease-related complications such as thrombosis. In addition, by testing at-risk relatives for EEC formation, it may be possible to identify additional asymptomatic individuals.[113,123] Furthermore, with the possible exception of anticipation,[130] the natural history of familial MPN does not differ from that of sporadic MPN, and consequently, treatment recommendations are similar.[121,123] There are data from 1 study to suggest that relatives of patients with MPN may also be at increased risk for other malignancies, specifically, CLL, malignant melanoma, and brain tumors (RR 1.3–1.6).[122]

ALL

ALL is the most common malignancy of childhood, accounting for approximately 20% of all pediatric cancers, with a peak incidence between the ages of 2 and 5 years.[131,132] Although its cause remains unclear, reports of ALL in nontwin siblings and from cancer registry data suggest a possible heritable component.[133,134] Unlike CLL, large family pedigrees with multiple affected individuals are not common. Several genetic syndromes include ALL among those cancers to which mutation carriers are predisposed. The genes implicated in these syndromes are diverse, and include genes involved in the DNA damage response and maintenance of genomic stability such as *TP53* in Li-Fraumeni syndrome and *ATM* in ataxia telangiectasia, and immune system function such as *WASP* in Wiskott-Aldrich syndrome. Individuals with Down syndrome have a 20-fold increased risk of ALL[135] in addition to a 400-fold increased risk of acute megakaryoblastic leukemia.[2] Ten percent of Down syndrome newborns develop a transient myeloproliferative disorder that may be associated with myeloid malignancy in as many as 30% of cases.[136] The mechanism of this increased risk of ALL remains unknown, but recent work has identified a gain-of function mutation in *JAK2* (R683) in 20% of Down syndrome-associated ALL.[135,137]

In sporadic ALL, several groups have undertaken large genome-wide analyses to identify recurrent acquired mutations associated with either the development of ALL or treatment resistance. Using Affymetrix genotyping arrays, Mullighan and colleagues[138] found an average of 6.5 acquired copy number alterations per patient in blasts from nearly 250 pediatric cases of ALL. They identified mutations in several genes regulating B-cell development, including *PAX5*, *IKZF1* (*IKAROS*), and *E2A*, in 40% of cases. *IKZF1* deletions appeared particularly important in Philadelphia chromosome positive ALL and were found in 84% of these patients.[139] This, again, highlights the importance in genetic studies of minimizing interindividual heterogeneity among cases to uncover cooperating genetic alterations influencing disease in specific patient subsets. Deletions in B-cell development pathways were confirmed in 2 other studies,[140,141] and abnormalities in cell cycle control, lymphocyte signaling, and apoptosis pathways were also identified.[138,141] Thus, genome-wide analyses provided important insights into genes under selective pressure for mutation acquisition in sporadic ALL, but similar insights into germline variants that may predispose individuals to ALL are only beginning to emerge.

Until recently, only a handful of candidate gene studies had been undertaken to identify ALL susceptibility variants. The results of these studies have been intriguing but difficult to replicate, with some implicating polymorphisms in folate metabolism (*MTHFR*),[142] drug resistance genes (*MDR1*),[143] cell cycle control (*CDKN2A*, *CDKN2B*, and *CDKN1B*),[144] DNA repair, xenobiotic metabolism (*MLH1* + *GSTT1* null + *CYP* variants),[145] and perforin-mediated cytotoxicity.[146–148] Two GWAS have been conducted. The first examined nearly 300,000 SNPs in 907 cases of ALL and 2398 controls and identified 10 SNPs in 3 separate loci significantly associated with ALL.[149] The strongest associations were found in SNPs mapping near *IKZF1* (*IKAROS*), a gene, as already discussed, often somatically mutated in high-risk ALL. Other risk loci mapped near *ARID5B*, a transcription factor involved in embryonic development and cell growth regulation, and *CEBPE*, a transcription factor important in granulocyte differentiation.[149] The second GWAS examined more than 300,000 SNPs in a cohort of 317 children with high-risk ALL and nearly 18,000 controls, and identified 18 SNPs near 12 separate genes significantly associated with ALL risk.[150] The 2 most significantly associated loci identified in their analysis were again *IKZF1* and *ARID5B*.

Both of these GWAS also examined whether these risk loci could be used to distinguish among ALL subtypes. In 1 study, 2 independent SNPs in *ARID5B* were associated with B-lineage hyperdiploid ALL but not other subtypes.[150] In the other study, a different SNP in *ARID5B* was associated with hyperdiploidy, and an SNP in *OR2C3* was associated with TEL-AML1 ALL.[150] The mechanisms accounting for the increased risk at the loci identified are not yet clearly established, but these GWAS illustrate the usefulness of unbiased genome-wide techniques for the identification of risk loci, and they further underscore the importance of examining biologically homogenous subsets. At the same time, the differing results obtained in these studies highlight the need for replication in even large and well-powered genomic studies.

MYELOID LEUKEMIA, MYELODYSPLASTIC SYNDROME, AND THERAPY-RELATED MYELOID NEOPLASMS
Myeloid Leukemia and Myelodysplastic Syndrome

Acute myelogenous leukemia (AML) and myelodysplastic syndrome (MDS) are a biologically heterogeneous group of clonal hematopoietic malignancies that can be subdivided into diagnostic and prognostic subgroups based on several clinical, cytogenetic, and molecular features. AML and MDS are generally diseases of older adults with an average age of onset of 65 years, although a small percentage of cases occur in younger adults and children.[151] Overall, the survival of those diagnosed with AML remains low with only 20% of affected individuals surviving 5 years.[151]

Familial AML and/or MDS are extremely rare; as a result, whereas some studies report as much as a 13-fold increased risk of myeloid leukemia in first-degree relatives of a proband,[38] others show no excess risk.[4,14] Although the heritability of sporadic myeloid malignancies has not been clearly established, there are several genetic syndromes associated with a dramatically increased risk of myeloid malignancy as well as a small number of familial myeloid malignancies pedigrees. These observations suggest that inherited genetic factors contribute to myeloid malignancies susceptibility.

Of the syndromes associated with myeloid malignancies, most have other associated phenotypes and many feature bone marrow failure (see **Table 1**). The genes mutated in these syndromes comprise diverse pathways including DNA repair (eg, Fanconi anemia and Bloom syndrome), tumor suppression (eg, Li-Fraumeni syndrome and neurofibromatosis), telomere maintenance (eg, dyskeratosis congenita), the RAS/ MAPK pathway (eg, Noonan syndrome), and RNA processing and ribosome biogenesis (eg, Shwachman-Diamond and Diamond-Blackfan).[1,2,152,153] Two other syndromes resulting from abnormalities of chromosome number, Down syndrome and trisomy 8 mosaicism, are also associated with a predisposition toward myeloid malignancies.[2,152] As a group, these disorders have provided insight into the pathogenesis of myeloid malignancies by highlighting pathways that would not have been intuitively thought of as predisposing to myeloid malignancies (eg, ribosome biogenesis).[153] In addition, they have shed light on genes that, when altered, cause overt leukemia. For example, studies in patients with Down syndrome identified somatic loss of function GATA1 mutations in those who developed acute megakaryoblastic leukemia[154] and transient myeloproliferative disorder.[155] Furthermore, somatic mutations in PTPN11, the gene mutated in Noonan syndrome (NS) have been identified in sporadic cases of juvenile myelomonocytic leukemia, MDS and AML (reviewed in Ref.[152,156]), suggesting that the study of these rare syndromes can contribute to our understanding of sporadic disease.

Through linkage analysis of rare myeloid malignancy pedigrees, 2 distinct familial leukemia syndromes, both with an autosomal dominant inheritance pattern, have been identified. The first, familial platelet disorder with propensity to myeloid malignancy (FPD/AML), is characterized by mild to moderate thrombocytopenia, clinical bleeding as a result of platelet dysfunction, and a propensity toward myeloid malignancy. To date, more than 30 families have been described in which nearly all affected members have heterozygous mutations of RUNX1, a transcription factor involved in regulation of hematopoiesis, on chromosome 21q22.[157,158] Significant clinical heterogeneity exists among families with RUNX1 mutations, and even within a single family, affected individuals can be phenotypically distinct, suggesting that modifiers of *RUNX1* remain undiscovered. For example, despite mutations in the same gene, some families have low platelet counts whereas others do not, and affected individuals in different families have different risks of progression to myeloid malignancy (range 11%–100%; median 50%).[152] Furthermore, within a single family, affected individuals often develop different myeloid malignancies.[152] Functionally, some of these familial *RUNX1* mutations show evidence of haploinsufficiency, whereas others seem to act in a dominant negative fashion.[159] As *RUNX1* is commonly mutated in sporadic AML/MDS, this syndrome provides a unique opportunity to study the contribution of *RUNX1* to leukemogenesis.[160]

The second familial myeloid malignancy syndrome, familial leukemia with *CEBPA* mutation, has only been identified in 5 families to date.[152,161,162] *CEBPA* encodes a transcription factor involved in granulocytic differentiation and is located on chromosome 19q13. Affected individuals across these families are clinically more homogenous than are individuals with FPD/AML, and develop AML, usually FAB subtypes M1 or M2 with prominent Auer rods and a normal karyotype. They are born with 1 mutated copy of *CEBPA* and somatically acquire a mutation on the remaining wild-type allele, suggesting that loss of *CEBPA* function is required for overt leukemia.[161] In addition, although only a small number of families have been described, this disorder is nearly 100% penetrant and is associated with a favorable prognosis, as 9 of 11 known affected individuals are alive and in complete remission despite multiple relapses in some individuals.[161] *CEBPA* mutations have been identified in sporadic AML as well, and confer a similarly favorable prognosis.[163]

Additional familial leukemia pedigrees have been reported that do not have either of these mutations. Linkage analysis in a handful of cases has suggested that a locus on chromosome 16q22 may be causative but no mutation has thus far been identified.[164] Familial AML/MDS featuring monosomy 7 with onset in childhood has also been described in 12 pedigrees, but so far the causative mutation has not been identified. Microsatellite analysis of chromosome 7 in 2 sisters with this disorder demonstrated that 1 had inherited chromosome 7 from their mother and the other had inherited it from their father, suggesting that monosomy 7 is a secondary occurrence.[165] Clinically, an awareness of these familial myeloid malignancy syndromes is important, as bone marrow transplant from an unsuspected affected matched sibling may have disastrous consequences.[166]

Candidate gene studies to identify inherited predisposing variants in AML and MDS have been undertaken mostly in therapy-related AML and/or MDS (discussed later), and have not yielded consistent results.[167] In sporadic disease, recent advances in next-generation sequencing (NGS) technology has allowed investigators to undertake whole-genome and whole-transcriptome sequencing studies to catalog the entire spectrum of acquired mutations in AML. In 2008, Ley and colleagues[168] sequenced the genome of an individual with normal karyotype AML and discovered only 10 acquired mutations in leukemic blasts that would disrupt the amino acid sequence of genes. Of these, 2 were in genes known to be mutated in sporadic AML (*FLT3* and *NPM1*) and 8 were in genes not previously shown to be mutated in AML. Four of these genes, *CDH24*, *SLC15A1*, *PTPRT*, and, *PCLKC*, have been associated with other cancers. The remaining 4, *KNDC1 GRINL1B*, *GPR123*, *EBI2*, are involved in metabolic pathways but have not been previously implicated in cancer. Subsequently, this group has sequenced another AML genome and identified 12 more somatic coding region mutations and an additional 52 mutations within other highly conserved regions, such as regulatory regions.[169] In addition, they showed that 1 of these newly identified mutations, located in *IDH1*, which encodes a cytoplasmic enzyme involved in NADPH production, is present in 16% of normal karyotype AML. Further work is needed to determine whether any of the newly identified mutations are required for leukemogenesis and to evaluate the mechanism by which they contribute to the development of leukemia. Thus, the use of NGS has provided significant insight into novel acquired mutations in AML. Furthermore, it has also led to the discovery of several rare inherited variants in patients with AML, the significance of which remains to be determined. As bioinformatics methods improve and the prohibitive cost of NGS continues to plummet, this technology may become a routine component of the clinical work-up in newly diagnosed patients, as well as an important research tool to discover acquired and inherited sources of genetic variation associated with myeloid and other malignancies.

Therapy-Related Myeloid Neoplasms

Therapy-related myeloid neoplasms (t-MN) are myeloid malignancies (ie, AML, myelodysplastic syndrome, and myelodysplastic/myeloproliferative neoplasms) associated with antecedent exposure to cytotoxic therapy for a previous malignancy or non-neoplastic disorder, and account for 10% to 20% of all myeloid malignancies.[60] Traditionally, 2 subtypes of t-MN have been recognized, each of which is associated with different clinical characteristics. T-MN following exposure to alkylating agents is characterized by a latency of 3 to 10 years, a preceding myelodysplastic phase, deletions of chromosomes 5 and/or 7, and loss of *TP53*.[170] T-MN following exposure to topoisomerase II inhibitors is characterized by a shorter latency of 2 to 3 years, no preceding myelodysplastic phase, and balanced chromosomal translocations often involving chromosome 11q23.[170] Although only a minority of patients receiving cytotoxic therapy develop t-MN, the diagnosis is devastating, with an average survival of only 8 to 9 months.[170,171] An understanding of the cause of t-MN may help to identify the subgroup of at-risk patients so that therapy can be altered to minimize this risk. Here, the evidence that implicates inherited genetic factors in t-MN susceptibility is reviewed.

Genetic syndromes associated with t-MN have pointed toward pathways in which genetic variation may contribute to an increased risk.[172] In particular, patients with neurofibromatosis, Fanconi anemia, and Li-Fraumeni syndrome, all syndromes characterized by defects in either DNA repair or tumor suppressor pathways, have a propensity for t-MN after cytotoxic treatment.[171,173] Candidate gene studies have also provided evidence to suggest that inherited polymorphisms in DNA repair and drug metabolism pathways are associated with t-MN. Because of the rarity of t-MN, however, most of these studies were undertaken on small cohorts of patients without consideration of the nature of the antecedent cytotoxic exposure; that is, whether the patients were exposed to alkylating agents or topoisomerase inhibitors. Thus, results have often been inconclusive (reviewed extensively in Ref.[171]). However, a small number of associations have been consistently replicated. Polymorphisms in NAD(P)H:quinone oxidoreductase (NQO1), an inducible enzyme that reduces substrates such as hematotoxic benzene metabolites to prevent the formation of damaging reactive oxygen species, and the glutathione *S*-transferase (GST) family, a group of enzymes that detoxify electrophiles (including metabolites of alkylating agents), have been implicated in t-MN risk in multiple studies.[171] In 1 study, for example, the NQO1 C609T allele was enriched 1.4-fold among patients with t-MN compared with healthy controls and 1.6-fold in the subset of t-MN patients with abnormalities of chromosomes 5 and/or 7.[174] In a second study, individuals homozygous for this polymorphism were found to be at a 2.6-fold increased risk of t-MN.[175] Likewise, the GSTT1 variant, a complete gene deletion polymorphism, was found to confer a 1.8- to 4.6-fold increased risk of t-MN in those homozygous for the GSTT1 polymorphism in 2 separate studies.[176,177]

Many other polymorphisms in other candidate genes have been assessed, but were not found to be reproducibly associated with t-MN. In combination, however, some variants have been associated with a dramatically increased risk of t-MN.[171] In 1 study, comprised of 51 t-MN patients and 186 controls, for example, individuals who carried at least 1 risk variant in each of 2 genes involved in homologous recombination, RAD51 and XRCC3, were found to have an 8-fold increased risk of t-MN, suggesting synergistic effects.[167] Other dramatic risks of t-MN development have been identified with the presence of risk alleles in both RAD51 and HLX1 (OR 9.5)[178] and the presence of risk alleles in 3 detoxification genes, NQO1*2, GSTT1, and CYP1A1*2A (OR 18.4).[179] These results all await replication in independent cohorts.

Because loss of TP53 is common in t-MN, our group assessed the association of the TP53 codon 72 SNP and the MDM2 SNP309 with t-MN. Although neither was individually associated with t-MN, the authors found that they functionally interact to result in a 1.8- and 2-fold increased risk of t-MN in individuals either homozygous for the TP53 codon 72Arg allele and the MDM2 SNP309T allele, or who carried at least 1 MDM2 309G allele and 1 TP53 72Pro allele, respectively.[180] Unlike the previous studies, these results were confirmed in an independent patient cohort. Because loss of TP53 is associated with both the subset of patients with antecedent exposure to alkylators and with acquired abnormalities of chromosomes 5 and/or 7, this cytogenetic abnormality could be a surrogate biomarker for t-MN as a result of alkylator exposure. If so, the effect of these variants on risk would be greatest in patients with this abnormality. Indeed, the interactive effect of these 2 genes on t-MN risk was most pronounced in those previously exposed to chemotherapy compared with radiotherapy alone, and in the subset of patients with abnormalities of chromosome 5 and/or 7. These results suggest that different exposures are likely to be associated with different genetic predispositions to t-MN.

To identify other risk alleles contributing to t-MN risk, investigators are turning to genome-wide strategies. In 1 study, for example, germline and tumor DNA from 13 patients with t-MN following treatment of ALL was compared with germline DNA from 156 patients similarly treated for ALL but who did not develop t-MN.[181] Global gene expression from a partially overlapping cohort was also analyzed. All patients had been exposed to etoposide, a topoisomerase inhibitor, and most patients with t-MN had acquired MLL rearrangements. Analysis of these patient-derived samples along with follow-up in vitro studies implicated mutations in adhesion as contributing to leukemogenesis in these cases of t-MN.[181]

The authors hypothesized that because exposure to cytotoxic therapy was shared by all patients who developed t-MN, the confounding effect of the variable contribution of nongenetic factors to cancer risk would be minimized among our cases. Furthermore, we predicted that because this exposure was potent and acute, it would potentiate the effect sizes of associated genetic variants.[182] Consequently, to identify germline variants associated with increased t-MN risk, we undertook a GWAS in 80 patients with t-MN and 150 healthy controls in whom more than 10,000 SNPs were genotyped.[182] We attempted to validate our most significant associations in an independent cohort of 70 patients with t-MN and 95 controls. Although they did not replicate in the entire cohort, we found that by limiting our analysis to only patients with acquired abnormalities of chromosomes 5 and/or 7, again using this as a biomarker for susceptibility to alkylator-induced t-MN, we were able to replicate 30% of our top associations, despite the modest sizes of both our discovery and replication cohorts.[182] By minimizing nongenetic variability and defining a cytogenetic surrogate for the mechanism of oncogenesis, we were able to identify and replicate t-MN associated variants with significant effect sizes. Thus, this study again underscores the importance of defining homogenous patient groups for analysis. These observations may be of clinical use not only in identifying patients at risk for t-MN but also in identifying patients at risk for sporadically occurring disease, because gene × chemotherapy can be thought of as just a specialized case of gene × environment interactions that underlie virtually all cancers.

SUMMARY

It is incontrovertible that there is a genetic component of risk to hematologic malignancies. Recognizing rare families with an inherited predisposition toward hematologic malignancies has important implications for these families, and investigations into the genetic basis of their increased risk has led to numerous insights into the pathways deranged in these disorders. As the studies discussed in this review demonstrate, however, risk alleles for familial disease only rarely translate into risk alleles for sporadic disease. The discovery of clinically useful prognostic markers for sporadic hematologic malignancies requires the use of new high-throughput genomic tools and novel investigative strategies. The advent of technologies such as GWAS and NGS offer enormous opportunities to catalog the entire spectrum of acquired and inherited genetic variation associated with disease, as the recent sequencing of an AML genome makes clear. NGS also provides opportunities to identify rare highly penetrant mutations in familial hematologic malignancies that have thus far eluded detection. These technologies, however, mandate the development of both new infrastructure to maintain securely the wealth of patient-derived data they yield, and new bioinformatics tools to analyze the data efficiently and in a timely manner.

Our investigations into t-MN susceptibility may suggest strategies to minimize intradisease heterogeneity, interindividual heterogeneity, and the variable contribution of nongenetic factors that can be applied to the study of a variety of other hematologic disorders. One consequence of our observations is that if different exposures elicit different cellular responses, each with its own cohort of genetic determinants, then an individualized assessment of genetic risk factors for malignancy can only be undertaken in association with an individualized assessment of nongenetic risk factors. Thus, although much remains unknown, investigations into the genetics of hematologic malignancies are at the forefront of the movement toward personalized medicine and the integration of the genome into clinical practice.

REFERENCES

1. Segel GB, Lichtman MA. Familial (inherited) leukemia, lymphoma, and myeloma: an overview. Blood Cells Mol Dis 2004;32(1):246–61.
2. Horwitz M. The genetics of familial leukemia. Leukemia 1997;11(8):1347–59.
3. Gunz FW, Gunz JP, Veale AM, et al. Familial leukaemia: a study of 909 families. Scand J Haematol 1975;15(2):117–31.
4. Goldgar DE, Easton DF, Cannon-Albright LA, et al. Systematic population-based assessment of cancer risk in first-degree relatives of cancer probands. J Natl Cancer Inst 1994;86(21):1600–8.
5. Goldin LR, Landgren O, McMaster ML, et al. Familial aggregation and heterogeneity of non-Hodgkin lymphoma in population-based samples. Cancer Epidemiol Biomarkers Prev 2005;14(10):2402–6.

6. Gunz F, Dameshek W. Chronic lymphocytic leukemia in a family, including twin brothers and a son. J Am Med Assoc 1957;164(12):1323–5.
7. Fraumeni JF Jr, Vogel CL, DeVita VT. Familial chronic lymphocytic leukemia. Ann Intern Med 1969;71(2):279–84.
8. Dameshek W, Savitz HA, Arbor B. Chronic Lymphatic leukemia in Twin Brothers Aged 56. JAMA 1929;92:1348–9.
9. Sellick GS, Goldin LR, Wild RW, et al. A high-density SNP genome-wide linkage search of 206 families identifies susceptibility loci for chronic lymphocytic leukemia. Blood 2007;110(9):3326–33.
10. Jonsson V, Houlston RS, Catovsky D, et al. CLL family 'Pedigree 14' revisited: 1947–2004. Leukemia 2005;19(6):1025–8.
11. Fuller SJ, Papaemmanuil E, McKinnon L, et al. Analysis of a large multi-generational family provides insight into the genetics of chronic lymphocytic leukemia. Br J Haematol 2008;142(2):238–45.
12. Goldin LR, Bjorkholm M, Kristinsson SY, et al. Elevated risk of chronic lympho-cytic leukemia and other indolent non-Hodgkin's lymphomas among relatives of patients with chronic lymphocytic leukemia. Haematologica 2009;94(5): 647–53.
13. Pottern LM, Linet M, Blair A, et al. Familial cancers associated with subtypes of leukemia and non-Hodgkin's lymphoma. Leuk Res 1991;15(5):305–14.
14. Amundadottir LT, Thorvaldsson S, Gudbjartsson DF, et al. Cancer as a complex phenotype: pattern of cancer distribution within and beyond the nuclear family. PLoS Med 2004;1(3):e65.
15. Raval A, Tanner SM, Byrd JC, et al. Downregulation of death-associated protein kinase 1 (DAPK1) in chronic lymphocytic leukemia. Cell 2007;129(5):879–90.
16. Goldin LR, Ishibe N, Sgambati M, et al. A genome scan of 18 families with chronic lymphocytic leukaemia. Br J Haematol 2003;121(6):866–73.
17. Sellick GS, Webb EL, Allinson R, et al. A high-density SNP genomewide linkage scan for chronic lymphocytic leukemia-susceptibility loci. Am J Hum Genet 2005;77(3):420–9.
18. Ng D, Marti GE, Fontaine L, et al. High-density mapping and follow-up studies on chromosomal regions 1, 3, 6, 12, 13 and 17 in 28 families with chronic lymphocytic leukaemia. Br J Haematol 2006;133(1):59–61.
19. Dohner H, Stilgenbauer S, Benner A, et al. Genomic aberrations and survival in chronic lymphocytic leukemia. N Engl J Med 2000;343(26):1910–6.
20. Reddy KS. Chronic lymphocytic leukaemia profiled for prognosis using a fluores-cence in situ hybridisation panel. Br J Haematol 2006;132(6):705–22.
21. Rush LJ, Raval A, Funchain P, et al. Epigenetic profiling in chronic lymphocytic leukemia reveals novel methylation targets. Cancer Res 2004;64(7):2424–33.
22. Raval A, Byrd JC, Plass C. Epigenetics in chronic lymphocytic leukemia. Semin Oncol 2006;33(2):157–66.
23. Enjuanes A, Benavente Y, Bosch F, et al. Genetic variants in apoptosis and immunoregulation-related genes are associated with risk of chronic lymphocytic leukemia. Cancer Res 2008;68(24):10178–86.
24. Rudd MF, Sellick GS, Webb EL, et al. Variants in the ATM-BRCA2-CHEK2 axis predispose to chronic lymphocytic leukemia. Blood 2006;108(2):638–44.
25. Zintzaras E, Kitsios GD. Synopsis and synthesis of candidate-gene association studies in chronic lymphocytic leukemia: the CUMAGAS-CLL information system. Am J Epidemiol 2009;170(6):671–8.
26. Crowther-Swanepoel D, Houlston RS. The molecular basis of familial chronic lymphocytic leukemia. Haematologica 2009;94(5):606–9.

27. Di Bernardo MC, Crowther-Swanepoel D, Broderick P, et al. A genome-wide association study identifies six susceptibility loci for chronic lymphocytic leukemia. Nat Genet 2008;40(10):1204–10.
28. Yendamuri S, Calin GA. The role of microRNA in human leukemia: a review. Leukemia 2009;23(7):1257–63.
29. Croce CM. Causes and consequences of microRNA dysregulation in cancer. Nat Rev Genet 2009;10(10):704–14.
30. Calin GA, Ferracin M, Cimmino A, et al. A MicroRNA signature associated with prognosis and progression in chronic lymphocytic leukemia. N Engl J Med 2005;353(17):1793–801.
31. Calin GA, Dumitru CD, Shimizu M, et al. Frequent deletions and down-regulation of micro- RNA genes miR15 and miR16 at 13q14 in chronic lymphocytic leukemia. Proc Natl Acad Sci U S A 2002;99(24):15524–9.
32. Dasanu CA, Alexandrescu DT. Risk for second nonlymphoid neoplasms in chronic lymphocytic leukemia. MedGenMed 2007;9(4):35.
33. Rawstron AC, Bennett FL, O'Connor SJ, et al. Monoclonal B-cell lymphocytosis and chronic lymphocytic leukemia. N Engl J Med 2008;359(6):575–83.
34. Rawstron AC, Yuille MR, Fuller J, et al. Inherited predisposition to CLL is detectable as subclinical monoclonal B-lymphocyte expansion. Blood 2002;100(7): 2289–90.
35. Gribben JG. How I treat CLL upfront. Blood 2010;115(2):187–97.
36. Punnett A, Tsang RW, Hodgson DC. Hodgkin lymphoma across the age spectrum: epidemiology, therapy, and late effects. Semin Radiat Oncol 2010;20(1):30–44.
37. Goldin LR, Pfeiffer RM, Gridley G, et al. Familial aggregation of Hodgkin lymphoma and related tumors. Cancer 2004;100(9):1902–8.
38. Kerber RA, O'Brien E. A cohort study of cancer risk in relation to family histories of cancer in the Utah population database. Cancer 2005;103(9):1906–15.
39. Mack TM, Cozen W, Shibata DK, et al. Concordance for Hodgkin's disease in identical twins suggesting genetic susceptibility to the young-adult form of the disease. N Engl J Med 1995;332(7):413–8.
40. Grufferman S, Cole P, Smith PG, et al. Hodgkin's disease in siblings. N Engl J Med 1977;296(5):248–50.
41. Kerzin-Storrar L, Faed MJ, MacGillivray JB, et al. Incidence of familial Hodgkin's disease. Br J Cancer 1983;47(5):707–12.
42. Altieri A, Hemminki K. The familial risk of Hodgkin's lymphoma ranks among the highest in the Swedish family-cancer database. Leukemia 2006;20(11):2062–3.
43. Goldin LR, McMaster ML, Ter-Minassian M, et al. A genome screen of families at high risk for Hodgkin lymphoma: evidence for a susceptibility gene on chromosome 4. J Med Genet 2005;42(7):595–601.
44. Horwitz M, Wiernik PH. Pseudoautosomal linkage of Hodgkin disease. Am J Hum Genet 1999;65(5):1413–22.
45. Horwitz MS, Mealiffe ME. Further evidence for a pseudoautosomal gene for Hodgkin's lymphoma: reply to 'The familial risk of Hodgkin's lymphoma ranks among the highest in the Swedish Family-Cancer Database' by Altieri A and Hemminki K. Leukemia 2007;21(2):351.
46. Shears DJ, Endris V, Gokhale DA, et al. Pseudoautosomal linkage of familial Hodgkin's lymphoma: molecular analysis of a unique family with Leri-Weill dyschondrosteosis and Hodgkins lymphoma. Br J Haematol 2003;121(2):377–9.
47. Kim SH, Choi EY, Shin YK, et al. Generation of cells with Hodgkin's and Reed-Sternberg phenotype through downregulation of CD99 (Mic2). Blood 1998; 92(11):4287–95.

48. Oudejans JJ, Jiwa NM, Kummer JA, et al. Analysis of major histocompatibility complex class I expression on Reed-Sternberg cells in relation to the cytotoxic T-cell response in Epstein-Barr virus-positive and -negative Hodgkin's disease. Blood 1996;87(9):3844–51.

49. Diepstra A, Niens M, te Meerman GJ, et al. Genetic susceptibility to Hodgkin's lymphoma associated with the human leukocyte antigen region. Eur J Haematol Suppl 2005;(66):34–41.

50. Harty LC, Lin AY, Goldstein AM, et al. HLA-DR, HLA-DQ, and TAP genes in familial Hodgkin disease. Blood 2002;99(2):690–3.

51. Klitz W, Aldrich CL, Fildes N, et al. Localization of predisposition to Hodgkin disease in the HLA class II region. Am J Hum Genet 1994;54(3):497–505.

52. Diepstra A, Niens M, Vellenga E, et al. Association with HLA class I in Epstein-Barr-virus-positive and with HLA class III in Epstein-Barr-virus-negative Hodgkin's lymphoma. Lancet 2005;365(9478):2216–24.

53. Cozen W, Gill PS, Ingles SA, et al. IL-6 levels and genotype are associated with risk of young adult Hodgkin lymphoma. Blood 2004;103(8):3216–21.

54. Cozen W, Gill PS, Salam MT, et al. Interleukin-2, interleukin-12, and interferon-gamma levels and risk of young adult Hodgkin lymphoma. Blood 2008;111(7):3377–82.

55. Straus SE, Jaffe ES, Puck JM, et al. The development of lymphomas in families with autoimmune lymphoproliferative syndrome with germline Fas mutations and defective lymphocyte apoptosis. Blood 2001;98(1):194–200.

56. Baumler C, Duan F, Onel K, et al. Differential recruitment of caspase 8 to cFlip confers sensitivity or resistance to Fas-mediated apoptosis in a subset of familial lymphoma patients. Leuk Res 2003;27(9):841–51.

57. Salipante SJ, Mealiffe ME, Wechsler J, et al. Mutations in a gene encoding a mid-body kelch protein in familial and sporadic classical Hodgkin lymphoma lead to binucleated cells. Proc Natl Acad Sci U S A 2009;106(35):14920–5.

58. Jaffe ES, Harris NL, Stein H, et al. Classification of lymphoid neoplasms: the microscope as a tool for disease discovery. Blood 2008;112(12):4384–99.

59. Anderson JR, Armitage JO, Weisenburger DD. Epidemiology of the non-Hodgkin's lymphomas: distributions of the major subtypes differ by geographic locations. Non-Hodgkin's lymphoma classification project. Ann Oncol 1998;9(7):717–20.

60. Swerdlow SH, Campo E, Harris NL, et al, editors. WHO classification of tumours of haematopoietic and lymphoid tissues. Lyon (France): IARC; 2008.

61. Alexander DD, Mink PJ, Adami HO, et al. The non-Hodgkin lymphomas: a review of the epidemiologic literature. Int J Cancer 2007;120(Suppl 12):1–39.

62. Linet MS, Pottern LM. Familial aggregation of hematopoietic malignancies and risk of non-Hodgkin's lymphoma. Cancer Res 1992;52(Suppl 19):5468s–73s.

63. Iscovich J, Parkin DM. Risk of cancer in migrants and their descendants in Israel: I. Leukaemias and lymphomas. Int J Cancer 1997;70(6):649–53.

64. Au WY, Gascoyne RD, Klasa RD, et al. Incidence and spectrum of non-Hodgkin lymphoma in Chinese migrants to British Columbia. Br J Haematol 2005;128(6):792–6.

65. Grulich AE, Swerdlow AJ, Head J, et al. Cancer mortality in African and Caribbean migrants to England and Wales. Br J Cancer 1992;66(5):905–11.

66. Wang SS, Slager SL, Brennan P, et al. Family history of hematopoietic malignancies and risk of non-Hodgkin lymphoma (NHL): a pooled analysis of 10 211 cases and 11 905 controls from the International Lymphoma Epidemiology Consortium (InterLymph). Blood 2007;109(8):3479–88.

67. Chatterjee N, Hartge P, Cerhan JR, et al. Risk of non-Hodgkin's lymphoma and family history of lymphatic, hematologic, and other cancers. Cancer Epidemiol Biomarkers Prev 2004;13(9):1415–21.
68. Lichtenstein P, Holm NV, Verkasalo PK, et al. Environmental and heritable factors in the causation of cancer–analyses of cohorts of twins from Sweden, Denmark, and Finland. N Engl J Med 2000;343(2):78–85.
69. Goldin LR, Bjorkholm M, Kristinsson SY, et al. Highly increased familial risks for specific lymphoma subtypes. Br J Haematol 2009;146(1):91–4.
70. Morton LM, Wang SS, Cozen W, et al. Etiologic heterogeneity among non-Hodgkin lymphoma subtypes. Blood 2008;112(13):5150–60.
71. Scott RH, Homfray T, Huxter NL, et al. Familial T-cell non-Hodgkin lymphoma caused by biallelic MSH2 mutations. J Med Genet 2007;44(7):e83.
72. Steffen J, Varon R, Mosor M, et al. Increased cancer risk of heterozygotes with NBS1 germline mutations in Poland. Int J Cancer 2004;111(1):67–71.
73. Chrzanowska KH, Piekutowska-Abramczuk D, Popowska E, et al. Carrier frequency of mutation 657del5 in the NBS1 gene in a population of Polish pediatric patients with sporadic lymphoid malignancies. Int J Cancer 2006;118(5): 1269–74.
74. Cerosaletti KM, Morrison VA, Sabath DE, et al. Mutations and molecular variants of the NBS1 gene in non-Hodgkin lymphoma. Genes Chromosomes Cancer 2002;35(3):282–6.
75. Siddiqui R, Onel K, Facio F, et al. The genetics of familial lymphomas. Curr Oncol Rep 2004;6(5):380–7.
76. Pineda M, Castellsague E, Musulen E, et al. Non-Hodgkin lymphoma related to hereditary nonpolyposis colorectal cancer in a patient with a novel heterozygous complex deletion in the MSH2 gene. Genes Chromosomes Cancer 2008;47(4): 326–32.
77. Skibola CF, Curry JD, Nieters A. Genetic susceptibility to lymphoma. Haematologica 2007;92(7):960–9.
78. Wang SS, Purdue MP, Cerhan JR, et al. Common gene variants in the tumor necrosis factor (TNF) and TNF receptor superfamilies and NF-kB transcription factors and non-Hodgkin lymphoma risk. PLoS One 2009;4(4):e5360.
79. Rothman N, Skibola CF, Wang SS, et al. Genetic variation in TNF and IL10 and risk of non-Hodgkin lymphoma: a report from the InterLymph Consortium. Lancet Oncol 2006;7(1):27–38.
80. Cerhan JR, Liu-Mares W, Fredericksen ZS, et al. Genetic variation in tumor necrosis factor and the nuclear factor-kappaB canonical pathway and risk of non-Hodgkin's lymphoma. Cancer Epidemiol Biomarkers Prev 2008;17(11): 3161–9.
81. Wang SS, Cerhan JR, Hartge P, et al. Common genetic variants in proinflammatory and other immunoregulatory genes and risk for non-Hodgkin lymphoma. Cancer Res 2006;66(19):9771–80.
82. Purdue MP, Lan Q, Kricker A, et al. Polymorphisms in immune function genes and risk of non-Hodgkin lymphoma: findings from the New South Wales non-Hodgkin Lymphoma Study. Carcinogenesis 2007;28(3):704–12.
83. Liang XS, Caporaso N, McMaster ML, et al. Common genetic variants in candidate genes and risk of familial lymphoid malignancies. Br J Haematol 2009; 146(4):418–23.
84. Novak AJ, Slager SL, Fredericksen ZS, et al. Genetic variation in B-cell-activating factor is associated with an increased risk of developing B-cell non-Hodgkin lymphoma. Cancer Res 2009;69(10):4217–24.

85. Zhang Y, Lan Q, Rothman N, et al. A putative exonic splicing polymorphism in the BCL6 gene and the risk of non-Hodgkin lymphoma. J Natl Cancer Inst 2005;97(21):1616–8.

86. Morton LM, Purdue MP, Zheng T, et al. Risk of non-Hodgkin lymphoma associated with germline variation in genes that regulate the cell cycle, apoptosis, and lymphocyte development. Cancer Epidemiol Biomarkers Prev 2009;18(4): 1259–70.

87. Lan Q, Morton LM, Armstrong B, et al. Genetic variation in caspase genes and risk of non-Hodgkin lymphoma: a pooled analysis of 3 population-based case-control studies. Blood 2009;114(2):264–7.

88. Purdue MP, Lan Q, Wang SS, et al. A pooled investigation of Toll-like receptor gene variants and risk of non-Hodgkin lymphoma. Carcinogenesis 2009;30(2): 275–81.

89. Skibola CF, Nieters A, Bracci PM, et al. A functional TNFRSF5 gene variant is associated with risk of lymphoma. Blood 2008;111(8):4348–54.

90. International Myeloma Working Group. Criteria for the classification of monoclonal gammopathies, multiple myeloma and related disorders: a report of the International Myeloma Working Group. Br J Haematol 2003;121(5):749–57.

91. McMaster ML. Familial Waldenstrom's macroglobulinemia. Semin Oncol 2003; 30(2):146–52.

92. Kristinsson SY, Bjorkholm M, Goldin LR, et al. Risk of lymphoproliferative disorders among first-degree relatives of lymphoplasmacytic lymphoma/Waldenstrom macroglobulinemia patients: a population-based study in Sweden. Blood 2008;112(8):3052–6.

93. McMaster ML, Goldin LR, Bai Y, et al. Genomewide linkage screen for Waldenstrom macroglobulinemia susceptibility loci in high-risk families. Am J Hum Genet 2006;79(4):695–701.

94. Landgren O, Weiss BM. Patterns of monoclonal gammopathy of undetermined significance and multiple myeloma in various ethnic/racial groups: support for genetic factors in pathogenesis. Leukemia 2009;23(10):1691–7.

95. Kyle RA, Therneau TM, Rajkumar SV, et al. A long-term study of prognosis in monoclonal gammopathy of undetermined significance. N Engl J Med 2002; 346(8):564–9.

96. Coleman EA, Lynch H, Enderlin C, et al. Initial report of a family registry of multiple myeloma. Cancer Nurs 2009;32(6):456–64.

97. Eriksson M, Hallberg B. Familial occurrence of hematologic malignancies and other diseases in multiple myeloma: a case-control study. Cancer Causes Control 1992;3(1):63–7.

98. Brown LM, Linet MS, Greenberg RS, et al. Multiple myeloma and family history of cancer among blacks and whites in the U.S. Cancer 1999;85(11): 2385–90.

99. Kristinsson SY, Bjorkholm M, Goldin LR, et al. Patterns of hematologic malignancies and solid tumors among 37,838 first-degree relatives of 13,896 patients with multiple myeloma in Sweden. Int J Cancer 2009;125(9):2147–50.

100. Landgren O, Linet MS, McMaster ML, et al. Familial characteristics of autoimmune and hematologic disorders in 8,406 multiple myeloma patients: a population-based case-control study. Int J Cancer 2006;118(12):3095–8.

101. Landgren O, Kristinsson SY, Goldin LR, et al. Risk of plasma cell and lymphoproliferative disorders among 14621 first-degree relatives of 4458 patients with monoclonal gammopathy of undetermined significance in Sweden. Blood 2009;114(4):791–5.

102. Vachon CM, Kyle RA, Therneau TM, et al. Increased risk of monoclonal gammopathy in first-degree relatives of patients with multiple myeloma or monoclonal gammopathy of undetermined significance. Blood 2009;114(4):785–90.
103. Lynch HT, Watson P, Tarantolo S, et al. Phenotypic heterogeneity in multiple myeloma families. J Clin Oncol 2005;23(4):685–93.
104. Shoenfeld Y, Berliner S, Shaklai M, et al. Familial multiple myeloma. A review of thirty-seven families. Postgrad Med J 1982;58(675):12–6.
105. Grosbois B, Jego P, Attal M, et al. Familial multiple myeloma: report of fifteen families. Br J Haematol 1999;105(3):768–70.
106. Deshpande HA, Hu XP, Marino P, et al. Anticipation in familial plasma cell dyscrasias. Br J Haematol 1998;103(3):696–703.
107. Kristinsson SY, Goldin LR, Bjorkholm M, et al. Risk of solid tumors and myeloid hematological malignancies among first-degree relatives of patients with monoclonal gammopathy of undetermined significance. Haematologica 2009;94(8): 1179–81.
108. Cao J, Hong CH, Rosen L, et al. Deletion of genetic material from a poly (ADP-ribose) polymerase-like gene on chromosome 13 occurs frequently in patients with monoclonal gammopathies. Cancer Epidemiol Biomarkers Prev 1995; 4(7):759–63.
109. Grass S, Preuss KD, Ahlgrimm M, et al. Association of a dominantly inherited hyperphosphorylated paraprotein target with sporadic and familial multiple myeloma and monoclonal gammopathy of undetermined significance: a case-control study. Lancet Oncol 2009;10(10):950–6.
110. Keats JJ, Fonseca R, Chesi M, et al. Promiscuous mutations activate the noncanonical NF-kappaB pathway in multiple myeloma. Cancer Cell 2007;12(2): 131–44.
111. Gilbert HS. Familial myeloproliferative disease. Baillieres Clin Haematol 1998; 11(4):849–58.
112. Perez-Encinas M, Bello JL, Perez-Crespo S, et al. Familial myeloproliferative syndrome. Am J Hematol 1994;46(3):225–9.
113. Kralovics R, Stockton DW, Prchal JT. Clonal hematopoiesis in familial polycythemia vera suggests the involvement of multiple mutational events in the early pathogenesis of the disease. Blood 2003;102(10):3793–6.
114. Levine RL, Wadleigh M, Cools J, et al. Activating mutation in the tyrosine kinase JAK2 in polycythemia vera, essential thrombocythemia, and myeloid metaplasia with myelofibrosis. Cancer Cell 2005;7(4):387–97.
115. Kralovics R, Passamonti F, Buser AS, et al. A gain-of-function mutation of JAK2 in myeloproliferative disorders. N Engl J Med 2005;352(17):1779–90.
116. James C, Ugo V, Le Couedic JP, et al. A unique clonal JAK2 mutation leading to constitutive signalling causes polycythaemia vera. Nature 2005;434(7037): 1144–8.
117. Baxter EJ, Scott LM, Campbell PJ, et al. Acquired mutation of the tyrosine kinase JAK2 in human myeloproliferative disorders. Lancet 2005;365(9464): 1054–61.
118. Skoda R. The genetic basis of myeloproliferative disorders. Hematology Am Soc Hematol Educ Program 2007;1–10.
119. Tefferi A, Vardiman JW. Classification and diagnosis of myeloproliferative neoplasms: the 2008 World Health Organization criteria and point-of-care diagnostic algorithms. Leukemia 2008;22(1):14–22.
120. Prchal JF, Axelrad AA. Letter: bone-marrow responses in polycythemia vera. N Engl J Med 1974;290(24):1382.

121. Rumi E, Passamonti F, Della Porta MG, et al. Familial chronic myeloproliferative disorders: clinical phenotype and evidence of disease anticipation. J Clin Oncol 2007;25(35):5630–5.
122. Landgren O, Goldin LR, Kristinsson SY, et al. Increased risks of polycythemia vera, essential thrombocythemia, and myelofibrosis among 24,577 first-degree relatives of 11,039 patients with myeloproliferative neoplasms in Sweden. Blood 2008;112(6):2199–204.
123. Bellanne-Chantelot C, Chaumarel I, Labopin M, et al. Genetic and clinical implications of the Val617Phe JAK2 mutation in 72 families with myeloproliferative disorders. Blood 2006;108(1):346–52.
124. Rumi E, Passamonti F, Pietra D, et al. JAK2 (V617F) as an acquired somatic mutation and a secondary genetic event associated with disease progression in familial myeloproliferative disorders. Cancer 2006;107(9):2206–11.
125. Olcaydu D, Harutyunyan A, Jager R, et al. A common JAK2 haplotype confers susceptibility to myeloproliferative neoplasms. Nat Genet 2009;41(4):450–4.
126. Jones AV, Chase A, Silver RT, et al. JAK2 haplotype is a major risk factor for the development of myeloproliferative neoplasms. Nat Genet 2009;41(4): 446–9.
127. Kilpivaara O, Mukherjee S, Schram AM, et al. A germline JAK2 SNP is associated with predisposition to the development of JAK2 (V617F)-positive myeloproliferative neoplasms. Nat Genet 2009;41(4):455–9.
128. Delhommeau F, Dupont S, Della Valle V, et al. Mutation in TET2 in myeloid cancers. N Engl J Med 2009;360(22):2289–301.
129. Saint-Martin C, Leroy G, Delhommeau F, et al. Analysis of the ten-eleven translocation 2 (TET2) gene in familial myeloproliferative neoplasms. Blood 2009; 114(8):1628–32.
130. Rumi E, Passamonti F, Picone C, et al. Disease anticipation in familial myeloproliferative neoplasms. Blood 2008;112(6):2587–8 [author reply 2588–9].
131. Jemal A, Siegel R, Ward E, et al. Cancer statistics, 2009. CA Cancer J Clin 2009; 59(4):225–49.
132. Smith MA, Ries LA, Gurney JG, et al. Leukemia. Bethesda (MD): National Cancer Institute, SEER Program; 1999.
133. Greaves MF, Maia AT, Wiemels JL, et al. Leukemia in twins: lessons in natural history. Blood 2003;102(7):2321–33.
134. Hemminki K, Jiang Y. Risks among siblings and twins for childhood acute lymphoid leukaemia: results from the Swedish family-cancer database. Leukemia 2002;16(2):297–8.
135. Malinge S, Izraeli S, Crispino JD. Insights into the manifestations, outcomes, and mechanisms of leukemogenesis in Down syndrome. Blood 2009;113(12): 2619–28.
136. Klusmann JH, Creutzig U, Zimmermann M, et al. Treatment and prognostic impact of transient leukemia in neonates with Down syndrome. Blood 2008; 111(6):2991–8.
137. Bercovich D, Ganmore I, Scott LM, et al. Mutations of JAK2 in acute lymphoblastic leukaemias associated with Down's syndrome. Lancet 2008;372(9648): 1484–92.
138. Mullighan CG, Goorha S, Radtke I, et al. Genome-wide analysis of genetic alterations in acute lymphoblastic leukaemia. Nature 2007;446(7137): 758–64.
139. Mullighan CG, Miller CB, Radtke I, et al. BCR-ABL1 lymphoblastic leukaemia is characterized by the deletion of Ikaros. Nature 2008;453(7191):110–4.

140. Kawamata N, Ogawa S, Zimmermann M, et al. Molecular allelokaryotyping of pediatric acute lymphoblastic leukemias by high-resolution single nucleotide polymorphism oligonucleotide genomic microarray. Blood 2008;111(2):776–84.

141. Kuiper RP, Schoenmakers EF, van Reijmersdal SV, et al. High-resolution genomic profiling of childhood ALL reveals novel recurrent genetic lesions affecting pathways involved in lymphocyte differentiation and cell cycle progression. Leukemia 2007;21(6):1258–66.

142. Wiemels JL, Smith RN, Taylor GM, et al. Methylenetetrahydrofolate reductase (MTHFR) polymorphisms and risk of molecularly defined subtypes of childhood acute leukemia. Proc Natl Acad Sci U S A 2001;98(7):4004–9.

143. Urayama KY, Wiencke JK, Buffler PA, et al. MDR1 gene variants, indoor insecticide exposure, and the risk of childhood acute lymphoblastic leukemia. Cancer Epidemiol Biomarkers Prev 2007;16(6):1172–7.

144. Healy J, Belanger H, Beaulieu P, et al. Promoter SNPs in G1/S checkpoint regulators and their impact on the susceptibility to childhood leukemia. Blood 2007; 109(2):683–92.

145. Mathonnet G, Krajinovic M, Labuda D, et al. Role of DNA mismatch repair genetic polymorphisms in the risk of childhood acute lymphoblastic leukaemia. Br J Haematol 2003;123(1):45–8.

146. Muralitharan S, Wali Y, Pathare AV. Perforin A91V polymorphism and putative susceptibility to hematological malignancies. Leukemia 2006;20(12):2178.

147. Schnakenberg E, Mehles A, Cario G, et al. Polymorphisms of methylenetetrahydrofolate reductase (MTHFR) and susceptibility to pediatric acute lymphoblastic leukemia in a German study population. BMC Med Genet 2005;6:23.

148. Santoro A, Cannella S, Trizzino A, et al. A single amino acid change A91V in perforin: a novel, frequent predisposing factor to childhood acute lymphoblastic leukemia? Haematologica 2005;90(5):697–8.

149. Papaemmanuil E, Hosking FJ, Vijayakrishnan J, et al. Loci on 7p12.2, 10q21.2 and 14q11.2 are associated with risk of childhood acute lymphoblastic leukemia. Nat Genet 2009;41(9):1006–10.

150. Trevino LR, Yang W, French D, et al. Germline genomic variants associated with childhood acute lymphoblastic leukemia. Nat Genet 2009;41(9):1001–5.

151. Yamamoto JF, Goodman MT. Patterns of leukemia incidence in the United States by subtype and demographic characteristics, 1997–2002. Cancer Causes Control 2008;19(4):379–90.

152. Owen C, Barnett M, Fitzgibbon J. Familial myelodysplasia and acute myeloid leukaemia–a review. Br J Haematol 2008;140(2):123–32.

153. Dokal I, Vulliamy T. Inherited aplastic anaemias/bone marrow failure syndromes. Blood Rev 2008;22(3):141–53.

154. Wechsler J, Greene M, McDevitt MA, et al. Acquired mutations in GATA1 in the megakaryoblastic leukemia of Down syndrome. Nat Genet 2002;32(1):148–52.

155. Xu G, Nagano M, Kanezaki R, et al. Frequent mutations in the GATA-1 gene in the transient myeloproliferative disorder of Down syndrome. Blood 2003;102(8): 2960–8.

156. Tartaglia M, Niemeyer CM, Fragale A, et al. Somatic mutations in PTPN11 in juvenile myelomonocytic leukemia, myelodysplastic syndromes and acute myeloid leukemia. Nat Genet 2003;34(2):148–50.

157. Jongmans MC, Kuiper RP, Carmichael CL, et al. Novel RUNX1 mutations in familial platelet disorder with enhanced risk for acute myeloid leukemia: clues for improved identification of the FPD/AML syndrome. Leukemia 2009;24(1): 242–6.

158. Song WJ, Sullivan MG, Legare RD, et al. Haploinsufficiency of CBFA2 causes familial thrombocytopenia with propensity to develop acute myelogenous leukaemia. Nat Genet 1999;23(2):166–75.
159. Michaud J, Wu F, Osato M, et al. In vitro analyses of known and novel RUNX1/AML1 mutations in dominant familial platelet disorder with predisposition to acute myelogenous leukemia: implications for mechanisms of pathogenesis. Blood 2002;99(4):1364–72.
160. Harada H, Harada Y, Tanaka H, et al. Implications of somatic mutations in the AML1 gene in radiation-associated and therapy-related myelodysplastic syndrome/acute myeloid leukemia. Blood 2003;101(2):673–80.
161. Renneville A, Mialou V, Philippe N, et al. Another pedigree with familial acute myeloid leukemia and germline CEBPA mutation. Leukemia 2009;23(4):804–6.
162. Smith ML, Cavenagh JD, Lister TA, et al. Mutation of CEBPA in familial acute myeloid leukemia. N Engl J Med 2004;351(23):2403–7.
163. Preudhomme C, Sagot C, Boissel N, et al. Favorable prognostic significance of CEBPA mutations in patients with de novo acute myeloid leukemia: a study from the Acute Leukemia French Association (ALFA). Blood 2002;100(8):2717–23.
164. Escher R, Jones A, Hagos F, et al. Chromosome band 16q22-linked familial AML: exclusion of candidate genes, and possible disease risk modification by NQO1 polymorphisms. Genes Chromosomes Cancer 2004;41(3):278–82.
165. Minelli A, Maserati E, Giudici G, et al. Familial partial monosomy 7 and myelodysplasia: different parental origin of the monosomy 7 suggests action of a mutator gene. Cancer Genet Cytogenet 2001;124(2):147–51.
166. Buijs A, Poddighe P, van Wijk R, et al. A novel CBFA2 single-nucleotide mutation in familial platelet disorder with propensity to develop myeloid malignancies. Blood 2001;98(9):2856–8.
167. Seedhouse C, Faulkner R, Ashraf N, et al. Polymorphisms in genes involved in homologous recombination repair interact to increase the risk of developing acute myeloid leukemia. Clin Cancer Res 2004;10(8):2675–80.
168. Ley TJ, Mardis ER, Ding L, et al. DNA sequencing of a cytogenetically normal acute myeloid leukaemia genome. Nature 2008;456(7218):66–72.
169. Mardis ER, Ding L, Dooling DJ, et al. Recurring mutations found by sequencing an acute myeloid leukemia genome. N Engl J Med 2009;361(11):1058–66.
170. Godley LA, Larson RA. Therapy-related myeloid leukemia. Semin Oncol 2008;35(4):418–29.
171. Seedhouse C, Russell N. Advances in the understanding of susceptibility to treatment-related acute myeloid leukaemia. Br J Haematol 2007;137(6):513–29.
172. Perentesis JP. Genetic predisposition and treatment-related leukemia. Med Pediatr Oncol 2001;36(5):541–8.
173. Maris JM, Wiersma SR, Mahgoub N, et al. Monosomy 7 myelodysplastic syndrome and other second malignant neoplasms in children with neurofibromatosis type 1. Cancer 1997;79(7):1438–46.
174. Larson RA, Wang Y, Banerjee M, et al. Prevalence of the inactivating 609C→T polymorphism in the NAD(P)H: quinone oxidoreductase (NQO1) gene in patients with primary and therapy-related myeloid leukemia. Blood 1999;94(2):803–7.
175. Naoe T, Takeyama K, Yokozawa T, et al. Analysis of genetic polymorphism in NQO1, GST-M1, GST-T1, and CYP3A4 in 469 Japanese patients with therapy-related leukemia/myelodysplastic syndrome and de novo acute myeloid leukemia. Clin Cancer Res 2000;6(10):4091–5.

176. Sasai Y, Horiike S, Misawa S, et al. Genotype of glutathione S-transferase and other genetic configurations in myelodysplasia. Leuk Res 1999;23(11): 975–81.
177. Allan JM, Wild CP, Rollinson S, et al. Polymorphism in glutathione S-transferase P1 is associated with susceptibility to chemotherapy-induced leukemia. Proc Natl Acad Sci U S A 2001;98(20):11592–7.
178. Jawad M, Seedhouse CH, Russell N, et al. Polymorphisms in human homeobox HLX1 and DNA repair RAD51 genes increase the risk of therapy-related acute myeloid leukemia. Blood 2006;108(12):3916–8.
179. Bolufer P, Collado M, Barragan E, et al. Profile of polymorphisms of drug-metabolising enzymes and the risk of therapy-related leukaemia. Br J Haematol 2007;136(4):590–6.
180. Ellis NA, Huo D, Yildiz O, et al. MDM2 SNP309 and TP53 Arg72Pro interact to alter therapy-related acute myeloid leukemia susceptibility. Blood 2008;112(3): 741–9.
181. Hartford C, Yang W, Cheng C, et al. Genome scan implicates adhesion biological pathways in secondary leukemia. Leukemia 2007;21(10):2128–36.
182. Knight JA, Skol AD, Shinde A, et al. Genome-wide association study to identify novel loci associated with therapy-related myeloid leukemia susceptibility. Blood 2009;113(22):5575–82.
183. Yohay K. Neurofibromatosis type 1 and associated malignancies. Curr Neurol Neurosci Rep 2009;9(3):247–53.
184. Birch JM, Alston RD, McNally RJ, et al. Relative frequency and morphology of cancers in carriers of germline TP53 mutations. Oncogene 2001;20(34):4621–8.
185. Gonzalez KD, Noltner KA, Buzin CH, et al. Beyond Li Fraumeni syndrome: clinical characteristics of families with p53 germline mutations. J Clin Oncol 2009; 27(8):1250–6.
186. Alter BP, Giri N, Savage SA, et al. Cancer in dyskeratosis congenita. Blood 2009; 113(26):6549–57.
187. Dale DC, Bolyard AA, Schwinzer BG, et al. The Severe Chronic Neutropenia International Registry: 10-year follow-up report. Support Cancer Ther 2006; 3(4):220–31.
188. Rosenberg PS, Alter BP, Ebell W. Cancer risks in Fanconi anemia: findings from the German Fanconi Anemia Registry. Haematologica 2008;93(4):511–7.
189. German J. Bloom's syndrome. XX. The first 100 cancers. Cancer Genet Cytogenet 1997;93(1):100–6.
190. Seiter K, Qureshi A, Liu D, et al. Severe toxicity following induction chemotherapy for acute myelogenous leukemia in a patient with Werner's syndrome. Leuk Lymphoma 2005;46(7):1091–5.
191. Knoell KA, Sidhu-Malik NK, Malik RK. Aplastic anemia in a patient with Rothmund-Thomson syndrome. J Pediatr Hematol Oncol 1999;21(5):444–6.
192. Nijmegen breakage syndrome. The International Nijmegen Breakage Syndrome Study Group. Arch Dis Child 2000;82(5):400–6.
193. Germeshausen M, Ballmaier M, Welte K. MPL mutations in 23 patients suffering from congenital amegakaryocytic thrombocytopenia: the type of mutation predicts the course of the disease. Hum Mutat 2006;27(3):296.
194. Jorge AA, Malaquias AC, Arnhold IJ, et al. Noonan syndrome and related disorders: a review of clinical features and mutations in genes of the RAS/MAPK pathway. Horm Res 2009;71(4):185–93.
195. Dale DC, Link DC. The many causes of severe congenital neutropenia. N Engl J Med 2009;360(1):3–5.

196. Whitlock JA. Down syndrome and acute lymphoblastic leukaemia. Br J Haematol 2006;135(5):595–602.
197. Taylor AM, Metcalfe JA, Thick J, et al. Leukemia and lymphoma in ataxia telangiectasia. Blood 1996;87(2):423–38.
198. Sullivan KE, Mullen CA, Blaese RM, et al. A multiinstitutional survey of the Wiskott-Aldrich syndrome. J Pediatr 1994;125(6 Pt 1):876–85.
199. Mueller BU, Pizzo PA. Cancer in children with primary or secondary immunodeficiencies. J Pediatr 1995;126(1):1–10.

Genome-wide Association Studies of Cancer Predisposition

Zsofia K. Stadler, MD, Joseph Vijai, PhD, Peter Thom, MS,
Tomas Kirchhoff, PhD, Nichole A.L. Hansen, BS,
Noah D. Kauff, MD, Mark Robson, MD,
Kenneth Offit, MD, MPH*

KEYWORDS

- Cancer predisposition • Cancer susceptibility regions
- Clinical role • Genome-wide association study

Rare, high-penetrance cancer predisposition genes account for only a small component of the overall familial risk of cancer.[1] Recently, it has been recognized that polygenic inheritance, wherein heritability is determined by the joint action of multiple genes, probably better characterizes the complex genetic architecture of diseases such as cancer. With technological advances in the interrogation of the human genome, genome-wide association studies (GWAS) have helped to identify multiple germline genetic risk variants or susceptibility loci for most common cancer types. Using a hypothesis-neutral genome-based approach, GWAS are able to compare DNA variations, in the form of single-nucleotide polymorphisms (SNPs), in a large set of unrelated cases and controls and pinpoint genetic variants associated with cancer risk.

To date, more than 50 cancer GWAS incorporating more than 15 different malignancies have been reported identifying over 100 genomic cancer susceptibility regions. The rapid discovery of common genetic variants associated with cancer risk generated excitement that such markers may prove useful for cancer risk prediction, improve our understanding of carcinogenesis, and possibly result in the development of targeted treatments for patients. However, as the effect size of most genetic

Supported in part by The Robert and Kate Niehaus Clinical Cancer Genetics Initiative, The Lymphoma Foundation, and the Breast Cancer Research Foundation.
Clinical Genetics Service, Department of Medicine, Memorial Sloan-Kettering Cancer Center, 1275 York Avenue, New York, NY 10021, USA
* Corresponding author. Memorial Sloan-Kettering Cancer Center, Box 192, 1275 York Avenue, New York, NY 10021.
E-mail address: offitk@mskcc.org

Hematol Oncol Clin N Am 24 (2010) 973–996
doi:10.1016/j.hoc.2010.06.009
0889-8588/10/$ – see front matter © 2010 Elsevier Inc. All rights reserved.

hemonc.theclinics.com

variants is less than 1.5 and the biologic mechanisms underpinning most associations are unknown, significant scientific barriers must be overcome before GWAS results can be meaningfully translated into patient care. This review of reported cancer GWAS summarizes what has been learned regarding the loci mapped, the frequency and magnitude of the cancer risk observed, and the clinical role, if any, for individualized testing for these variants. A more detailed description of population genetics methodology, as well as a more detailed version of the data from which **Tables 1–5** of this paper are adapted, are provided in a separate report.[2]

BREAST CANCER
Genetics of Breast Cancer

Mutations in the well-characterized high-penetrance *BRCA1* and *BRCA2* cancer susceptibility genes account for less than 20% of the familial risk of breast cancer, with other rarely mutated genes (*TP53*, *STK11*, *PTEN*) accounting for only a small additional fraction of the risk. Several intermediate-penetrance cancer predisposition genes (*ATM*, *CHEK2*, *BRIP1*, and *PALB2*) have also been described with modest ~2.0-fold increases in relative risk of breast cancer. Together with the high-penetrance genes, known breast cancer predisposition genes account for only ~25% of the familial risk of breast cancer.

Breast Cancer GWAS

Breast cancer has been at the forefront of cancer GWAS with 10 published studies and at least 13 independent loci implicated in disease risk (see **Table 1**). The most strongly associated SNP, with an odds ratio of 1.26, is rs2981582 in intron 2 of *FGFR2*.[3] The protein encoded by this gene is a member of the fibroblast growth factor receptor

Table 1
GWAS for breast cancer

Locus	Implicated Gene	SNP	Per Allele OR Ranges[a]	References
1p11.2	Pericentric	rs11249433	1.16	18
2q35	Intergenic	rs13387042	1.2–1.25	18,21
3p24.1	SLC4A7	rs4973768	1.11	14
5p12	Intergenic (*MRPS30*)	rs4415084 rs10941679	1.16–1.19	22
5q11.2	*MAP3K1, MIER3, C5orf35*	rs889312	1.13	3
6q22.33	*ECHDC1, RNF146*	rs2180341	1.41	23
6q25.1	*ESR1*	rs2046210	1.29	25
8q24	Intergenic	rs13281615	1.08	3
10q26	*FGFR2*	rs2981582 rs1219648 rs1078806	1.20–1.29	3 17,22 23
11p15.5	*LSP1*	rs3817198	1.07	3
14q24.1	*RAD51L1*	rs999737	1.06	18
16q12	*TNRC9 (TOX3), LOC643714*	rs3803662	1.16–1.28	3,18,21
17q23	*STXBP4*	rs6504950	1.05	14

Abbreviations: OR, odds ratio; SNP, single nucleotide polymorphism.
   [a] ORs <1 in the original publication have been converted to ORs >1 for the alternate allele.

(FGFR) family, whose members share evolutionarily highly conserved amino acid sequences and gene structure.[4,5] *FGFR2* is overexpressed and amplified in 5% to 10% of breast tumors[4] and the FGF-signaling pathway has been implicated in early mammary gland development in murine models.[6] Although the precise mechanism(s) of *FGFR2* deregulation in breast cancer etiology remains unknown, fine mapping of the region suggests that the causative variants lie in intron 2 of *FGFR2*; by protein-DNA interaction analysis, 2 *cis*-regulatory SNPs that alter binding affinity for transcription factors have been identified.[7] Since the initial study, the 10q26 loci mapping to *FGFR2* has been implicated in several breast cancer GWAS using different patient populations and seems to be strongest in estrogen receptor–positive breast cancer.[8,9]

The other susceptibility loci identified in gene-containing regions have not been implicated in cancer previously. The 16q12 locus containing the *TOX3* gene encodes an HMG-box protein that may be involved in bending and unwinding DNA and altering chromatic structure.[10] The 5q11.2 locus contains 3 genes, *MIER3, MGC33648*, whose functions are unknown, and *MAP3K1*, a component of a protein kinase signal transduction cascade involved in activating the Erk/Jnk and NFκB pathways.[11,12] For the *MAP3K1* variant, an association was found with estrogen and progesterone receptor–positive, HER2/Neu–negative tumors in African American, but not European American women.[8] The 11p15.5 locus contains *LSP1*, a cytoskeletal targeting protein for the ERK/MAP kinase pathway expressed in lymphocytes and endothelial cells.[13] A fifth locus at 8q24, a gene desert, has also been associated in GWAS with prostate, colorectal, and urinary bladder cancers.

Using combined data from the Cancer Genetic Markers of Susceptibility group (CGEMS) and Breast Cancer Association Consortium (BCAC), 2 additional SNPs associated with breast cancer were indentified.[14] The 3p24.1 locus maps to *SLC4A7*, a sodium- and bicarbonate-dependent cotransporter that regulates intracellular pH. Expression analysis showed this gene was down-regulated in most breast cancer cell lines and tumors.[15] The 17q23 locus maps to intron 1 of *STXBP4*, a mediator of insulin's role in glucose transport not previously associated with neoplasms.[16]

A separate GWAS by CGEMS confirmed the *FGFR2* locus[17] and analyses of additional stages to the original study identified 2 additional SNPs[18]: an SNP at 1p11.2 resides in a linkage disequilibrium block neighboring *NOTCH2*, which plays a role in epithelial-mesenchymal transition[19]; an SNP at 17q23, localized to *RAD51L1*, is evolutionarily conserved and essential for DNA repair by homologous recombination.[20]

The DeCode group in Iceland, in 2 separate GWAS,[21,22] detected an association with an SNP near *TOX3* and found additional loci at 2q35 (an intergenic region with no known nearby genes), and 5p12, containing *MRPS30* (which codes for an evolutionarily, highly conserved, mitochondrial ribosomal protein).

A GWAS of Ashkenazi Jewish breast cancer cases by Gold and colleagues[23] confirmed susceptibility loci mapping to *FGFR2* and identified an additional locus at 6q22.33, which contains *ECHDC1*, encoding a protein involved in mitochondrial fatty oxidation, and *RNF146*, encoding a ubiquitin protein ligase. This locus showed significant but weaker association in non-Ashkenazi Jewish whites, and, like most GWAS-based associations to date, was correlated with estrogen receptor–positive breast cancer.[24] A Chinese GWAS[25] found an association at 6q25.1, ~60 kb upstream of *ESR1*, which codes for an estrogen receptor. This locus showed significant but weaker association with breast cancer in a European cohort.

Clinical Correlations

The magnitude of risk associated with each of the loci identified is modest, with odds ratios largely ranging from 1.1 to 1.4. Although the established independent breast cancer loci are believed to result in a joint population attributable risk (PAR) of more than 60%, the contribution of these loci to the familial risk of cancer is no more than ~8%[26] thereby leaving most of the familial risk of breast cancer unexplained. There has been significant interest in determining whether the presence of risk variants predict for a particular clinical outcome. In a study evaluating 5 breast cancer susceptibility loci, only 1 SNP was associated with overall survival after diagnosis, however, after adjusting for known prognostic factors, this association no longer proved significant.[10]

To date, 2 modeling studies predict that together the 7 most common breast cancer–associated SNPs would add little in terms of improved discriminatory accuracy when compared with, or when used in conjunction with, a standard clinical breast cancer risk model (eg, the Gail model).[27,28] In the first clinical study, based on more than 5000 breast cancer cases and nearly 6000 controls, the addition of 10 breast cancer SNPs to a standard clinical breast cancer risk model predicted the risk of breast cancer only slightly better than the clinical model alone suggesting that risk prediction based on currently identified risk SNPs is premature.[29] As the strongest associations have been found in estrogen receptor–positive disease, a GWAS for women with triple-negative breast cancer is ongoing and may demonstrate different genetic associations.

PROSTATE CANCER
Genetics of Prostate Cancer

Family studies show strong evidence for a genetic predisposition to prostate cancer, with a 2- to 3-fold increased risk of disease in first-degree relatives of affected men.[30] Germline mutations in genes such as *BRCA2* have been found to be associated with prostate cancer risk, however, such mutations explain less than 10% of the familial risk of prostate cancer.[31]

Prostate Cancer GWAS

Prostate cancer GWAS have identified more than 2 dozen SNPs associated with disease risk (see **Table 2**). Using a genome-wide linkage scan, the DeCode group previously identified the association of the 8q24 locus with prostate cancer risk in Icelandic patients.[32] In African Americans, a group with a high incidence of prostate cancer, a higher minor allele frequency of the associated 8q24 loci was demonstrated. A separate admixture mapping study, a method that screens through the genome of populations of recently mixed ancestry, also emphasized the importance of the 8q24 region.[33] Subsequently, 2 GWAS, by the CGEMS group[34] and the DeCode group,[35] confirmed the association between the 8q24 region and prostate cancer risk. This association has been replicated in subsequent GWAS and through fine mapping analyses of the region with allele-specific risks for prostate cancer ranging from 1.4 to 2.0.[36–42] In a multiethnic study, Haiman and colleagues,[36] identified 7 independent risk variants in the 8q24 region and observed that the risk variants were most common in the African American population possibly suggesting a partial explanation for the higher incidence of prostate cancer in African American men. Analysis by Ghoussaini and colleagues[43] identified at least 5 loci at 8q24.21 independently separated by recombination hotspots. The gene nearest this 8q24.21 region, mapping at least 116 kb distally, is *MYC*, aberrations of which have been linked to multiple cancers,[44] with evidence suggesting that the 8q24 predisposition locus may be involved in *MYC* regulation.[45–47]

Table 2
GWAS for prostate cancer

Locus	Implicated Gene	SNP	Per Allele OR Ranges[a]	References
2p15	EHBP1	rs721048	1.15	60
2p21	THADA	rs1465618	1.08	164
2q31	ITGA6	rs12621278	1.33	164
3p12	Intergenic	rs2260753	1.18	38
3q21	Intergenic	rs10934853	1.12	165
4q22	PDLIM5	rs17021918	1.11	164
		rs12500426	1.08	
4q24	TET2	rs7679673	1.10	164
6q25	SLC22A3	rs9364554	1.17	38
7p15	Intergenic	rs12155172	1.05	164
7p15.2-15.1	JAZF1	rs10486567	1.12–1.35	37
7q21.3	LMTK2	rs6465657	1.12	38
8p21	NKX3-1	rs2928679	1.05	164
		rs1512268	1.18	
8q24	Intergenic	HapC 14 SNPs	2.10	35
		rs16901979	1.79–1.80	35,165
		DG8S737	1.64	32
		rs1447295	1.36–1.60	32–35,165
		rs1016343	1.37	38
		rs6983267	1.26–1.42	34,37,38
		rs4242382	1.41–1.87	37,38
		rs1006908	1.15	166
		rs620861	1.17	167
		rs16902094	1.14	165
10q11.2	MSMB	rs10993994	1.16–1.25	37,38
10q26.13	CTBP2	rs4962416	1.17–1.20	37
11p15	IGF2, IGF2AS, INS, TH	rs7127900	1.22	164
11q13.2	Intergenic	rs10896449	1.10–1.28	37
		rs7931342	1.19	38
17q12	TCF2 (HNF1B)	rs4430796	1.18–1.38	37,48,165
		rs7501939	1.41	38
17q24.3	Intergenic	rs1859962	1.20–1.26	38,48
19q13.2	PPP1R14A	rs8102476	1.12	165
19q13.41	KLK2, KLK3	rs2735839	1.20	38
22q13	TTLL1, BIK, MCAT, PACSIN2	rs5759167	1.20	164
22q13	TNRC6B	rs9623117	1.18	61
Xp11.23-p11.22	NUDT10, NUDT11 LOC340602, GSPT2, MAGED1	rs5945619	1.19	38
		rs5945572	1.23	60

Abbreviations: OR, odds ratio; SNP, single nucleotide polymorphism.
[a] ORs <1 in the original publication have been converted to ORs >1 for the alternate allele.

Two distinct loci in chromosome 17 have been implicated in prostate cancer risk. The 17q12 locus containing the *HNF1B/TCF2* gene was identified in multiple GWAS.[37,38,48] *HNF1B* encodes a member of the transcription factor superfamily and is involved in nephrogenesis.[49] Heterozygous germline mutations in *HNF1B* cause maturity-onset diabetes of the young.[50,51] One of the SNPs at the 17q12 locus seems to be protective for type 2 diabetes,[48] consistent with epidemiologic data demonstrating an inverse relationship between diabetes and prostate cancer risk.[52,53] Family-based studies confirmed an association of *HNF1B* with increased risk for prostate cancer among Hispanic men diagnosed at less than 50 years of age,[54] and subsequent fine mapping uncovered evidence for 2 independent prostate cancer loci in *HNF1B*.[55]

An SNP in 10q11.2, near the *MSMB* gene, has been associated with prostate cancer in 2 separate GWAS.[37,38] *MSMB* codes for prostate secretory protein of 94 amino acids (PSP94), which is synthesized by prostatic epithelia and is underexpressed in prostate tumors.[56] Decreased serum levels of PSP94 have been associated with increased prostate cancer risk.[57] Prostate cancer was also associated with an SNP at 19q13.41[38] between *KLK3*, which codes for prostate-specific antigen protein, and *KLK2*, which is amplified and overexpressed in prostate carcinoma tissue.[58] The same study[38] identified the Xp11.23 locus, which falls between *NUDT10* and *NUDT11*, 2 genes believed to play a role in signal transduction and found to be highly expressed in prostate and testis tissue.[59] This association was confirmed in another GWAS by Gudmundsson and colleagues.[60] Sun and colleagues[61] used combined data from their previous study[55] and CGEMS public data to identify a locus at 22q13 associated with aggressive prostate cancer cases.

Clinical Correlations

As with breast cancer, the magnitude of risk associated with each of the prostate cancer risk loci is modest, with odds ratios ranging from 1.2 to 2.0. The joint contribution of identified loci to the familial risk of prostate cancer approaches 20%. Unfortunately, none of the prostate cancer risk SNPs consistently distinguish risk for more or less aggressive cancer,[62,63] nor are they associated with cancer-specific mortality.[64] In addition, a family history of prostate cancer still confers a greater risk than the presence of any individual risk allele,[62] thereby providing no evidence that changing screening recommendations in men carrying a prostate cancer–associated risk SNP would be warranted. The effect of carrying multiple risk alleles on prostate cancer risk has also been assessed with results demonstrating that men who carried 4 or more of 5 possible risk alleles had a 4.5-fold increased risk of disease.[65] There was no evidence that the risk alleles were associated with disease aggressiveness, earlier age at diagnosis, or presence or absence of family history. A subsequent analysis demonstrated that these 5 risk alleles do not improve prediction models for disease risk or disease-specific mortality once known risk factors (age, prostate-specific antigen [PSA], family history) or prognostic factors (Gleason score, diagnostic PSA, stage, age, primary treatment) are taken into account.[66] Thus, the clinical usefulness of using risk SNPs as a tool for risk stratification has remained limited. As an alternative to the case-control study design, a recent GWAS used a case-case design of more or less aggressive prostate cancer to identify a genetic variant that predisposes to aggressive but not indolent disease.[67] It is feasible that additional similar studies identifying genetic variants predisposing to more aggressive disease may help to risk stratify populations appropriate for screening, prevention, and more aggressive treatment.

COLORECTAL CANCER
Genetics of Colorectal Cancer

Analysis of phenotype concordance in monozygotic twins of cases, suggests that inherited susceptibility is responsible for ~35% of all colorectal cancers (CRCs).[68] However, only ~6% of CRCs occur in the setting of a known high-penetrance cancer predisposition syndrome, such as (familial adenomatous polyposis) or Lynch syndrome. Therefore, most of the genetic risk of CRC remains unexplained.

CRC GWAS

There have been 7 GWAS in CRC (see **Table 3**). The first GWAS of CRC identified the 8q24 locus, containing the rs6983267 SNP, with an associated ~1.2-fold increased risk of disease.[69] This same SNP was also associated with about a 1.2- to 1.4-fold increase in prostate cancer risk.[34,37,38] In addition to the risk of CRC, the rs6983267 SNP at 8q24 was also found to be associated with adenoma risk with an odds ratio of 1.16.[70] The nearby pseudogene, POU5F1P1, expressed in several human malignancies shows 95% homology to POU5F1, a candidate stem cell gene that encodes a transcription factor,[71] but despite close mapping, the causative variant has not yet been identified. Two recent publications suggest that, at least in CRC predisposition, the rs6983267 SNP at 8q24 may be connected to enhanced Wnt signaling and subsequent MYC regulation.[46,47] Two additional SNPs in the 8q24 region have been implicated with similarly modest risks of CRC.[72,73]

Nearly half of the susceptibility loci in CRC are in linkage disequilibrium or are nearby genes of the transforming growth factor beta (TGF-β) signaling pathway previously implicated in carcinogenesis.[74,75] Increased TGF-β1 expression has been linked to tumor progression and recurrence in CRC, and germline mutations in components of the TGF-β signaling pathway, namely SMAD4 and BMPR1A, are responsible for juvenile polyposis, a high-penetrance CRC susceptibility syndrome. The rs4939827 SNP lying in an intron of SMAD7 at 18q21 was associated with CRC risk in 2

Table 3
GWAS for colorectal cancer

Locus	Implicated Gene	SNP	Per Allele OR Ranges[a]	References
8q23.3	EIF3H	rs16892766	1.25	77
8q24.21	LOC727677, POU5F1P1	rs10505477	1.17	72
		rs6983267	1.17–1.27	69,77
		rs7014346	1.19	73
10p14	Intergenic	rs10795668	1.11	77
11q23	Intergenic	rs3802842	1.12	73
14q22-q23	BMP4	rs4444235	1.11	78
15q13	Intergenic	rs4779584	1.23–1.26	77,81
	GREM1	rs10318	1.19	81
16q22.11	CDH1	rs9929218	1.10	78
18q21.1	SMAD7	rs4939827	1.16–1.20	73,76
19q13.11	RHPN2	rs10411210	1.15	78
20p12.3	Intergenic	rs961253	1.12	78

Abbreviations: OR, odds ratio; SNP, single nucleotide polymorphism.
[a] ORs <1 in the original publication have been converted to ORs >1 for the alternate allele.

GWAS[73,76] with a third study indicating an opposite effect.[77] The COGENT study performed a meta-analysis of 2 prior GWAS in CRC and followed up with replication analyses in 8 case-control series totaling more than 20,000 cases and controls.[78] This study implicated 2 other components of the TGF-β signaling pathway: an SNP in 19q13.11 maps to *RHPN2*, a gene involved in regulating actin cytoskeleton organization and gene expression responses to TGF-β signaling[79] and an SNP in 14q22 is near the transcription start site of *BMP4*, a member of the TGF-β family that is overexpressed in colon cancer cells.[80] Possible other genes implicated along the TGF-β signaling pathway are *BMP2* and *GREM1*.[78,81] In addition, an SNP at 16q22 maps to an intron of *CDH1*, a gene with a well-established role in CRC etiology and in which germline mutations cause hereditary diffuse gastric cancer.[78] Risks at each of these loci were modest, in the range of 1.1 to 1.2.

Clinical Correlations

Overall, the 10 risk loci identified account for only ~6% of the excess familial risk of CRC.[78] There is currently no evidence that individual SNPs or panels of SNPs adds to the discriminatory accuracy of current clinical criteria based on age, personal and family history of adenomas or CRC, and preexisting inflammatory bowel disease. Nor is there convincing evidence that these SNPs correlate with survival, early age at onset, site of tumor, or a histologically more aggressive subset of disease[78,82] By comparison, the relative risk for CRC for an individual carrying the 8q24 variant is ~1.2 versus a 1.8-fold increased risk for the first-degree relatives of individuals with an adenoma[83] and a 2.5-fold increased risk for individuals with a first-degree relative with CRC.[84] Thus, at the current time, recommendations for CRC screening would not be altered from that of the general population based solely on the presence of a CRC-associated risk SNP.

GASTROINTESTINAL (NONCOLORECTAL) CANCERS

An estimated 10% of patients with pancreatic cancer have an inherited form of the disease. However, only a small fraction of the familial risk of pancreatic cancer is explained by mutations in *BRCA*, *p16*, *STK11* and the mismatch repair genes associated with Lynch syndrome. The first GWAS in pancreatic cancer identified SNPs mapping to the first intron of the *ABO* blood group gene on chromosome 9q34 to be associated with a 1.2-fold increased risk of pancreatic cancer.[85] Earlier epidemiologic data have pointed to an association between ABO blood type and pancreatic and gastric cancer risk.[86–88] A second pancreatic cancer GWAS identified 8 additional SNPs mapping to 3 loci (13q22.1, 1q32.1, and 5p15.33).[89] The 2 SNPs at 13q22.1 are in intergenic regions between 2 genes belonging to the family of kruppel-like transcription factors, *KLF5* and *KLF12*. Somatic deletions in this area of chromosome 13 have been found in a variety of cancers, including pancreatic cancer. The 1q32.1 region harbors the *NR5A2* gene, which encodes a nuclear receptor of the fushi tarazu subfamily and is predominantly expressed in the exocrine gland of the pancreas, liver, intestines, and ovaries. The third locus at 5p15.33 is in intron 13 of *CLPTM1L*, and is part of the *CLPTM1L-TERT* locus. *CLPTM1L* has been implicated in carcinogenesis and the 5p15.33 region has been identified in several cancer GWAS including brain tumors, lung cancer, basal cell cancer, and melanoma.[90]

A GWAS in Japanese patients with esophageal squamous cell carcinoma identified the 12q24 and 4q21-23 susceptibility regions with odds ratios of 1.67 and 1.79, respectively.[91] The 4q21-23 region includes 7 members of the alcohol dehydrogenase (ADH) family involved in alcohol metabolism. The 12q24 region is in linkage disequilibrium with

ALDH2, a gene that encodes a member of the ADH family and is 1 of the key enzymes in alcohol metabolism. Previous candidate gene studies of esophageal squamous cell cancer have identified risk variants at both the *ADH1B* and *ALDH2* genes.[92,93]

A gastric cancer GWAS in Japanese patients identified an SNP at 8q24.3 mapping to the *PSCA* gene and conferring an allele-specific risk of 1.62 specifically for diffuse-type gastric cancer.[94] PSCA was originally identified as a prostate-specific stem cell antigen[95,96] but has been reported in bladder, esophageal, and stomach cancers,[97] as well as in a recent GWAS of bladder cancer.[98]

LUNG CANCER

Multiple lung cancer GWAS[99–101] identified a region at 15q24-q25.1 containing *CHRNA3*, *CHRNA4*, *CHRNA5*, *PSM4*, *LOC123688*, and *IREB2* (see **Table 4**). The *CHRNA* genes code for subunits of nicotinic acetylcholine receptors, members of a pathway implicated in lung cancer etiology and progression[102,103] as well as nicotine dependence.[104] A variant (rs1051730) within *CHRNA3* was associated with higher quantity of smoking and an increased risk of peripheral artery disease.[105] The 15q24-q25 association was significant even with never-smokers and Liu and colleagues[106] noted the same association even after adjustment for smoking habits.

Three GWAS[101,107,108] identified the 5p15.33 locus, mapping to *CLPTM1L*, a gene amplified in NSCLC.[109] Additional SNPs at 5p15.33 have been identified, with 1 in *TERT*, a gene that induces immortality when constitutively expressed in transfected cells.[110] In a recent GWAS analyses by lung cancer histology, the rs2736100 (*TERT*) SNP at 5p15.33 was associated with a 1.23-fold increased risk of adenocarcinoma but not with other histologic subtypes of lung cancer.[111] Two GWAS implicated the 6p21.33 locus, which is associated with a large region of linkage dysequilibrium.[101,107] *BAT3* within this regions represents a strong candidate gene as it is implicated in apoptosis and is needed for acetylation of p53 in response to DNA damage.[112] A multicancer study of more than 30,000 cases and more than 45,000 controls identified an association between the 5p15.33 locus and risk of lung, urinary bladder, prostate, and cervical cancers with a protective effect for cutaneous melanoma.[90] The 5p15.33

Table 4
GWAS for lung cancer

Locus	Implicated Gene	SNP	per Allele OR Ranges[a]	References
5pter-p15.33	*CLPTM1L, TERT*	rs401681	1.16	107
		rs402710	1.18	108
	TERT	rs2736100	1.14	108
			1.23 (adenocarcinoma)	111
5p15.33		rs4975616	1.16	101
6p21.33-p21.3	*BAT3, MSH5*	rs3117582	1.24	101,107
15q24-q25	*CHRNA3, CHRNA5,*	rs8034191	1.30–1.38	99,100,106
	CHRNB4, PSMA4,	rs1051730	1.31–1.35	99,106,108
	LOC123688	rs8042374	1.33, NR	101,107
15q25.1	*CHRNA3*	rs938682	1.33	101
		rs12914385	1.29	101

Abbreviations: OR, odds ratio; SNP, single nucleotide polymorphism.
a ORs <1 in the original publication have been converted to ORs >1 for the alternate allele.

locus is thus the second locus, along with 8q24, to be associated with multiple cancers by GWAS.

Clinical Correlations

Compared with the 10- to 20-fold increase in risk of lung cancer in cigarette smokers, the risk associated with each of the lung cancer risk SNPs is much smaller with odds ratios ranging between 1.1 and 1.3. Moreover, the strongest susceptibility locus, 15q25, is also strongly linked to smoking, the main environmental risk factor for lung cancer, and it is possible that the effect of this loci on lung cancer risk is entirely mediated through its influence on nicotine dependence. Although some of the SNPs show a statistically significant association even after adjustment for smoking behavior,[99,100,106] in at least 1 study, extent of exposure correlated with risk in a particular SNP.[105]

BASAL CELL CARCINOMA AND CUTANEOUS MELANOMA

Several GWAS have been performed not just for basal cell carcinoma (BCC) and cutaneous melanoma (CM) (see **Table 5**) but also for known risk factors and predictors of melanoma including pigmentation phenotypes and precursor lesions. The first cancer GWAS for CM found a risk loci at the 20q11.22 locus to be associated with a 1.75-fold increased risk of melanoma.[113] Fine mapping identified variants affecting hair, eye, and skin pigmentation in Europeans, features known to affect CM and BCC risk.[114,115] Gudbjartsson and colleagues[114] found a haplotype near *ASIP*, and a nonsynonymous SNP in *TYR* that conferred increased risks of CM and BCC, and an eye-color variant in *TYRP1* associated with an increased risk of CM alone. Another GWAS[116] identified 2 regions on chromosome 1 associated with BCC but not CM, one near a gene involved in oocyte cytoskeletal organization[117] and the other near a gene involved in actin cytoskeleton regulation, adhesion turnover, and increased cell migration.[118] A follow-up study identified 3 more BCC risk loci including rs11170164 in the *KRT5* gene that codes for a basal cell keratin; rs2151280 at 9p21 near the CDKN2A/B locus and rs157935 on chromosome 7q32.[119] A recent melanoma GWAS identified 3 loci including 16q24, encompassing *MC1R*, involved in cell-cycle regulation.[120] This same 16q24 region was previously implicated in a GWAS of hair color and skin pigmentation.[115] The second loci, at 11q14, again implicated *TYR*; the third loci at 9p21, adjacent to *MTAP*, flanks *CDKN2A*, a well-known high-penetrance melanoma susceptibility gene. The 9p21 loci has also been implicated in a recent GWAS of cutaneous nevi development[121] in addition to being implicated in BCC susceptibility[116] and association to pigmentation phenotypes.

URINARY BLADDER CANCER

The first GWAS for bladder cancer identified 2 loci: the strongest association was an SNP at 8q24, 30 kb upstream of the *MYC* oncogene, conferring an allele-specific risk of 1.22.[122] Although the 8q24 loci has been implicated in cancer risk in multiple malignancies, this particular SNP (rs9642880) was not associated with breast cancer, prostate cancer, or CRC. Another SNP mapping to 3q28 is in a linkage dysequilibrium block containing *TP63* that codes for the p63 protein involved in regulating cell-cycle arrest and apoptosis. Loss of p63 protein expression in bladder tumors is associated with cancer progression and poor prognosis.[123,124] The second bladder cancer GWAS identified a single missense variant (rs2294008) in the *PSCA* gene conferring an allele-specific risk of 1.15.[98] PSCA, initially identified as a prostate-specific cell surface marker, is overexpressed in most bladder cancers.[95,96] Paradoxically, the missense variant alters the start codon leading to reduced promoter activity in vitro; consequences of the risk variant in vivo are unknown. The same locus was recently implicated in a GWAS of diffuse-type gastric cancer in Japan.[94]

HEMATOLOGICAL MALIGNANCIES

The first chronic lymphocytic leukemia (CLL) GWAS identified 6 SNPs all conferring a modest risk of disease, with odds ratios less than 1.6.[125] The strongest association was at 6p25.3 with an SNP in the 3' untranslated terminal region of *IRF4*, expression of which has been linked to CLL, multiple myeloma, and B-cell lymphoproliferative disorder development.[126,127] The SNP at 2q37.1 maps to *SP140*, putatively involved in the pathogenesis of acute promyelocytic leukemia and viral infection.[128] The association at 19q13.32 maps to *PRKD2*, decreased expression of which is seen in some B-cell tumors and ~50% of CLL or small lymphocytic lymphomas.[129] However, expression of *PRKD2* mRNA in lymphocytes was not associated with genotypes in this GWAS. In an expanded follow-up analysis,[130] 4 new susceptibility loci were reported with the strongest association at 8q24.21 (odd ratio 1.26), an area associated with multiple cancers. A second SNP at 2q37.3 maps to *FARP2*, a gene involved in signaling downstream of G protein-coupled receptors.[131] An additional SNP mapping to 16q24.1 implicates *IRF8* as a candidate gene, given that it is involved in B-cell lineage specification, immunoglobulin rearrangement, and regulation of germinal center reaction.[132] A risk loci at *IRF8* has been previously reported in multiple sclerosis, a disease that has been reported to be associated with CLL risk.[133] The last SNP at 15q21.3 is in a linkage dysequilibrium region flanked by *NEDD4*, involved in regulating viral latency and pathogenesis of Epstein-Barr virus (EBV). A GWAS of non-Hodgkin lymphoma including follicular, diffuse, large B-cell (DLBCL) and CLL/small lymphocytic lymphomas, found an SNP at 6p21.33 to be associated with a decreased risk of follicular lymphoma.[134] This SNP is just downstream of *C6orf15* (*STG*), near psoriasis susceptibility region 1 (*PSORS1*). No significant associations for other subtypes of lymphoma were found and SNPs implicated in the prior CLL GWAS were not confirmed, although the power of the study was limited by sample size. Two GWAS in childhood acute lymphoblastic leukemia (ALL) have been published[135,136] with both studies implicating a loci on chromosome 10 mapping to the *ARID5B* gene, which encodes a member of the ARID family of transcription factors important in embryogenesis and growth regulation[137] Some of the risk alleles at *ARID5B* seem to be selective for the subset of B-cell precursor ALL with hyperploidy that has a better response to methotrexate chemotherapy than other ALL subtypes.[138]

A GWAS in patients with myeloproliferative neoplasms (MPN), including polycythemia vera, essential thrombocythemia and primary myelofibrosis, identified an SNP (rs10974944) that maps to *JAK2*, a gene that harbors a somatic activating point mutation, *JAK2^V617F*, commonly seen in MPNs.[139] Further analysis found that germline alterations of rs10974944 were significantly associated with *JAK2^V617F*-positive subjects. Moreover, the non–wild-type SNP was far more likely to be in *cis* with *JAK2^V617F*, suggesting that the SNP predisposes to the development of the somatic mutation. In contrast to other GWAS findings, this SNP was associated with a 3-fold increase in MPN risk, and is believed to be associated with nearly 50% of MPN cases.

TESTICULAR GERM CELL TUMORS

Genetic susceptibility to testicular germ cell tumors (TGCTs) is supported by an 8- to 10-fold and a 4- to 6-fold increased risk of disease in brothers and fathers of affected

Table 5
GWAS for other cancers

Locus	Implicated Gene	SNP	Per Allele OR Ranges[a]	References
Basal cell carcinoma and Cutaneous melanoma				
1p36.13	PADI4, PADI6, RCC2, AHRGEF10L	rs7538876	1.28 BCC	[116]
1q42.11-q42.3	RHOU	rs801114	1.28 BCC	[116]
7q32	KLF14	rs157935	1.23 BCC	[119]
9p21	MTAP, CDKN2A	rs7023329	1.18 CM	[120]
9p21	CDKN2A, CDKN2B	rs2151280	1.19 BCC	[119]
9p23	TYRP1	rs1408799	1.15 CM	[114]
11q14-q21	TYR	rs1126809	1.21 CM	[114]
			1.14 BCC	[114]
		rs1393350	1.29 CM	[120]
12q12-q13	KRT5	rs11170164	1.35 BCC	[119]
16q24	MC1R	rs258322	1.67 CM	[120]
20q11.2-q12	ASIP	Hap rs1015362G rs4911414T	1.45 CM 1.35 BCC	[114]
20q11.22	CDC91L1 (PIGU)	rs910873 rs1885120	1.75 CM	[113]
Urinary Bladder				
3q28	TP63	rs710521	1.19	[122]
8q24.21	MYC, BC042052	rs9642880	1.22	[122]
8q24.2	PSCA	rs2294008	1.15	[98]
Neuroblastoma				
2q35	BARD1	rs3768716 rs6435862	1.68 1.68	[153]
6p22.3	FLJ22536, FLJ44180	rs4712653 rs9295536 rs6939340	1.35 1.32 1.37	[152]
Glioma				
5p15.33	TERT	rs2736100	1.27	[155]
8q24.21	CCDC26	rs4295627	1.36	[155]
9p21.3	CDKN2B	rs1412829 rs4977756	1.42 1.24	[161] [155]
11q23.3	PHLDB1	rs498872	1.18	[155]
20q13.33	RTEL1	rs6010620	1.51 1.28	[161] [155]
Acute lymphoblastic leukemia (childhood)				
7p12.2	IKZF1	rs4132601	1.69	[136]
10q21.2 maps to 10q11.22 by HGNC	ARID5B	rs10994982 rs10821936 rs7089424	1.62 1.91 1.65	[135] [135] [136]
14q11.2	CEBPE	rs2239633	1.34	[136]
Chronic lymphocytic leukemia				
2q13	ACOXL, BCL2L11	rs17483466	1.39	[125]
2q37.1	SP140	rs13397985	1.41	[125]
2q37.3	FARP2	rs757978	1.39	[130]
6p25-p23	IRF4	rs872071	1.54	[125]
8q24.21	Intergenic	rs2456449	1.26	[130]

(continued on next page)

Table 5
(continued)

Locus	Implicated Gene	SNP	Per Allele OR Ranges[a]	References
11q24.1	GRAMD1B	rs735665	1.45	[125]
15q21.3	NEDD4, RFX7	rs7169431	1.36	[130]
15q23	Intergenic	rs7176508	1.37	[125]
16q24.1	IRF8	rs305061	1.22	[130]
19q13.2-q13.3	PRKD2, STRN4	rs11083846	1.35	[125]
Follicular Lymphoma				
6p21.33	STG, PSORS1	rs6457327	1.69	[134]
Thyroid (Papillary and Follicular)				
9q22.33	Intergenic	rs965513	1.75	[150]
14q13.3	Intergenic	rs944289	1.37	[150]
Myeloproliferative Neoplasms				
9p24.1	JAK2	rs10974944	3.10	[139]
Testicular Germ Cell Cancer				
4q24	Intergenic	rs4699052	1.21	[144]
5q31.3	SPRY4	rs4324715	1.37	[143]
		rs4624820	1.37	[144]
		rs6897876	1.39	[143]
6p21.3	BAK1	rs210138	1.50	[144]
12q22	KITLG	rs995030	2.55	[144]
		rs3782179	3.08	[143]
		rs4474514	3.07	[143]
		rs1508595	2.69	[144]
Pancreatic				
1q32.1	NR5A2	rs3790844	1.30	[89]
5p15.33	TERT-CLPTM1L	rs401681	1.19	[89]
9q34	ABO	rs505922	1.20	[85]
13q22.1	Intergenic	rs9543325	1.26	[89]
Ovarian				
9p22	BNC2, CNTLN, LOC648570	rs3814113	1.22	[148]
Gastric (diffuse)				
8q24.3	PSCA	rs2976392	1.62 (Japan) 1.90 (Korea)	[94]
Esophageal (squamous)				
4q21-23	ADH1B	rs1229984	1.79	[91]
12q24	ALDH2	rs671	1.67	[91]
Single locus 5p15.33 multiple cancers	TERT-CLPTM1L	rs401681		[90]
Prostate			1.07	
Lung			1.15	
BCC			1.25	
Urinary bladder			1.12	
Cervical			1.31	

Abbreviations: BCC, basal cell carcinoma; CM, cutaneous melanoma; OR, odds ratio; SNP, single nucleotide polymorphism.

[a] ORs <1 in the original publication have been converted to ORs >1 for the alternate allele.

patients, respectively.[140–142] The genetic underpinnings of this strong familial risk have remained largely unexplained. The 2 TGCT GWAS[143,144] both identified SNPs at the 12q22 locus, associated with a 2.55- to 3-fold increased risk of TGCT. The 12q22 region contains *KITLG*, which encodes the ligand for the receptor tyrosine kinase, c-KIT. The KITLG-KIT signaling pathway has a role in gametogenesis with Kitl being necessary for primordial germ cell (PGC) development.[145] Studies have suggested that TGCTs arise from PGCs and delayed differentiation of PGCs has been linked to TGCT in situ in individuals with chromosomal abnormalities.[146,147]

OVARIAN CANCER

Although ovarian cancer is known to have a large hereditary component, less than half of the excess familial risk of ovarian cancer is explained by the high-penetrance *BRCA1* and *BRCA2* cancer predisposition genes. The first GWAS of ovarian cancer initially identified 12 SNPs, all in the same linkage disequilibrium block at the 9p22 locus, as being associated with a risk of ovarian cancer, however, after final analysis, only 1 of these SNPs (rs3814113) retained statistical significance.[148] Nearest genes are *BNC2*, encoding a DNA-binding zinc-finger protein possibly involved in DNA transcription regulation[149] and *CNTLN*, encoding a centrosomal protein. When evaluated by histologic subtype, the strength of the association was strongest for serous cases.

THYROID CANCER

Thyroid cancer has a strong hereditary component, however, little is known about the genetic variation underlying thyroid cancer predisposition. The single GWAS for thyroid cancer identified 2 significantly associated SNPs.[150] The SNP in region 9q22.33, associated with a 1.75-fold increased risk of disease, is near *FOXE1*, which is implicated in embryonic thyroid organogenesis.[151] The SNP at 14q13.3, in an intragenic region, is associated with a 1.37-fold increased risk of disease and is near *NKX2-1*, a gene known to play a role in embryonic thyroid differentiation.[151]

NEUROBLASTOMA

The first GWAS for neuroblastoma identified 3 associated SNPs, all in a linkage disequilibrium block at 6p22.3 containing 2 hypothetical genes, and conferring a 1.3-fold increased risk of disease.[152] A second analysis focusing only on high-risk neuroblastoma cases, found 2 SNPs at 2p35, mapping to the *BARD1* (*BRCA1*-associated RING domain-1) locus, with each SNP conferring an allele-specific risk of 1.68.[153] BARD1 forms a heterodimer with BRCA1 and is believed to be essential in the tumor suppressor function of BRCA1.[154]

GLIOMA

A meta-analysis from 2 glioma GWAS identified 5 susceptibility loci.[155] The strongest association at 8q24.21, with an allele-specific risk of 1.36, maps to an intron of *CCDC26*, encoding a retinoic acid modulator of differentiation and death. This glioma variation region is distinctly different from the 8q24.21 region implicated in colorectal, breast, prostate, and bladder cancer risk. Another loci at 9p21.3 maps to the *CDKN2A-CDKN2B* tumor suppressor genes in which germline mutations cause the melanoma-astrocytoma syndrome.[156,157] Somatic deletions in *CDKN2A* are detectable in ~50% of gliomas[158,159] with loss of expression correlating with poor prognosis.[160] A GWAS of high-grade gliomas confirmed an association with genetic variants localizing to 9p21.[161] Both glioma GWAS[155,161] found SNPs at 20q13.3, mapping to the *RTEL1* helicase gene, involved in maintaining genomic stability through suppression of homologous recombination.[162]

DISCUSSION

Cancer GWAS have identified over 100 low-penetrance cancer susceptibility loci associated with modest increases in disease risk, with odds ratios generally less than ~1.5. Exceptions are the risk alleles in *JAK2* in myeloproliferative neoplasms and the 12p22 locus mapping to *KITLG* in testicular cancer associated with a 3-fold increased risk of disease. Given the large size of the studies conducted and the use of high-density genotyping arrays, it is unlikely that new common genetic variants with much higher odd ratios will be identified for the cancers studied to date. The initial expectation that GWAS would explain much of the missing heritability of cancers has yet to be fulfilled. The common risk variants from GWAS explain only about 8%, 20%, and 6% of the familial risk of breast cancer, prostate cancer, and CRC, respectively. With advances in technology, additional common genetic variants with risks of ~1.1 will inevitably be found but, as has been observed by many in the field, a large number of such variants would need to be identified to explain the remaining genetic component of common cancers.[163] Although disregarded in prior GWAS, the role of rare genetic variants with allele frequencies less than 10% are just beginning to be explored, and alternative forms of genetic variations, such as genomic structural variations consisting of insertions, deletions, copy-number variations, translocations and inversions, may shed further light on the genetic risk of cancer.

As the biologic mechanisms underlying most of the associations remain unexplained, functional studies now need to be performed. However, first, resequencing and fine mapping of the implicated regions to identify the most likely causal variants will be necessary. Evaluation of more heterogeneous populations with different linkage disequilibrium structures may be especially useful in pinpointing the true causal variants and may also identify ethnicity- and race-specific risk alleles. Interactions between different genetic variants and known epidemiologic and environmental modifiers have yet to be revealed. Although GWAS have revolutionized our ability to study genetic variation across the human genome, a considerable translational effort remains before the results of GWAS can be responsibly incorporated into cancer risk prediction and preventive medicine.

REFERENCES

1. Easton DF. How many more breast cancer predisposition genes are there? Breast Cancer Res 1999;1:14–7.
2. Stadler ZK, Thom P, Robson ME, et al. Genome-Wide Association Studies of cancer. J Clin Oncol 2010. [Epub ahead of print]. DOI:10.1200/JCO. 2009.25.7816.
3. Easton DF, Pooley KA, Dunning AM, et al. Genome-wide association study identifies novel breast cancer susceptibility loci. Nature 2007;447:1087–93.
4. Adnane J, Gaudray P, Dionne CA, et al. BEK and FLG, two receptors to members of the FGF family, are amplified in subsets of human breast cancers. Oncogene 1991;6:659–63.
5. Ornitz DM, Itoh N. Fibroblast growth factors. Genome Biol 2001;2:12 Reviews3005.1–3005.
6. Grose R, Dickson C. Fibroblast growth factor signaling in tumorigenesis. Cytokine Growth Factor Rev 2005;16:179–86.

7. Meyer KB, Maia AT, O'Reilly M, et al. Allele-specific up-regulation of FGFR2 increases susceptibility to breast cancer. PLoS Biol 2008;6:e108.

8. Rebbeck TR, DeMichele A, Tran TV, et al. Hormone-dependent effects of FGFR2 and MAP3K1 in breast cancer susceptibility in a population-based sample of post-menopausal African-American and European-American women. Carcinogenesis 2009;30:269–74.

9. Garcia-Closas M, Hall P, Nevanlinna H, et al. Heterogeneity of breast cancer associations with five susceptibility loci by clinical and pathological characteristics. PLoS Genet 2008;4:e1000054.

10. O'Flaherty E, Kaye J. TOX defines a conserved subfamily of HMG-box proteins. BMC Genomics 2003;4:13.

11. Xia Y, Wu Z, Su B, et al. JNKK1 organizes a MAP kinase module through specific and sequential interactions with upstream and downstream components mediated by its amino-terminal extension. Genes Dev 1998;12: 3369–81.

12. Mokhtari D, Myers JW, Welsh N. MAPK kinase kinase-1 is essential for cytokine-induced c-Jun NH2-terminal kinase and nuclear factor-kappaB activation in human pancreatic islet cells. Diabetes 2008;57:1896–904.

13. Harrison RE, Sikorski BA, Jongstra J. Leukocyte-specific protein 1 targets the ERK/MAP kinase scaffold protein KSR and MEK1 and ERK2 to the actin cytoskeleton. J Cell Sci 2004;117:2151–7.

14. Ahmed S, Thomas G, Ghoussaini M, et al. Newly discovered breast cancer susceptibility loci on 3p24 and 17q23.2. Nat Genet 2009;41:585–90.

15. Chen Y, Choong LY, Lin Q, et al. Differential expression of novel tyrosine kinase substrates during breast cancer development. Mol Cell Proteomics 2007;6: 2072–87.

16. Min J, Okada S, Kanzaki M, et al. Synip: a novel insulin-regulated syntaxin 4-binding protein mediating GLUT4 translocation in adipocytes. Mol Cell 1999;3:751–60.

17. Hunter DJ, Kraft P, Jacobs KB, et al. A genome-wide association study identifies alleles in FGFR2 associated with risk of sporadic postmenopausal breast cancer. Nat Genet 2007;39:870–4.

18. Thomas G, Jacobs KB, Kraft P, et al. A multistage genome-wide association study in breast cancer identifies two new risk alleles at 1p11.2 and 14q24.1 (RAD51L1). Nat Genet 2009;41:579–84.

19. Grego-Bessa J, Díez J, Timmerman L, et al. Notch and epithelial-mesenchyme transition in development and tumor progression: another turn of the screw. Cell Cycle 2004;3:718–21.

20. Thacker J. The RAD51 gene family, genetic instability and cancer. Cancer Lett 2005;219:125–35.

21. Stacey SN, Manolescu A, Sulem P, et al. Common variants on chromosomes 2q35 and 16q12 confer susceptibility to estrogen receptor-positive breast cancer. Nat Genet 2007;39:865–9.

22. Stacey SN, Manolescu A, Sulem P, et al. Common variants on chromosome 5p12 confer susceptibility to estrogen receptor-positive breast cancer. Nat Genet 2008;40:703–6.

23. Gold B, Kirchhoff T, Stefanov S, et al. Genome-wide association study provides evidence for a breast cancer risk locus at 6q22.33. Proc Natl Acad Sci U S A 2008;105:4340–5.

24. Kirchhoff T, Chen ZQ, Gold B, et al. The 6q22.33 locus and breast cancer susceptibility. Cancer Epidemiol Biomarkers Prev 2009;18:2468–75.

25. Zheng W, Long J, Gao YT, et al. Genome-wide association study identifies a new breast cancer susceptibility locus at 6q25.1. Nat Genet 2009;41:324–8.

26. Hemminki K, Försti A, Lorenzo Bermejo J. New cancer susceptibility loci: population and familial risks. Int J Cancer 2008;123:1726–9.

27. Gail MH. Discriminatory accuracy from single-nucleotide polymorphisms in models to predict breast cancer risk. J Natl Cancer Inst 2008;100:1037–41.

28. Gail MH. Value of adding single-nucleotide polymorphism genotypes to a breast cancer risk model. J Natl Cancer Inst 2009;101:959–63.

29. Wacholder S, Hartge P, Prentice R, et al. Performance of common genetic variants in breast-cancer risk models. N Engl J Med 2010;362:986–93.

30. Bruner DW, Moore D, Parlanti A, et al. Relative risk of prostate cancer for men with affected relatives: systematic review and meta-analysis. Int J Cancer 2003;107:797–803.

31. Edwards SM, Kote-Jarai Z, Meitz J, et al. Two percent of men with early-onset prostate cancer harbor germline mutations in the BRCA2 gene. Am J Hum Genet 2003;72:1–12.

32. Amundadottir LT, Sulem P, Gudmundsson J, et al. A common variant associated with prostate cancer in European and African populations. Nat Genet 2006;38:652–8.

33. Freedman ML, Haiman CA, Patterson N, et al. Admixture mapping identifies 8q24 as a prostate cancer risk locus in African-American men. Proc Natl Acad Sci U S A 2006;103:14068–73.

34. Yeager M, Orr N, Hayes RB, et al. Genome-wide association study of prostate cancer identifies a second risk locus at 8q24. Nat Genet 2007;39:645–9.

35. Gudmundsson J, Sulem P, Manolescu A, et al. Genome-wide association study identifies a second prostate cancer susceptibility variant at 8q24. Nat Genet 2007;39:631–7.

36. Haiman CA, Patterson N, Freedman ML, et al. Multiple regions within 8q24 independently affect risk for prostate cancer. Nat Genet 2007;39:638–44.

37. Thomas G, Jacobs KB, Yeager M, et al. Multiple loci identified in a genome-wide association study of prostate cancer. Nat Genet 2008;40:310–5.

38. Eeles RA, Kote-Jarai Z, Giles GG, et al. Multiple newly identified loci associated with prostate cancer susceptibility. Nat Genet 2008;40:316–21.

39. Severi G, Hayes VM, Padilla EJ, et al. The common variant rs1447295 on chromosome 8q24 and prostate cancer risk: results from an Australian population-based case-control study. Cancer Epidemiol Biomarkers Prev 2007;16:610–2.

40. Schumacher FR, Feigelson HS, Cox DG, et al. A common 8q24 variant in prostate and breast cancer from a large nested case-control study. Cancer Res 2007;67:2951–6.

41. Suuriniemi M, Agalliu I, Schaid DJ, et al. Confirmation of a positive association between prostate cancer risk and a locus at chromosome 8q24. Cancer Epidemiol Biomarkers Prev 2007;16:809–14.

42. Zheng SL, Sun J, Cheng Y, et al. Association between two unlinked loci at 8q24 and prostate cancer risk among European Americans. J Natl Cancer Inst 2007;99:1525–33.

43. Ghoussaini M, Song H, Koessler T, et al. Multiple loci with different cancer specificities within the 8q24 gene desert. J Natl Cancer Inst 2008;100:962–6.

44. Dalla-Favera R, Bregni M, Erikson J, et al. Human c-myc onc gene is located on the region of chromosome 8 that is translocated in Burkitt lymphoma cells. Proc Natl Acad Sci U S A 1982;79:7824–7.

45. Solé X, Hernández P, de Heredia ML, et al. Genetic and genomic analysis modeling of germline c-MYC overexpression and cancer susceptibility. BMC Genomics 2008;9:12.
46. Pomerantz MM, Ahmadiyeh N, Jia L, et al. The 8q24 cancer risk variant rs6983267 shows long-range interaction with MYC in colorectal cancer. Nat Genet 2009;41:882–4.
47. Tuupanen S, Turunen M, Lehtonen R, et al. The common colorectal cancer predisposition SNP rs6983267 at chromosome 8q24 confers potential to enhanced Wnt signaling. Nat Genet 2009;41:885–90.
48. Gudmundsson J, Sulem P, Steinthorsdottir V, et al. Two variants on chromosome 17 confer prostate cancer risk, and the one in TCF2 protects against type 2 diabetes. Nat Genet 2007;39:977–83.
49. Dudziak K, Mottalebi N, Senkel S, et al. Transcription factor HNF1beta and novel partners affect nephrogenesis. Kidney Int 2008;74:210–7.
50. Horikawa Y, Iwasaki N, Hara M, et al. Mutation in hepatocyte nuclear factor-1 beta gene (TCF2) associated with MODY. Nat Genet 1997;17:384–5.
51. Fajans SS, Bell GI, Polonsky KS. Molecular mechanisms and clinical pathophysiology of maturity-onset diabetes of the young. N Engl J Med 2001; 345:971–80.
52. Kasper JS, Giovannucci E. A meta-analysis of diabetes mellitus and the risk of prostate cancer. Cancer Epidemiol Biomarkers Prev 2006;15:2056–62.
53. Waters KM, Henderson BE, Stram DO, et al. Association of diabetes with prostate cancer risk in the multiethnic cohort. Am J Epidemiol 2009;169:937–45.
54. Levin AM, Machiela MJ, Zuhlke KA, et al. Chromosome 17q12 variants contribute to risk of early-onset prostate cancer. Cancer Res 2008;68:6492–5.
55. Sun J, Zheng SL, Wiklund F, et al. Evidence for two independent prostate cancer risk-associated loci in the HNF1B gene at 17q12. Nat Genet 2008;40:1153–5.
56. Liu AY, Bradner RC, Vessella RL. Decreased expression of prostatic secretory protein PSP94 in prostate cancer. Cancer Lett 1993;74:91–9.
57. Nam RK, Reeves JR, Toi A, et al. A novel serum marker, total prostate secretory protein of 94 amino acids, improves prostate cancer detection and helps identify high grade cancers at diagnosis. J Urol 2006;175:1291–7.
58. Herrala AM, Porvari KS, Kyllönen AP, et al. Comparison of human prostate specific glandular kallikrein 2 and prostate specific antigen gene expression in prostate with gene amplification and overexpression of prostate specific glandular kallikrein 2 in tumor tissue. Cancer 2001;92:2975–84.
59. GeneCards. Available at: http://www.genecards.org/cgi-bin/carddisp.pl?gene=NUDT10&search=NUDT10&suff=txt. Accessed February 25, 2009.
60. Gudmundsson J, Sulem P, Rafnar T, et al. Common sequence variants on 2p15 and Xp11.22 confer susceptibility to prostate cancer. Nat Genet 2008;40:281–3.
61. Sun J, Zheng SL, Wiklund F, et al. Sequence variants at 22q13 are associated with prostate cancer risk. Cancer Res 2009;69:10–5.
62. Fitzgerald LM, Kwon EM, Koopmeiners JS, et al. Analysis of recently identified prostate cancer susceptibility loci in a population-based study: associations with family history and clinical features. Clin Cancer Res 2009;15:3231–7.
63. Kader AK, Sun J, Isaacs SD, et al. Individual and cumulative effect of prostate cancer risk-associated variants on clinicopathologic variables in 5,895 prostate cancer patients. Prostate 2009;69:1195–205.
64. Wiklund FE, Adami HO, Zheng SL, et al. Established prostate cancer susceptibility variants are not associated with disease outcome. Cancer Epidemiol Biomarkers Prev 2009;18:1659–62.

65. Zheng SL, Sun J, Wiklund F, et al. Cumulative association of five genetic variants with prostate cancer. N Engl J Med 2008;358:910–9.
66. Salinas CA, Koopmeiners JS, Kwon EM, et al. Clinical utility of five genetic variants for predicting prostate cancer risk and mortality. Prostate 2009;69: 363–72.
67. Xu J, Zheng SL, Isaacs SD, et al. Inherited genetic variant predisposes to aggressive but not indolent prostate cancer. Proc Natl Acad Sci U S A 2010; 107:2136–40.
68. Lichtenstein P, Holm NV, Verkasalo PK, et al. Environmental and heritable factors in the causation of cancer–analyses of cohorts of twins from Sweden, Denmark, and Finland. N Engl J Med 2000;343:78–85.
69. Tomlinson I, Webb E, Carvajal-Carmona L, et al. A genome-wide association scan of tag SNPs identifies a susceptibility variant for colorectal cancer at 8q24.21. Nat Genet 2007;39:984–8.
70. Berndt SI, Potter JD, Hazra A, et al. Pooled analysis of genetic variation at chromosome 8q24 and colorectal neoplasia risk. Hum Mol Genet 2008;17:2665–72.
71. Panagopoulos I, Möller E, Collin A, et al. The POU5F1P1 pseudogene encodes a putative protein similar to POU5F1 isoform 1. Oncol Rep 2008;20:1029–33.
72. Zanke BW, Greenwood CM, Rangrej J, et al. Genome-wide association scan identifies a colorectal cancer susceptibility locus on chromosome 8q24. Nat Genet 2007;39:989–94.
73. Tenesa A, Farrington SM, Prendergast JG, et al. Genome-wide association scan identifies a colorectal cancer susceptibility locus on 11q23 and replicates risk loci at 8q24 and 18q21. Nat Genet 2008;40:631–7.
74. Roberts AB, Wakefield LM. The two faces of transforming growth factor beta in carcinogenesis. Proc Natl Acad Sci U S A 2003;100:8621–3.
75. Siegel PM, Massagué J. Cytostatic and apoptotic actions of TGF-beta in homeostasis and cancer. Nat Rev Cancer 2003;3:807–21.
76. Broderick P, Carvajal-Carmona L, Pittman AM, et al. A genome-wide association study shows that common alleles of SMAD7 influence colorectal cancer risk. Nat Genet 2007;39:1315–7.
77. Tomlinson IP, Webb E, Carvajal-Carmona L, et al. A genome-wide association study identifies colorectal cancer susceptibility loci on chromosomes 10p14 and 8q23.3. Nat Genet 2008;40:623–30.
78. Houlston RS, Webb E, Broderick P, et al. Meta-analysis of genome-wide association data identifies four new susceptibility loci for colorectal cancer. Nat Genet 2008;40:1426–35.
79. Peck JW, Oberst M, Bouker KB, et al. The RhoA-binding protein, rhophilin-2, regulates actin cytoskeleton organization. J Biol Chem 2002;277:43924–32.
80. Kim JS, Crooks H, Dracheva T, et al. Oncogenic beta-catenin is required for bone morphogenetic protein 4 expression in human cancer cells. Cancer Res 2002;62:2744–8.
81. Jaeger E, Webb E, Howarth K, et al. Common genetic variants at the CRAC1 (HMPS) locus on chromosome 15q13.3 influence colorectal cancer risk. Nat Genet 2008;40:26–8.
82. Curtin K, Lin WY, George R, et al. Meta association of colorectal cancer confirms risk alleles at 8q24 and 18q21. Cancer Epidemiol Biomarkers Prev 2009;18: 616–21.
83. Winawer SJ, Zauber AG, Gerdes H, et al. Risk of colorectal cancer in the families of patients with adenomatous polyps. National Polyp Study Workgroup. N Engl J Med 1996;334:82–7.

84. Johns LE, Houlston RS. A systematic review and meta-analysis of familial colo-rectal cancer risk. Am J Gastroenterol 2001;96:2992–3003.
85. Amundadottir L, Kraft P, Stolzenberg-Solomon RZ, et al. Genome-wide associa-tion study identifies variants in the ABO locus associated with susceptibility to pancreatic cancer. Nat Genet 2009;41:986–90.
86. Aird I, Bentall HH, Roberts JA. A relationship between cancer of stomach and the ABO blood groups. Br Med J 1953;1:799–801.
87. Aird I, Lee DR, Roberts JA. ABO blood groups and cancer of oesophagus, cancer of pancreas, and pituitary adenoma. Br Med J 1960;1:1163–6.
88. Marcus DM. The ABO and Lewis blood-group system. Immunochemistry, genetics and relation to human disease. N Engl J Med 1969;280:994–1006.
89. Petersen GM, Amundadottir L, Fuchs CS, et al. A genome-wide association study identifies pancreatic cancer susceptibility loci on chromosomes 13q22.1, 1q32.1 and 5p15.33. Nat Genet 2010;42:224–8.
90. Rafnar T, Sulem P, Stacey SN, et al. Sequence variants at the TERT-CLPTM1L locus associate with many cancer types. Nat Genet 2009;41:221–7.
91. Cui R, Kamatani Y, Takahashi A, et al. Functional variants in ADH1B and ALDH2 coupled with alcohol and smoking synergistically enhance esophageal cancer risk. Gastroenterology 2009;137:1768–75.
92. Wu MT, Lee JM, Wu DC, et al. Genetic polymorphisms of cytochrome P4501A1 and oesophageal squamous-cell carcinoma in Taiwan. Br J Cancer 2002;87:529–32.
93. Yokoyama A, Muramatsu T, Omori T, et al. Alcohol and aldehyde dehydroge-nase gene polymorphisms and oropharyngolaryngeal, esophageal and stomach cancers in Japanese alcoholics. Carcinogenesis 2001;22:433–9.
94. Study Group of Millennium Genome Project for Cancer, Sakamoto H, Yoshimura K, et al. Genetic variation in PSCA is associated with susceptibility to diffuse-type gastric cancer. Nat Genet 2008;40:730–40.
95. Reiter RE, Gu Z, Watabe T, et al. Prostate stem cell antigen: a cell surface marker overexpressed in prostate cancer. Proc Natl Acad Sci U S A 1998;95:1735–40.
96. Amara N, Palapattu GS, Schrage M, et al. Prostate stem cell antigen is overexpressed in human transitional cell carcinoma. Cancer Res 2001;61:4660–5.
97. Bahrenberg G, Brauers A, Joost HG, et al. Reduced expression of PSCA, a member of the LY-6 family of cell surface antigens, in bladder, esophagus, and stomach tumors. Biochem Biophys Res Commun 2000;275:783–8.
98. Wu X, Ye Y, Kiemeney LA, et al. Genetic variation in the prostate stem cell antigen gene PSCA confers susceptibility to urinary bladder cancer. Nat Genet 2009;41:991–5.
99. Amos CI, Wu X, Broderick P, et al. Genome-wide association scan of tag SNPs iden-tifies a susceptibility locus for lung cancer at 15q25.1. Nat Genet 2008;40:616–22.
100. Hung RJ, McKay JD, Gaborieau V, et al. A susceptibility locus for lung cancer maps to nicotinic acetylcholine receptor subunit genes on 15q25. Nature 2008;452:633–7.
101. Broderick P, Wang Y, Vijayakrishnan J, et al. Deciphering the impact of common genetic variation on lung cancer risk: a genome-wide association study. Cancer Res 2009;69:6633–41.
102. Minna JD. Nicotine exposure and bronchial epithelial cell nicotinic acetylcholine receptor expression in the pathogenesis of lung cancer. J Clin Invest 2003;111:31–3.

103. Zhang Q, Tang X, Zhang ZF, et al. Nicotine induces hypoxia-inducible factor-1alpha expression in human lung cancer cells via nicotinic acetylcholine receptor-mediated signaling pathways. Clin Cancer Res 2007;13:4686–94.

104. Saccone SF, Hinrichs AL, Saccone NL, et al. Cholinergic nicotinic receptor genes implicated in a nicotine dependence association study targeting 348 candidate genes with 3713 SNPs. Hum Mol Genet 2007;16:36–49.

105. Thorgeirsson TE, Geller F, Sulem P, et al. A variant associated with nicotine dependence, lung cancer and peripheral arterial disease. Nature 2008;452:638–42.

106. Liu P, Vikis HG, Wang D, et al. Familial aggregation of common sequence variants on 15q24-25.1 in lung cancer. J Natl Cancer Inst 2008;100:1326–30.

107. Wang Y, Broderick P, Webb E, et al. Common 5p15.33 and 6p21.33 variants influence lung cancer risk. Nat Genet 2008;40:1407–9.

108. McKay JD, Hung RJ, Gaborieau V, et al. Lung cancer susceptibility locus at 5p15.33. Nat Genet 2008;40:1404–6.

109. Kang JU, Koo SH, Kwon KC, et al. Gain at chromosomal region 5p15.33, containing TERT, is the most frequent genetic event in early stages of non-small cell lung cancer. Cancer Genet Cytogenet 2008;182:1–11.

110. Armanios M, Chen JL, Chang YP, et al. Haploinsufficiency of telomerase reverse transcriptase leads to anticipation in autosomal dominant dyskeratosis congenita. Proc Natl Acad Sci U S A 2005;102:15960–4.

111. Landi MT, Chatterjee N, Yu K, et al. A genome-wide association study of lung cancer identifies a region of chromosome 5p15 associated with risk for adenocarcinoma. Am J Hum Genet 2009;85:679–91.

112. Sasaki T, Gan EC, Wakeham A, et al. HLA-B-associated transcript 3 (Bat3)/Scythe is essential for p300-mediated acetylation of p53. Genes Dev 2007;21:848–61.

113. Brown KM, Macgregor S, Montgomery GW, et al. Common sequence variants on 20q11.22 confer melanoma susceptibility. Nat Genet 2008;40:838–40.

114. Gudbjartsson DF, Sulem P, Stacey SN, et al. ASIP and TYR pigmentation variants associate with cutaneous melanoma and basal cell carcinoma. Nat Genet 2008;40:886–91.

115. Han J, Kraft P, Nan H, et al. A genome-wide association study identifies novel alleles associated with hair color and skin pigmentation. PLoS Genet 2008;4:e1000074.

116. Stacey SN, Gudbjartsson DF, Sulem P, et al. Common variants on 1p36 and 1q42 are associated with cutaneous basal cell carcinoma but not with melanoma or pigmentation traits. Nat Genet 2008;40:1313–8.

117. Esposito G, Vitale AM, Leijten FP, et al. Peptidylarginine deiminase (PAD) 6 is essential for oocyte cytoskeletal sheet formation and female fertility. Mol Cell Endocrinol 2007;273:25–31.

118. UniProtKB/Swiss-Prot Q7L0Q8 (RHOU_HUMAN). Available at: http://www.uniprot.org/uniprot/Q7L0Q8#section_comments. Accessed March 4, 2009.

119. Stacey SN, Sulem P, Masson G, et al. New common variants affecting susceptibility to basal cell carcinoma. Nat Genet 2009;41:909–14.

120. Bishop DT, Demenais F, Iles MM, et al. Genome-wide association study identifies three loci associated with melanoma risk. Nat Genet 2009;41:920–5.

121. Falchi M, Bataille V, Hayward NK, et al. Genome-wide association study identifies variants at 9p21 and 22q13 associated with development of cutaneous nevi. Nat Genet 2009;41:915–9.

122. Kiemeney LA, Thorlacius S, Sulem P, et al. Sequence variant on 8q24 confers susceptibility to urinary bladder cancer. Nat Genet 2008;40:1307–12.

123. Urist MJ, Di Como CJ, Lu ML, et al. Loss of p63 expression is associated with tumor progression in bladder cancer. Am J Pathol 2002;161:1199–206.
124. Koga F, Kawakami S, Fujii Y, et al. Impaired p63 expression associates with poor prognosis and uroplakin III expression in invasive urothelial carcinoma of the bladder. Clin Cancer Res 2003;9:5501–7.
125. Di Bernardo MC, Crowther-Swanepoel D, Broderick P, et al. A genome-wide association study identifies six susceptibility loci for chronic lymphocytic leukemia. Nat Genet 2008;40:1204–10.
126. Shapiro-Shelef M, Calame K. Regulation of plasma-cell development. Nat Rev Immunol 2005;5:230–42.
127. Klein U, Dalla-Favera R. Germinal centres: role in B-cell physiology and malignancy. Nat Rev Immunol 2008;8:22–33.
128. UniProtKB/Swiss-Prot Q13342 (LY10_HUMAN). Available at: http://www.uniprot.org/uniprot/Q13342#section_comments. Accessed March 4, 2009.
129. Kovalevska LM, Yurchenko OV, Shlapatska LM, et al. Immunohistochemical studies of protein kinase D (PKD) 2 expression in malignant human lymphomas. Exp Oncol 2006;28:225–30.
130. Crowther-Swanepoel D, Broderick P, Di Bernardo MC, et al. Common variants at 2q37.3, 8q24.21, 15q21.3 and 16q24.1 influence chronic lymphocytic leukemia risk. Nat Genet 2010;42:132–6.
131. Miyamoto Y, Yamauchi J, Itoh H. Src kinase regulates the activation of a novel FGD-1-related Cdc42 guanine nucleotide exchange factor in the signaling pathway from the endothelin A receptor to JNK. J Biol Chem 2003;278:29890–900.
132. Wang H, Morse HC. IRF8 regulates myeloid and B lymphoid lineage diversification. Immunol Res 2009;43:109–17.
133. De Jager PL, Jia X, Wang J, et al. Meta-analysis of genome scans and replication identify CD6, IRF8 and TNFRSF1A as new multiple sclerosis susceptibility loci. Nat Genet 2009;41:776–82.
134. Skibola CF, Bracci PM, Halperin E, et al. Genetic variants at 6p21.33 are associated with susceptibility to follicular lymphoma. Nat Genet 2009;41:873–5.
135. Treviño LR, Yang W, French D, et al. Germline genomic variants associated with childhood acute lymphoblastic leukemia. Nat Genet 2009;41:1001–5.
136. Papaemmanuil E, Hosking FJ, Vijayakrishnan J, et al. Loci on 7p12.2, 10q21.2 and 14q11.2 are associated with risk of childhood acute lymphoblastic leukemia. Nat Genet 2009;41:1006–10.
137. Wilsker D, Patsialou A, Dallas PB, et al. ARID proteins: a diverse family of DNA binding proteins implicated in the control of cell growth, differentiation, and development. Cell Growth Differ 2002;13:95–106.
138. Paulsson K, Mörse H, Fioretos T, et al. Evidence for a single-step mechanism in the origin of hyperdiploid childhood acute lymphoblastic leukemia. Genes Chromosomes Cancer 2005;44:113–22.
139. Kilpivaara O, Mukherjee S, Schram AM, et al. A germline JAK2 SNP is associated with predisposition to the development of JAK2(V617F)-positive myeloproliferative neoplasms. Nat Genet 2009;41:455–9.
140. Forman D, Oliver RT, Brett AR, et al. Familial testicular cancer: a report of the UK family register, estimation of risk and an HLA class 1 sib-pair analysis. Br J Cancer 1992;65:255–62.
141. Hemminki K, Chen B. Familial risks in testicular cancer as aetiological clues. Int J Androl 2006;29:205–10.
142. Han S, Peschel RE. Father-son testicular tumors: evidence for genetic anticipation? A case report and review of the literature. Cancer 2000;88:2319–25.

143. Kanetsky PA, Mitra N, Vardhanabhuti S, et al. Common variation in KITLG and at 5q31.3 predisposes to testicular germ cell cancer. Nat Genet 2009;41:811–5.
144. Rapley EA, Turnbull C, Al Olama AA, et al. A genome-wide association study of testicular germ cell tumor. Nat Genet 2009;41:807–10.
145. Mahakali Zama A, Hudson FP, Bedell MA. Analysis of hypomorphic KitlSl mutants suggests different requirements for KITL in proliferation and migration of mouse primordial germ cells. Biol Reprod 2005;73:639–47.
146. Oosterhuis JW, Looijenga LH. Testicular germ-cell tumours in a broader perspective. Nat Rev Cancer 2005;5:210–22.
147. Rajpert-de Meyts E, Hoei-Hansen CE. From gonocytes to testicular cancer: the role of impaired gonadal development. Ann N Y Acad Sci 2007;1120:168–80.
148. Song H, Ramus SJ, Tyrer J, et al. A genome-wide association study identifies a new ovarian cancer susceptibility locus on 9p22.2. Nat Genet 2009;41:996–1000.
149. Vanhoutteghem A, Djian P. Basonuclin 2: an extremely conserved homolog of the zinc finger protein basonuclin. Proc Natl Acad Sci U S A 2004;101:3468–73.
150. Gudmundsson J, Sulem P, Gudbjartsson DF. Common variants on 9q22.33 and 14q13.3 predispose to thyroid cancer in European populations. Nat Genet 2009;41:460–4.
151. Parlato R, Rosica A, Rodriguez-Mallon A, et al. An integrated regulatory network controlling survival and migration in thyroid organogenesis. Dev Biol 2004;276:464–75.
152. Maris JM, Mosse YP, Bradfield JP, et al. Chromosome 6p22 locus associated with clinically aggressive neuroblastoma. N Engl J Med 2008;358:2585–93.
153. Capasso M, Devoto M, Hou C, et al. Common variations in BARD1 influence susceptibility to high-risk neuroblastoma. Nat Genet 2009;41:718–23.
154. Wu LC, Wang ZW, Tsan JT, et al. Identification of a RING protein that can interact in vivo with the BRCA1 gene product. Nat Genet 1996;14:430–40.
155. Shete S, Hosking FJ, Robertson LB, et al. Genome-wide association study identifies five susceptibility loci for glioma. Nat Genet 2009;41:899–904.
156. Bahuau M, Vidaud D, Jenkins RB, et al. Germ-line deletion involving the INK4 locus in familial proneness to melanoma and nervous system tumors. Cancer Res 1998;58:2298–303.
157. Randerson-Moor JA, Harland M, Williams S, et al. A germline deletion of p14(ARF) but not CDKN2A in a melanoma-neural system tumour syndrome family. Hum Mol Genet 2001;10:55–62.
158. The Cancer Genome Atlas Research Network, Tissue Source Sites: Duke University Medical School, McLendon R, et al. Comprehensive genomic characterization defines human glioblastoma genes and core pathways. Nature 2008;455:1061–8.
159. Parsons DW, Jones S, Zhang X, et al. An integrated genomic analysis of human glioblastoma multiforme. Science 2008;321:1807–12.
160. Wager M, Menei P, Guilhot J, et al. Prognostic molecular markers with no impact on decision-making: the paradox of gliomas based on a prospective study. Br J Cancer 2008;98:1830–8.
161. Wrensch M, Jenkins RB, Chang JS, et al. Variants in the CDKN2B and RTEL1 regions are associated with high-grade glioma susceptibility. Nat Genet 2009;41:905–8.
162. Barber LJ, Youds JL, Ward JD, et al. RTEL1 maintains genomic stability by suppressing homologous recombination. Cell 2008;135:261–71.

163. Goldstein DB. Common genetic variation and human traits. N Engl J Med 2009; 360:1696–8.

164. Eeles RA, Kote-Jarai Z, Al Olama AA, et al. Identification of seven new prostate cancer susceptibility loci through a genome-wide association study. Nat Genet 2009;41:1116–21.

165. Gudmundsson J, Sulem P, Gudbjartsson DF, et al. Genome-wide association and replication studies identify four variants associated with prostate cancer susceptibility. Nat Genet 2009;41:1122–6.

166. Al Olama AA, Kote-Jarai Z, Giles GG, et al. Multiple loci on 8q24 associated with prostate cancer susceptibility. Nat Genet 2009;41:1058–60.

167. Yeager M, Chatterjee N, Ciampa J, et al. Identification of a new prostate cancer susceptibility locus on chromosome 8q24. Nat Genet 2009;41:1055–7.

Index

Note: Page numbers of article titles are in **boldface** type.

A

Acute lymphocytic leukemia, heritability of, 955–957
Adenocarcinoma, esophageal, association with familial Barrett esophagus, 817

B

Barrett esophagus, familial, association with esophageal adenocarcinoma, 817
Basal cell carcinoma, genome-wide association studies, 982
Birt-Hogg-Dubé syndrome, hereditary kidney cancer in, 870
Bladder. *See* Urinary bladder.
BRCA1 mutations, in breast cancer predisposition syndromes, **799–814**
    in pancreatic cancer predisposition syndromes, 822–823
BRCA2 mutations, in breast cancer predisposition syndromes, **799–814**
    in pancreatic cancer predisposition syndromes, 822–823
    linkage with esophageal squamous cell carcinoma, 816
Breast cancer, genome-wide association studies, 974–976
    predisposition syndromes, **799–814**
        Cowden syndrome, 802–805
        hereditary breast and ovarian cancer syndrome, 805–810
        Li Fraumeni syndrome, 799–802

C

Cancer predisposition. *See* Genetic predisposition.
Cancer susceptibility regions, in genome-wide association studies, **973–996**
Chemoprevention, for Lynch syndrome, 845–846
Chemotherapy, for Lynch syndrome, 845
Chronic lymphocytic leukemia, heritability of, 940–946
Clinical applications, of genome-wide association studies, 975–976, 978, 980, 982
Colorectal cancer, hereditary, clinical genetics of, **837–859**
        familial adenomatous polyposis, 846–848
            attenuated, 847–848
            genetic testing and management, 846–847
        familial cancer type X, 851–852
        genome-wide association studies, 852, 979–980
        hamartomatous polyposis syndromes, 849–851
            Cowden syndrome, 850–851
            juvenile polyposis syndrome, 850
            others, 851
            Peutz-Jeghers syndrome, 849–850
        hyperplastic polyposis, 851
        Lynch syndrome, 838–846

Hematol Oncol Clin N Am 24 (2010) 997–1004
doi:10.1016/S0889-8588(10)00130-9
0889-8588/10/$ – see front matter © 2010 Elsevier Inc. All rights reserved.

hemonc.theclinics.com

United States Postal Service

Statement of Ownership, Management, and Circulation
(All Periodicals Publications Except Requestor Publications)

1. Publication Title
Hematology/Oncology Clinics of North America

2. Publication Number
0 0 2 - 4 7 1 3

3. Filing Date
9/15/10

4. Issue Frequency
Feb, Apr, Jun, Aug, Oct, Dec

5. Number of Issues Published Annually
6

6. Annual Subscription Price
$306.00

7. Complete Mailing Address of Known Office of Publication (Not printer) (Street, city, county, state, and ZIP+4®)
Elsevier Inc.
360 Park Avenue South
New York, NY 10010-1710

Contact Person: Stephen Bushing

Telephone (Include area code): 215-239-3688

8. Complete Mailing Address of Headquarters or General Business Office of Publisher (Not printer)
Elsevier Inc., 360 Park Avenue South, New York, NY 10010-1710

9. Full Names and Complete Mailing Addresses of Publisher, Editor, and Managing Editor (Do not leave blank)

Publisher (Name and complete mailing address)
Kim Murphy, Elsevier, Inc., 1600 John F. Kennedy Blvd. Suite 1800, Philadelphia, PA 19103-2899

Editor (Name and complete mailing address)
Kerry Holland, Elsevier, Inc., 1600 John F. Kennedy Blvd. Suite 1800, Philadelphia, PA 19103-2899

Managing Editor (Name and complete mailing address)
Catherine Bewick, Elsevier, Inc., 1600 John F. Kennedy Blvd. Suite 1800, Philadelphia, PA 19103-2899

10. Owner (Do not leave blank. If the publication is owned by a corporation, give the name and address of the corporation immediately followed by the names and addresses of all stockholders owning or holding 1 percent or more of the total amount of stock. If not owned by a corporation, give the names and addresses of the individual owners. If owned by a partnership or other unincorporated firm, give its name and address as well as those of each individual owner. If the publication is published by a nonprofit organization, give its name and address.)

Full Name	Complete Mailing Address
Wholly owned subsidiary of	4520 East-West Highway
Reed/Elsevier, US holdings	Bethesda, MD 20814

11. Known Bondholders, Mortgagees, and Other Security Holders Owning or Holding 1 Percent or More of Total Amount of Bonds, Mortgages, or Other Securities. If none, check box. ☐ None

Full Name	Complete Mailing Address
N/A	

12. Tax Status (For completion by nonprofit organizations authorized to mail at nonprofit rates) (Check one)
The purpose, function, and nonprofit status of this organization and the exempt status for federal income tax purposes:
☐ Has Not Changed During Preceding 12 Months
☐ Has Changed During Preceding 12 Months (Publisher must submit explanation of change with this statement)

PS Form 3526, September 2007 (Page 1 of 3 (Instructions Page 3)) PSN 7530-01-000-9931 PRIVACY NOTICE: See our Privacy policy in www.usps.com

13. Publication Title
Hematology/Oncology Clinics of North America

14. Issue Date for Circulation Data Below
June 2010

15. Extent and Nature of Circulation		Average No. Copies Each Issue During Preceding 12 Months	No. Copies of Single Issue Published Nearest to Filing Date
a. Total Number of Copies (Net press run)		1713	1676
b. Paid Circulation (By Mail and Outside the Mail)	(1) Mailed Outside-County Paid Subscriptions Stated on PS Form 3541. (Include paid distribution above nominal rate, advertiser's proof copies, and exchange copies)	522	462
	(2) Mailed In-County Paid Subscriptions Stated on PS Form 3541 (Include paid distribution above nominal rate, advertiser's proof copies, and exchange copies)		
	(3) Paid Distribution Outside the Mails Including Sales Through Dealers and Carriers, Street Vendors, Counter Sales, and Other Paid Distribution Outside USPS®	422	392
	(4) Paid Distribution by Other Classes Mailed Through the USPS (e.g. First-Class Mail®)		
c. Total Paid Distribution (Sum of 15b (1), (2), (3), and (4))		944	854
d. Free or Nominal Rate Distribution (By Mail and Outside the Mail)	(1) Free or Nominal Rate Outside-County Copies Included on PS Form 3541	135	128
	(2) Free or Nominal Rate In-County Copies Included on PS Form 3541		
	(3) Free or Nominal Rate Copies Mailed at Other Classes Through the USPS (e.g. First-Class Mail)		
	(4) Free or Nominal Rate Distribution Outside the Mail (Carriers or other means)		
e. Total Free or Nominal Rate Distribution (Sum of 15d (1), (2), (3) and (4))		135	128
f. Total Distribution (Sum of 15c and 15e)		1079	982
g. Copies not Distributed (See instructions to publishers #4 (page #3))		634	694
h. Total (Sum of 15f and g)		1713	1676
i. Percent Paid (15c divided by 15f times 100)		87.49%	86.97%

16. Publication of Statement of Ownership
☐ If the publication is a general publication, publication of this statement is required. Will be printed in the **October 2010** issue of this publication. ☐ Publication not required.

17. Signature and Title of Editor, Publisher, Business Manager, or Owner

Stephen R. Bushing

Stephen R. Bushing – Fulfillment/Inventory Specialist

Date: September 15, 2010

I certify that all information furnished on this form is true and complete. I understand that anyone who furnishes false or misleading information on this form or who omits material or information requested on the form may be subject to criminal sanctions (including fines and imprisonment) and/or civil sanctions (including civil penalties).

PS Form 3526, September 2007 (Page 2 of 3)

Moving?

Make sure your subscription moves with you!

To notify us of your new address, find your **Clinics Account Number** (located on your mailing label above your name), and contact customer service at:

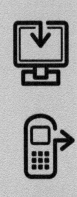

Email: **journalscustomerservice-usa@elsevier.com**

800-654-2452 (subscribers in the U.S. & Canada)
314-447-8871 (subscribers outside of the U.S. & Canada)

Fax number: **314-447-8029**

Elsevier Health Sciences Division
Subscription Customer Service
3251 Riverport Lane
Maryland Heights, MO 63043

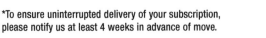

Printed and bound by CPI Group (UK) Ltd, Croydon, CR0 4YY

03/10/2024

01040447-0002